AF181360

Cardiac Arrhythmias

Diagnosis Prognosis Therapy

Proceedings 1st International
Rytmonorm-Congress

Edited by
M. Schlepper and B. Olsson

With 91 Figures and 67 Tables

Springer-Verlag
Berlin Heidelberg New York 1983

Professor Dr. M. Schlepper
Kerckhoff-Klinik
of the Max-Planck-Society
Benekestraße 4–6
D-6350 Bad Nauheim

Dr. B. Olsson
Department of Cardiology
Sahlgrenska University Hospital
S-41345 Göteborg

ISBN-13: 978-3-642-68928-4 e-ISBN-13: 978-3-642-68926-0
DOI:10/1007/978-3-642-68926-0

Library of Congress Cataloging in Publication Data
International Rytmonorm-Congress (1st:)
Cardiac arrhythmias.
1. Arrhythmia--Congresses. 2. Arrhythmia--Chemotherapy--Congresses. 3. Propafenone--Testing--Congresses. I. Schlepper, M. (Martin), 1928– . II. Olsson, B. (Bertil), 1941– III. Title. [DNLM: 1. Arrhythmias. WG 330 C2649] RC685.A65156 1983 616.1'28 83-350

This work is subject to copyright. All rights are reserved, whether the whole or part of the material is concerned, specifically those of translation, reprinting, re-use of illustrations. broadcasting, reproduction by photocopying machine or similar means, and storage in data banks. Under § 54 of the German Copyright Law where copies are made for other than private use a fee is payable to "Verwertungsgesellschaft Wort", Munich.
©Springer-Verlag Berlin Heidelberg 1983
Softcover reprint of the hardcover 1st edition 1983

The use of general descriptive names, trade marks, etc. in this publication, even if the former are not especially identified, is not be taken as a sign that such names, as understood by the Trade Marks and Merchandise Marks Act, may accordingly by used freely by anyone.
Type-setting and book binding: G. Appl, Wemding
Printing: aprinta, Wemding
2121/3140-543210

Preface

Asked to organize an international meeting on Propafenone (Rytmonorm) we had to question ourselves, whether to accept this offer just as interested physicians or in our capacity as chairmen of the study group on arrhythmias and intracardiac electrography of the European Society of Cardiology.

Considerung the "pros and contras" and well aware that one can easily be regarded as "product promoter" we, nevertheless, choose to organize the Symposion in association with the study group. We felt justified to do so for a number of reasons: Arrhythmias and their treatment as well as the tools to detect the first and to control the latter are well within the scope of the study group. An international symposion provided the opportunity to have the "state of the art" in arrhythmias and antiarrhythmic treatment thoroughly reviewed by internationally renowned investigators, thus serving an educational purpose.

Furthermore it was the intention and aim of the meeting to have what is known about a fairly new drug presented in a critical manner and to point out what is not known, but should be known.

It is in that context the presentations of the free session should be judged. To the careful reader it will become apparent that much which was not said, can be read "between the lines".

To "set the stage" it is of utmost importance for the organizers not to be influenced in any way by the sponsors. It is gratefully acknowledged that Knoll AG was not only a generous sponsor as far as the scientific program is concerned but at no time tried to influence or even manage contents and proceedings of the symposion.

It is our sincere wish for the proceedings of the symposion to stimulate the interest in arrhythmias and their treatment, to provide more information about a fairly new drug, its potential efficacy and the indwelling danger of this and similar remedies and to help the physician to find its proper place in a rational and, may be, live-saving treatment for the benefit of the patients.

Martin Schlepper, MD
Kerckhoff-Klinik of the
Max-Planck-Society
Bad Nauheim/FRG

Bertil Olsson, MD
Sahrgrenska University Hospital
Göteborg/Sweden

Table of Contens

Introduction
(D. Krikler) 1

Differentiation Between "Normal" and "Abnormal" in Ambulatory Electrocardiography
(P. Bjerregaard) 3

Identification of the Patient at High Risk of Sudden Cardiac Death
(J. Morganroth) 13

Efficacy of Oral Propafenone in Supraventricular and Ventricular Arrhythmias: Experience with 47 Cases
(P. Coumel and J.-F. Leclercq) 21

The Possible Relevance of Late Potentials for the Identification of Patients Needing Antiarrhythmic Treatment
(G. Breithardt, M. Borggrefe, U. Karbenn, K. Haerten, J. Ostermeyer and L. Seipel) 37

Simulation Studies for the Interpretation of Delayed Potentials
(R. Frank, G. Fontaine, M. Pierfitte and Y. Grosgogeat) 53

Electrophysiologic Testing in Patients with Ventricular Tachycardia
(E. N. Prystowsky, G. V. Naccarelli, J. J. Heger and D. P. Zipes) 63

Results of Invasive Methods
(H. J. Wellens) 71

Specific Antiarrhythmic Drugs for Specific Arrhythmias
(R. W. F. Campbell) 75

Sudden Cardiac Death: Prognosis of Long-term Antiarrhythmic Therapy
(M. Manz, G. Steinbeck and B. Lüderitz) 83

Basic Electrophysiological Actions of Propafenone in Heart Muscle
(M. Kohlhardt) 91

The Pharmacology of Propafenone
(H. Scholz) 103

Clinical Pharmacology of Propafenone
(H. Neuss and M. Schlepper) 113

Pharmacokinetic and Metabolic Studies on Propafenone in Volunteers
(M. Hollmann, H. G. Hege, E. Brode, V. Bühler, D. Hotz, S. Kaumeier, O. H. Kehrhahn, H. Lietz, J. A. Schwarz, B. Stieren and J. Weymann) 125

Effects of Propafenone on Hemodynamics and Cardiac Inotropy
(M. Schlepper and H. Neuss) 133

Interaction Between Propafenone and Other Drugs
(K. Steinbach, K. Frohner, F. Meisl and G. Unger) 141

Comparison of the Efficacy of Propafenone and Lidocaine in Patients with Acute Myocardial Infarction and Ventricular Extrasystoles: Result of a 24-h Holter Monitoring
(N. Rehnqvist) 149

Observations on the Antiarrhythmic Effects of Rytmonorm
(Ku Fu-sheng, Lin Jui-Chin, Liu Pei-Tsun, Li Qing-lang, Chang Jang-thi, Shen Lu-hua and Yang Shi Hau) 151

Comparative Study of the Therapeutic Effect of Propafenone and Disopyramide in the Oral Treatment of Chronic Ventricular Premature Beats
(J. Clementy, M. Dallocchio and H. Bricaud) 159

Propafenone, Flecainide and Mexiletine in the Treatment of Stable Ventricular Premature Beats
(H.-W. Klempt and A. Nayebagha) 171

Long-term Prognosis for Patients with Complex Ventricular Arrhythmias of Lown Grades IVa and IVb
(F. Theisen, K. Theisen and H. Jahrmärker) 179

Experience with Propafenone in the Treatment of Arrhythmias in Pediatric Patients
(H. Weber, G. Eigster and H. Wesselhoeft) 185

Electrophysiologic Effects and Antiarrhythmic Efficacy of Rytmonorm Evaluated with Programmed Electrical Stimulation of the Heart in Patients with Recurrent Reentrant Supraventricular Tachycardia
(A. Waleffe and H. Kulbertus) 191

Antiarrhythmic Effect and Study of Segmentary Contractility Following the Administration of Propafenone in Coronary Patients with Ventricular Arrhythmias
(J. L. Palma, A. Bayés de Luna, M. Fiol, P. Yuste, V. Aza, J. Sadurni, C. E. R. y Cajal, R. Son Dureta and H. San Pablo) 199

Propafenone in Office Use: Results of an Open, Multicenter Study
(H.-F. Spies and F. Sesto) 211

The Safety and Efficacy of Propafenone in Suppressing Ventricular Ectopy
(N. de Soyza, M. Murphy, M. Sakhaii and L. Treat) 217

Dose-Response Effect of Propafenone in Patients with Ventricular Arrhythmias
(P. Larochelle, L. Belanger, F. Lemire, D. Phaneuf and R. Huot) 221

Treatment of Severe Ventricular Arrhythmias with Propafenone
(L. Ledain, N. Sourdille, J. P. Colle, J. Ohayon and P. Besse) . 231

Use of Propafenone for the Prevention of Ventricular Hyperkinetic Arrhythmias in the Mitral Valve Prolapse Syndrome
(F. Furlanello, G. B. Durante, P. Dal Forno, L. Frisanco, G. Mosna, R. Bettini, M. Disertori, G. Vergara, A. Del Favero and E. Stirpe) 237

List of Authors

V. Aza
Servicio de Cardiol., Hôspital de la Santa Cruz y San Pablo, Av. San Antonia Ma Claret 167, Barcelona 13, Spain

A. Bayés de Luna
Servicio de Cardiol., Hospital de la Santa Cruz y San Pablo, Av. San Antonia Ma Claret 167, Barcelona 13, Spain

L. Belanger
Institut de Recherches Cliniques de Montréal, 110 avenue des Pins ouest, Montréal, QC, H2W 1R7, Canada

P. Besse
Hôpital Cardiologique, 208, avenue de Magellan, 33604 Pessac, France

P. Bjerregaard
University Department of Cardiology, Aarhus Kommunehospital, 8000 Aarhus C, Denmark

M. Borggrefe
Medizinische Klinik B, Universität Düsseldorf, Moorenstr. 5, 4000 Düsseldorf, W. Germany

G. Breithardt
Medizinische Klinik B, Universität Düsseldorf, Moorenstr. 5, 4000 Düsseldorf, W. Germany

H. Bricaud
Clinique Médicale Cardiologique, Hôpital Cardiologique de Bordeaux, 33604 Pessac, France

E. Brode
Knoll AG, Knollstraße 50, 6700 Ludwigshafen, W. Germany

V. Bühler
Knoll AG, Knollstraße 50, 6700 Ludwigshafen, W. Germany

R. W. F. Campbell
University Department of Cardiology, Freeman Hospital, Newcastle upon Tyne, England, NE7 7DN

Chang Jang-thi
Beijing Friendship Hospital, Beijing, Peoples Republic of China

J. Clementy
Clinique Médicale Cardiologique, Hôpital Cardiologique de Bordeaux, 33604 Pessac, France

J. P. Colle
Hôpital Cardiologique, 208, avenue de Magellan, 33604 Pessac, France

P. Coumel
Hôpital Lariboisiere, 2 rue Ambroise-Pare, 75010 Paris, France

M. Dallocchio
Clinique Médicale Cardiologique, Hôpital Cardiologique de Bordeaux, 33604 Pessac, France

N. de Soyza
1238 Taransay Dr. Henderson, KY 42420, USA

G. Eigster
Kinderklinik und Poliklinik, Waldweg 33, 3400 Göttingen, W. Germany

M. Fiol
Servicio de Cardiol, Hospital de la Santa Cruz y San Pablo, Av. San Antonia Ma Claret 167, Barcelona 13, Spain

G. Fontaine
Hôpital Jean Rostand, 39 rue le Galleu, 94200 Ivry, France

R. Frank
Hôpital Jean Rostand, 39 rue le Galleu, 94200 Ivry, France

K. Frohner
III. Medizinische Abteilung (Kardiologie und Nephrologie), Montlearstr. 37, 1160 Wien, Austria

F. Furlanello
Division of Cardiology and Arrhythmologie Center, S. Chiara Hospital, Trento, Italy

Y. Grosgogeat
Hôpital Jean Rostand, 39 rue le Galleu, 94200 Ivry, France

K. Haerten
Medizinische Klinik B, Universität Düsseldorf, Moorenstr. 5, 4000 Düsseldorf, W. Germany

H. G. Hege
Knoll AG, Knollstr. 50, 6700 Ludwigshafen, W. Germany

J. J. Heger
Krannert Institute of Cardiology, Indiana University School of Medicine, 1100 West Michigan Street, Indianapolis, Indiana 46223, U. S. A.

M. Hollmann
Knoll AG, Knollstraße 50, 6700 Ludwigshafen, W. Germany

D. Hotz
Knoll AG, Knollstraße 50, 6700 Ludwigshafen, W. Germany

R. Huot
Institut de Recherches Cliniques de Montréal, 110 avenue des Pins ouest, Montréal, QC, H2W 1R7, Canada

H. Jahrmärker
Medizinische Klinik, Innenstadt der Universität München, Ziemssenstr. 1, 8000 München 20, W. Germany

U. Karbenn
Medizinische Klinik B, Universität Düsseldorf, Moorenstr. 5, 4000 Düsseldorf, W. Germany

S. Kaumeier
Knoll AG, Knollstr. 50, 6700 Ludwigshafen, W. Germany

O. H. Kehrhahn
Knoll AG, Knollstr. 50, 6700 Ludwigshafen, W. Germany

Ku Fu-sheng
Beijing Friendship Hospital, Beijing, Peoples Republik of China

H. Kulbertus
University of Liège Medical School, Institute of Medicine, Cardiology Division, Laboratory of Cardiac Clinical Electrophysiology and Pharmacology, Hôpital de Bavière, 4020 Liège, Belgium

H.-W. Klempt
Klinik Martinusquelle, An der Martinusquelle 10, 4792 Bad Lippspringe, W. Germany

M. Kohlhardt
Physiologisches Institut, Universität Freiburg, 7800 Freiburg, W. Germany

D. Krikler
Cardiovascular Division, Royal Postgraduate Medical School, Hammersmith Hospital, London W12 0H2, Great Britain

P. Larochelle
Institut de Recherches Cliniques de Montréal, 110 avenue des Pins ouest, Montréal, QC, H2W 1R7, Canada

J.-F. Leclercq
Hôpital Lariboisière, 2 rue Ambroise-Pare, 75010 Paris, France

L. Ledain
Hôpital Cardiologique, 208 avenue de Magellan, 33604 Pessac, France

F. Lemire
Institut de Recherches Cliniques de Montréal, 110 avenue des Pins ouest, Montréal, QC, H2W 1R7, Canada

H. Lietz
Knoll AG, Knollstr. 50, 6700 Ludwigshafen, W. Germany

Lin Jui-Chin
Beijing Friendship Hospital, Beijing, Peoples Rebublic of China

Li Qing-lang
Beijing Friendship Hospital, Beijing, Peoples Republic of China

Liu Pei-Tsun
Beijing Friendship Hospital, Beijing, Peoples Republic of China

B. Lüderitz
Medizinische Klinik I der Universität München, Klinikum Grosshadern, Marchioninistr. 15, 8000 München 70, W. Germany

M. Manz
Medizinische Klinik I der Universität, Klinikum Grosshadern, Marchioninistr. 15, 8000 München 70, W. Germany

F. Meisl
III. Medizinische Abteilung (Kardiologie und Nephrologie), Montlearstr. 37, 1160 Wien, Austria

J. Morganroth
Hahnemann University, Likoff Cardiovascular Institute, Philadelphia, PA 19102, U.S.A.

M. Murphy
Veterans Administration Medical Center, 300 E. Roosevelt Rd., Little Rock, Arkansas 72206, U.S.A.

G. V. Naccarelli
Indiana University School of Medicine, Krannert Institute of Cardiology, 1100 West Michigan Street, Indianapolis, Indiana 46223, U.S.A.

A. Nayebagha
Klinik Martinusquelle, An der Martinusquelle 10, 4792 Bad Lippspringe, W. Germany

H. Neuss
Kerckhoff-Klinik, Benekestr. 4–6, 6350 Bad Nauheim, W. Germany

J. Ohayon
Hôpital Cardiologique, 208 avenue de Magellan, 33604 Pessac, France

J. Ostermeyer
Chirurgische Klinik B, Universität Düsseldorf, Moorenstr. 5, 4000 Düsseldorf, W. Germany

J. L. Palma
Servicio de Cardiol., Hospital de la Santa Cruz y San Pablo, Av. San Antonia Ma Claret 167, Barcelona 13, Spain

D. Phaneuf
Institut de Recherches Cliniques de Montréal, 110 avenue des Pins ouest, Montréal, QC, H2W 1R7, Canada

M. Pierfitte
Hôpital Jean Rostand, 39 rue le Galleu, 94200 Ivry, France

E. N. Prystowsky
Indiana University School of Medicine, Krannert Institute of Cardiology, 1100 West Michigan Street, Indianapolis, Indiana 46223, U.S.A.

N. Rehnqvist
Department of Medicine, Danderyd's Hospital, 18288 Danderyd, Sweden

J. Sadurni
Servicio de Cardiol., Hospital de la Santa Cruz y San Pablo, Av. San Antonia Ma Claret 167, Barcelona 13, Spain

M. Sakhaii
1962 W. Alex Bell Rd. Dayton, OH 45459

H. San Pablo
Servicio de Cardiol., Hospital de la Santa Cruz y San Pablo, Av. San Antonia Ma Claret, 167, Barcelona 13, Spain

M. Schlepper
Kerckhoff-Klinik der Max-Planck-Gesellschaft, Benekestr. 4–6, 6350 Bad Nauheim, W. Germany

H. Scholz
Abteilung Allgemeine Pharmakologie, Universitäts-Krankenhaus Eppendorf, 2000 Hamburg 20, W. Germany

J. A. Schwarz
Knoll AG, Knollstr. 50, 6700 Ludwigshafen, W. Germany

L. Seipel
Medizinische Universitätsklinik III, Ottfried-Müller Straße, 7400 Tübingen, W. Germany

F. Sesto
Knoll AG, Knollstr. 50, 6700 Ludwigshafen, W. Germany

Shen Lu-hua
Beijing Friendship Hospital, Beijing, Peoples Republic of China

R. Son Dureta
Servicio de Cardiol., Hospital de la Santa Cruz y San Pablo, Av. San Antonia Ma Claret 167, Barcelona 13, Spain

N. Sourdille
Hôpital Cardiologique, 208 avenue de Magellan, 33604 Pessac, France

H.-F. Spies
Knoll AG, Knollstr. 50, 6700 Ludwigshafen, W. Germany

K. Steinbach
III. Medizinische Abteilung (Kardiologie und Nephrologie), Montlearstr. 37, 1160 Wien, Austria

G. Steinbeck
Medizinische Klinik I der Universität München, Klinikum Grosshadern, Marchioninistr. 15, 8000 München 70, W. Germany

B. Stieren
Knoll AG, Knollstr. 50, 6700 Ludwigshafen, W. Germany

F. Theisen
Medizinische Klinik, Innenstadt der Universität München, Ziemssenstr. 1, 8000 München 20, W. Germany

K. Theisen
Medizinische Klinik, Innenstadt der Universität München, Ziemssenstr. 1, 8000 München 20, W. Germany

L. Treat
Veterans Administration Medical Center, 300 E. Roosevelt Rd., Little Rock, Arkansas, 72206, U. S. A.

G. Unger
III. Medizinische Abteilung (Kardiologie und Nephrologie), Montlearstr. 37, 1160 Wien, Austria

A. Waleffe
University of Liège Medical School, Institute of Medicine, Cardiology Division, Laboratory of Cardiac Clinical Electrophysiology and Pharmacology, Hôpital de Bavière, 4020 Liège, Belgium

H. Weber
Kinderklinik und Poliklinik, Waldweg 33, 3400 Göttingen, W. Germany

H. J. Wellens
Head Department of Cardiology, Hospital Maastricht, Netherlands

H. Wesselhoeft
Kinderklinik und Poliklinik, Waldweg 33, 3400 Göttingen, W. Germany

J. Weymann
Knoll AG, Knollstr. 50, 6700 Ludwigshafen, W. Germany

C. E. R. y Cajal
Servicio de Cardiol., Hospital de la Santa Cruz y San Pablo, Av. San Antonia Ma Claret 167, Barcelona 13, Spain

Yang Shi Hau
Beijing Friendship Hospital, Beijing, Peoples Republic of China

P. Yuste
Servicio de Cardiol., Hospital de la Santa Cruz y San Pablo, Av. San Antonia Ma Claret 167, Barcelona 13, Spain

D. P. Zipes
Indiana University School of Medicine, Krannert Institute of Cardiology, 1100 West Michigan Street, Indianapolis, Indiana 46223, U. S. A.

Introduction

This meeting, organised in association with the working party on arrhythmias of the European Society of Cardiology, provided one-and-a-half days of fruitful interchange between workers from various European countries, the United States, Canada, and China. An essential prerequisite of the proper management of arrhythmia is the careful understanding of mechanisms, incidence and specific features, which was provided by the first half day. It is important to appreciate the incidence of arrhythmias in the apparently healthy population, and to compare it with that seen in patients. In addition to the conventional electrocardiographic tracing we now, from many centres, have further information obtained by long-term ambulatory monitoring. From these data we can correlate aspects of biological variability in arrhythmias, including the influence of the autonomic nervous system. Delayed conduction is often an important marker of a tendency to develop arrhythmias and the possibility of recording late potentials from the surface of the body is a great step forward from having always to depend on invasive investigations. Nevertheless, the precise determination of the nature of certain arrhythmias and the assessment of possible therapeutic benefit still depends on programmed electric stimulation of the heart with appropriate recordings. We are thus usefully reminded of the fact that different information may be obtained from different sites. While we would like to be able to tailor antiarrhythmic therapy precisely to the type of rhythm disorder that has been recorded, this has not yet been achieved with anything like the degree of confidence that one knows from other clinical situations e.g. antibacterial therapy. Indeed, we still need to agree on the definition of high risk regarding the development of arrhythmias including those likely to cause sudden death, whether in the context of ischaemic or other heart disease.

In general terms, Propafenone falls within the first class of antiarrhythmic agents as defined by Vaughan Williams. Its antiarrhythmic properties may depend to a considerable extent upon its ability to impede fast-channel conduction across the myocardial cell membrane. There are many such agents but none is perfect. We have considerable knowledge about Propafenone which enables us to look at its potential efficacy in comparison with agents accepted as working along these lines. In conventional doses as used clinically its potential to cause negative inotropic action is gratifyingly slight, though it is useful to remember that higher doses such as may be used in animal studies, may have such effects.

The free sessions offered a variety of expositions on the efficacy of Propafenone under a number of circumstances. In common with a number of other agents it has the ability to decrease the number of ventricular extrasystoles, and can be used for this and other ventricular arrhythmias by intravenous or longterm oral use. One should not forget its potential benefit in patients with supraventricular arrhythmias, especially arrhythmias associated with atrioventricular reentry as well as preexcitation syndromes.

This symposium and the book on its proceedings provide us with useful information not only about Propafenone but also on the current state of our knowledge of arrhythmias, including their investigation and assessment. From the proceedings it is quite clear that

Propafenone has an important role to play in the management of arrhythmias and that its introduction into clinical use offers great advantages over many other agents: we have a sound characterization not only of its properties but also of its potential interactions. Our own limited studies over the last few years have accorded entirely with the favourable results reported. We thus consider Propafenone a much-needed agent which, in addition to its undoubted efficacy, has the great virtue of good tolerance.

Dennis Krikler MD FRCP
Consultant Cardiologist
Hammersmith Hospital
London W12 OHS

Differentiation Between "Normal" and "Abnormal" in Ambulatory Electrocardiography

P. Bjerregaard

The establishment of normal limits for electrocardiographic features is based on a statistical description of a healthy population sample, but neither "normal" nor "healthy" has been unambiguously defined. At the tenth Bethesda Conference on Optimal Electrocardiography in 1977 (Abildskov 1978) a healthy population sample was defined as a representative sample of ambulatory noninstitutionalized persons without medical complaints or evidence by history or examination of any disease or dysfunction that may impair health or affect the electrocardiogram. None of the studies concerning ambulatory ECG recording in healthy subjects have been performed on representative healthy population samples, but there are several good reasons why. Healthy subjects are not immediately accessible, but must be drawn from a general population sample. This means that a lot of subjects would have to be examined and excluded from the study because they did not fulfil the requirements for healthy. "Nonhealthy" subjects are prevalent especially in higher age groups (Hinkle et al. 1969; Camm et al. 1978). Another problem is the high number of refusals, with approximately every third subject unwilling to participate (Raftery and Cashman 1976; Camm et al. 1978; Goulding 1978), making the requirement of a representative sample illusory. Many reports in the literature concerning healthy subjects therefore deal with subjects drawn from selected populations with a low incidence of disease and a low number of refusals (medical students, hospital staff, company employees, etc.). In studies concerning electrocardiographic features unknown to the subject himself such an approach may in most cases be acceptable, but it does involve a certain risk of not being sufficiently representative.

A problem in the establishment of comparable healthy population samples is the difference in number and types of investigative procedures performed in various studies in order to identify healthy subjects, and differences in this respect may have had some bearing on differences in the results obtained. In all studies (where the criteria for inclusion have been mentioned) absence of history of cardiovascular disease or symptoms, normal physical examination, and normal resting ECG have been required unanimously. Unfortunately the definition of a normal ECG ist not unequivocal in terms of, for example, premature beats. In the study of 50 young women by Sobotka et al. (1981) two subjects with ventricular premature beats on resting 12-lead ECG and one with a single atrial premature beat were excluded. Since these subjects very likely would have had a high number of premature beats during a 24-h period, their exclusion from the study may have influenced the reported results significantly. In the study by Bjerregaard (1982 b) subjects with premature beats in the resting ECG were included, and were those who had the highest number of premature beats during the subsequent 24-h recording period. In a study of the prevalence of ECG features in a healthy population the ECG should only be used for exclusion of subjects with certain well-established ECG patterns of abnormality, such as myocardial infarct (Simonson 1961). If subjects with arrhythmias not normally connected to any particular disease are excluded from a study of the heart rhythm, the study is severely limited, and less relevant for an estimate of the prevalence of arrhythmias. In four studies (Engel and Burckhardt 1975; Kostis et al. 1979; Leitner et al. 1979; Møller and Thayssen 1980) a normal exercise tolerance test was a prerequisite for inclusion in a study of healthy subjects, and four (Brodsky et al. 1977; Djiane et al. 1977; Kostis et al. 1979; Sobotka et al. 1981) required a normal echocardiogram. In only one study (Kostis et al. 1979) were invasive studies (right and left heart catheterization and coronary arteriography) performed. It is an open question, however, how far in diagnostic testing one should go in order to exclude "nonhealthy" subjects. It may be stated that "healthy" subjects are only underinvestigated people, and by using very sensitive diagnostic tests one may end up with a "disappearing" group of subjects. In spite of all precautions, it is probable that any large healthy group will include some individuals with latent disease.

These problems in selecting healthy population samples must be kept in mind when results of 17 studies involving 1427 healthy subjects (Table 1) are used in this paper to differentiate between "normal" and "abnormal" in ambulatory electrocardiography.

Minimal Heart Rate

The heart rate in healthy subjects shows a typical day-and-night pattern, with the highest rates during the daytime and the lowest at night. This means that the minimal heart rate in a 24-h ambulatory ECG usually occurs during sleep, beyond the control of the individual subject, and very likely with some important diagnostic information attached to its level. The establishment of clear-cut limits for the minimal heart rate in humans during a 24-h period has hitherto been difficult, however, partially owing to the lack of a generally accepted method of determining heart rate. In the study by Bjerregaard (1982a) these methodological problems were illustrated by comparison of figures for minimal heart rate obtained by four different methods in a subgroup of healthy subjects characterized by R-R intervals in excess of 1.5 s. When only three consecutive beats were used for heart rate determination, the mean minimal heart rate was 41 beats/min compared with a mean of 49 beats/min when the actual number of beats in a 1-min period was used. It was also shown that the lowest value on a heart rate trend curve with a time constant of 1 min real time, used in many cardiological centers in Europe, provides an acceptable estimate of the minimal number of beats/min. Available data on minimal heart rates in healthy adult subjects are given in Table 2. It is important to note that the data from the studies by Brodsky et al. (1977) and Sobotka et al. (1981) are based on periods of six consecutive beats, whereas the other three studies used 1-min periods. A lower minimal heart rate in young males compared with young females is evident, and a similar sex difference was found among subjects 40–79 years of age by Bjerregaard (1982a). The data presented show that a minimal heart rate of less than 40 beats/min determined from a 1-min period is extremely unusual in an adult subject above 40 years of age. Figures for minimal heart rate in younger subjects determined from 1-min periods are lacking, but the data from the study by Brodsky et al. (1977) suggest that even in subjects below the age of 40, a minimal heart rate of less than 40 beats/min determined from a 1-min period is rare.

Table 1. Studies concerning ambulatory ECG recording in healthy adult subjects

Author (year of publication)	Characteristics of subjects studied	Recording h	Arrhythmias searched for		
			SA	A	AV
Kleiger and Senior (1974)	51 nonsmoking, normal subjects, aged 35–65 years (control group)	10		x	
Engel and Burckhardt (1975)	35 (13 female, 22 male) healthy volunteers, mean age 24±4 years	7.5	x	x	
Clarke et al. (1976)	86 (45 female, 41 male) company employees, aged 16–65 years	48	(x)	(x)	x
Raftery and Cashman (1976)	53 (24 female, 29 male) healthy volunteers, aged 20–79 years	24	(x)	x	
Brodsky et al. (1977)	50 male medical students, aged 23–27 years	24	x	x	x
Djiane et al. (1977)	50 (13 female, 37 male) healthy volunteers, aged 22–57 years	24	x	x	x
Kennedy et al. (1977)	23 (1 female, 22 male) healthy volunteers, aged 35–66 years (control group)	24			
Federman et al. (1978)	21 (4 female, 17 male) hospital staff or their relatives, aged 40–66 years (control group)	24			
Goulding (1978)	100 (50 female, 50 male) healthy volunteers, aged 25–74 years	24	(x)	x	
Verbaan et al. (1978)	74 (39 female, 35 male) healthy volunteers, aged 20–80 years	24	(x)	x	
Kostis et al. (1979)	100 (45 female, 55 male) healthy volunteers, aged 16–68 years	24	(x)		x
Leitner et al. (1979)	100 healthy volunteers, aged 40–69 years	24	x	x	x
Møller and Thayssen (1980)	24 healthy volunteers, mean age 53±10 (control group)	24			
Orth-Gomér (1980)	50 healthy male subjects, aged 40–65 years (control group)	24			
Cats et al. (1981)	300 actively employed men aged 40–59 years, without symptomatic coronary heart disease	24			
Sobotka et al. (1981)	50 female volunteers, aged 22–28 years	24	x	x	x
Bjerregaard (1982a)	260 (90 female, 170 male) healthy volunteers, aged 40–79 years	24	x	x	x

SA, x sinoatrial; A, x atrial; AV, x atrioventricular
In connection with SA arrhythmias (x) denotes that only the mean heart rate (as a manifestation of the sinus node function) has been evaluated.
In connection with A arrhythmias (x) denotes that only the occurrence of supraventricular tachycardia (and not atrial premature beats) has been evaluated.

Table 2. Studies on minimal heart rate during ambulatory ECG in healthy adult subjects

Author (year of publication)	Age range (years)	Minimal heart rate		Heart rate < 40 beats/min (% of subjects)
		Mean ± SD (Beats/min)	Range (Beats/min)	
Brodsky et al. (1977)	23–27	43±5	33–55	24
Sobotka et al. (1981)	22–28	48±6	37–59	8
Djiane et al. (1977)	32±9	56±7	45–74	None
Leitner et al. (1979)	40–65		44–	None
Bjerregaard (1982a)	40–79	56±8	36–78	1

Table 3. Studies of the longest pauses in the ambulatory ECG in healthy adult subjects

Author (year of publication)	Subjects		Longest pauses			Duration of longest pause	
	Sex	Age range (years)	≥ 1 500 ms No. (%) of subjects	≥ 1 750 ms No. (%) of subjects	≥ 2 000 ms No. (%) of subjects	Mean ±SD (ms)	Range (ms)
Brodsky et al. (1977)	Male	23–27	34 (68)	14 (28)	2 (4)	1.62±0.20	1.20–2.06
Sobotka et al. (1981)	Female	22–28			None	1.47±0.20	1.08–1.92
Djiane et al. (1977)	Male and female	22–57	24 (48)	8 (16)	2 (4)		–2.52
Bjerregaard (1982 a)	Male and female	40–49	36 (37)	3 (3)	1 (1)		–2.04
Bjerregaard (1982 a)	Male and female	50–59	27 (31)	4 (5)	1 (1)		–2.02
Bjerregaard (1982 a)	Male and female	60–79	14 (18)	5 (7)	None		–1.92

Pauses

As long as there is no generally accepted definition for a pause in the ECG, any such definition will be arbitrary, and every interval between two consecutive ventricular depolarizations (R-R interval or ventricular gap) is in fact a pause. Some authors (Djiane et al. 1977; Bjerregaard, 1982 a) regard only R-R intervals ≥1 500 ms as pauses, and most authors exclude AV block.

Available data concerning the duration of the longest pauses in the ambulatory ECG in healthy adult subjects are shown in Table 3. Pauses ≥1 500 ms are seen in approximately half of the subjects (30%–68%), but with an inverse relationship between age and the proportion of subjects with pauses. The longest pause in a 24-h ambulatory ECG usually occurs during sleep (Brodsky et al. 1977; Sobotka et al. 1981), and in the study by Bjerregaard (1982 a) 96% occurred between 10 p.m. and 8 a.m. In most studies no attempt has been made to give a more detailed electrocardiographic interpretation of these pauses, which have mostly been diagnosed as sinus arrhythmia (Brodsky et al. 1977; Leitner et al. 1979; Sobotka et al. 1981), and marked sinus arrhythmia with adjacent R-R intervals varying by more than 100% has been reported in 50% of young men (Brodsky et al. 1977) and in 34% of young women (Sobotka et al. 1981). In the preliminary report of a study which will later be published in more detail (Bjerregaard, 1982 a), Bjerregaard (1980) introduced the descriptive term "postacceleration pause" for 60% of the pauses. Following a period with only minimal variation in the R-R intervals, an acceleration in heart rate for a few beats (usually 5–10) is replaced by a sudden deceleration for two beats, forming a pause prior to a gradual return in heart rate to the prepause level. In the same study sinus arrest was diagnosed in 16% of the sinus pauses, but only present in 5% of the total number of subjects studied.

Table 4. Electrocardiographic changes during sleep in healthy adult subjects

Time of day	Heart rate Mean ± SD (Beats/min)	P-R interval Mean ± SD (s)	Q-T interval Mean ± SD (s)
8 a.m.–8 p.m.	76 ± 15	0.16 ± 0.02	0.37 ± 0.03
Midnight	65 ± 15	0.17 ± 0.02	0.40 ± 0.02
4 a.m.	60 ± 15	0.18 ± 0.02	0.41 ± 0.03

Until more precise information about pauses in healthy subjects and in subjects with sinus node disease is available, it seems reasonable to consider pauses in the ambulatory ECG $\geqslant$ 1750 ms – seen in only 5% of healthy subjects 40–79 years of age – an "abnormal" finding within this age group. For younger subjects the corresponding figure is somewhere between 1750 ms and 2000 ms. In all age groups, pauses greater than 2000 ms are extremely rare.

Atrioventricular Block

Since many factors known to influence AV conduction operate in healthy subjects during a 24-h period, changes in the P-R interval are to be expected in the ambulatory ECG. In a study by Bjerregaard (unpublished data) 10-s ECG samples were obtained from ambulatory ECG recordings in 28 healthy subjects every 4 h and the R-R, P-R and Q-T intervals measured (Table 4). Slowing of the heart rate during sleep was accompanied by a modest increase in the P-R interval. In subjects with borderline prolongation of the P-R interval the increase might possibly be more pronounced.

Of the studies of healthy subjects presented in Table 1, AV conduction disturbances were searched for in seven, involving 696 subjects; 12 cases (1.7%) of first degree AV block and nine (1.3%) of second degree AV block were observed. All cases of second degree AV block were of the Wenckebach type, and they all occurred during sleep. Only two subjects also had second degree AV block in the daytime.

Atrial Premature Beats

This category of ectopic depolarizations includes atrial, as well as atrioventricular or junctional premature beats (APBs). Exact figures for APBs in a 24-h ambulatory ECG in healthy adult subjects have been reported in only a few studies (Table 5). It is obvious from these studies, however, that APBs occur in most healthy adult subjects, but with a great variation in the number of APBs per 24-h period among different age groups, with a statistically significant increase in the number of APBs/1000 QRS as well as in APBs/h with increasing age, as shown for the age range 40–79 years (Bjerregaard, 1982b). All seven subjects with more than 10 APBs/24 h in the study by Goulding (1978)

Table 5. Studies of APBs in a 24-h ambulatory ECG in healthy adult subjects

Author (year of publication)	Age range (years)	Atrial premature beats			
		< 10/24 h	> 10/24 h	> 100/24 h	> 1 000/24 h
		Subjects studied			
Brodsky et al. (1977)	23–27	56	8	2	0
Sobotka et al. (1981)	22–28	64	4		
Djiane et al. (1977)	22–57	22	4	2	0
Goulding (1978)	25–74	12	7	7	5
Raftery and Cashman (1976)	20–79	17	15	11	0
Verbaan et al. (1978)	20–80	73			
Bjerregaard (1982b)	40–49	78	41	2	1
Leitner et al. (1979)	40–65	61	38	5	1
Bjerregaard (1982b)	50–59	89	58	9	2
Bjerregaard (1982b)	60–79	97	76	21	5

were above the age of 45 years and five were 65 years or more. Similarly, all the subjects in the study by Raftery and Cashman (1976) who had more than 100 APBs/24 h were 50 years of age or older. The relatively high incidence of APBs in the study by Verbaan et al. (1978) likewise may be accounted for by the fact that two-thirds of the subjects were above 40 years of age. Complex forms of APBs in terms of couplets or APB as bigeminy have been reported only as isolated events (Brodsky et al. 1977; Djiane et al. 1977; Sobotka et al. 1981; Bjerregaard 1982b), but APBs with marked variability in P-wave morphology, suggesting multifocal origin, were seen in 52% of subjects 40–79 years of age studied by Bjerregaard (to be published b).

It may be concluded that an APB in a 24-h ambulatory ECG in a healthy adult subject is normal. If events occurring in approximately 5% of a healthy population sample are "normal", a rough estimate of the upper limit of "normal" for APBs/24 h based on the data in Table 5 would be ten within the age range 20–40 years, 100 within the age range 40–60 years, and 1 000 above the age of 60.

Atrial Tachycardia

Just as with other complex forms of APBs, the occurrence of more than two consecutive APBs with an instantaneous heart rate above 100 beats/min (atrial tachycardia, AT) has hitherto been considered rare in a healthy adult subject. Recent data have shown, however, that it is seen in approximately half of the subjects above the age of 60 years studied (Table 6). It is nevertheless important to stress the fact that even in older subjects AT usually occurs as isolated events, and the highest number of episodes reported in any one subject has been four. In the study by Bjerregaard (1982b) a total of 92 episodes of AT were registered in 57 subjects, and more than two episodes in only 13 subjects (5%), with more than ten beats per episode in only six subjects.

Even though the amount of data concerning AT, especially in the older age group, is still sparse, the overall data currently available suggest that AT as isolated events of short duration are "normal" in adult subjects. Repeated episodes, especially in more sustained form, are, on the other hand, not seen in asymptomatic subjects.

Table 6. Studies of AT in the ambulatory ECG in healthy adult subjects

Author (year of publication)	Age range (years)	Atrial tachycardia No. (%) of subjects	Highest number of beats per episode
Brodsky et al. (1977)	23–27	1 (2)	12
Sobotka et al. (1981)	22–28	1 (2)	6
Djiane et al. (1977)	22–57	1 (2)	3
Clarke et al. (1976)	16–65	4 (5)	
Goulding (1978)	25–74	0	
Raftery and Cashman (1976)	20–79	2 (4)	34
Verbaan et al. (1978)	20–80	7 (9)	
Bjerregaard (1982b)	40–49	5 (5)	7
Bjerregaard (1982b)	50–59	17 (20)	23
Bjerregaard (1982b)	60–79	35 (46)	18

Table 7. Studies of VPBs in a 24-h ambulatory ECG in healthy adult subjects

Author (year of publication)	Age range (years)	Ventricular premature beats			
		< 10/24 h	> 10/24 h	> 100/24 h	> 1000/24 h
		Subjects studied			
Brodsky et al. (1977)	23–27	50	12	0	0
Sobotka et al. (1981)	22–28	54	10	4	2
Djiane et al. (1977)	22–57	22	2	0	0
Kostis et al. (1979)	16–68	46	20	5	
Clarke et al. (1976)	16–65	73		8	2
Raftery and Cashman (1976)	20–79	15	10	2	
Verbaan et al. (1978)	20–80	76	13	4	2
Bjerregaard (1982b)	40–49	57	13	4	2
Cats et al. (1981)	40–49	71		7	
Leitner et al. (1979)	40–65	63	34	7	
Bjerregaard (1982b)	50–59	73	22	10	2
Cats et al. (1981)	50–59	81		19	
Bjerregaard (1982b)	60–79	79	27	12	1

Ventricular Premature Beats

Of all the disturbances of rhythm and conduction, none has engendered as much interest during ambulatory ECG recording as the ventricular premature beat (VPB) (Table 7). A slight increase in the proportion of subjects with VPBs with age has been observed, but even below 28 years of age, half of the subjects have at least one VPB during a 24-h period. Bjerregaard (1982b) showed a statistically significant increase in both the number of VPBs per hour and per 1000 QRS with age, but more than 200 VPBs per 24-h period were seen in only 5% of 260 healthy subjects 40–79 years of age. Below the age of 50 years it is unusual to have more than 100 VPBs per 24 h – a figure proposed by Kostis et al. (1979) as the upper limit of "normal" for VPBs in healthy adult subjects. Available

Table 8. Studies of complex VPBs in a 24-h ambulatory ECG in healthy adult subjects

Author (year of publication)	Age range (years)	Complex ventricular premature beats				
		Multiform	Couplets	Coupled	R-on-T	Ventricular tachycardia
		Subjects studied				
Brodsky et al. (1977)	23–27	12	0	2	6	2
Sobotka et al. (1981)	22–28	10	0		4	2
Djiane et al. (1977)	22–57	8	6			2
Clarke et al. (1976)	16–65	15		3	5	2
Verbaan et al. (1978)	20–80	38	9	3	5	1
Bjerregaard (1982b)	40–49	12	3	2	1	3
Cats et al. (1981)	40–49	26	7	2		1
Leitner et al. (1979)	40–65	22	2	4		3
Orth-Gomér (1980)	40–65	22	14		2	0
Bjerregaard (1982b)	50–59	28	10	3	1	1
Cats et al. (1981)	50–59	39	17	9		2
Bjerregaard (1982b)	60–79	32	11	1	0	1

data seem, however, to indicate a somewhat higher limit for subjects above 50 years of age.

Any of the complex forms of VPBs seen in patients with heart disease may appear as an incidental finding in a 24-h ambulatory ECG in a healthy subject, but with great variability in prevalence among the various forms (Table 8). Approximately half of the subjects with more than one VPB have VPBs with variable contour (multiform), but VPBs of more than two different configurations are "abnormal". VPBs in couplets, coupled, or as R-on-T are seen in less than 5% of subjects, except in those above 50 years of age, where VPB couplets have been observed in 10%–17%. Ventricular tachycardia is a rare finding in a healthy subject and has always been reported as isolated events.

Final Remarks

With the exception of sustained forms of tachyarrhythmias, most arrhythmias seen in patients with heart disease can occur in healthy subjects, but usually in low number. For a proper evaluation of arrhythmias in a particular subject in terms of "normal" or "abnormal" it is therefore important to quantitate the various arrhythmias separately; the

Table 9. Differentiation between "normal" and "abnormal" in the ambulatory ECG

"normal"	"abnormal"
minimal HR < 50 beats/min pauses > 1 500 ms post-acceleration pauses	minimal HR < 40 beats/min pauses > 1750 ms (> 2000 ms) sinus arrest
	AV-block
atrial premature beats (APBs) multiform APBs > 50 years of age: paroxysmal atrial tachycardia (PAT)	20–40 years of age: > 10 APBs/24 h 40–60 years of age: > 100 APBs/24 h 60–80 years of age: > 1 000 APBs/24 h > 2 different forms of APBs < 50 years of age: PAT > 2 episodes of PAT/24 h PAT of > 10 beats/episode
ventricular premature beats (VPBs) multiform VPBs > 50 years of age: single episodes of VPB couplets	< 50 years of age: > 100 VPBs/24 h > 50 years of age: > 200 VPBs/24 h > 2 different forms of VPBs < 50 years of age: VPB couplets VPB as bigeminy R-on-T VPB ventricular tachycardia

use of grading systems such as the one proposed by Lown and Wolf (1971) should be discouraged, since they do not consider quantitation of individual arrhythmias sufficiently.

The available data on incidence and variability of cardiac arrhythmias in healthy adult subjects here presented do not allow establishment of normal limits for the ambulatory ECG based on statistical descriptions, but enough data have accumulated for a rough differentiation between "normal" and "abnormal". Such a differentiation is shown in Table 9.

The next step is the establishment of the prognostic significance of an "abnormal" finding in a healthy subject in order to obtain a more rational basis for therapeutical interventions.

References

Abildskov JA (1978) Tenth Bethesda conference on optimal electrocardiography. Am J Cardiol 41: 130–132

Bjerregaard P (1980) The longest pauses observed during ambulatory electrocardiography in healthy subjects. Proceedings of the VIIIth European Congress of Cardiology, Paris, Abstr 1041

Bjerregaard P (1982a) Mean 24 hour heart rate, minimal heart rate and pauses in healthy subjects 40–79 years of age. Eur Heart J (Accepted for publication)

Bjerregaard P (1982b) Premature beats in healthy subjects 40–79 years of age. Eur Heart J (Accepted for publication)

Brodsky M, Wu D, Denes P, Kanakis C, Rosen KM (1977) Arrhythmias documented by 24 hour continuous electrocardiographic monitoring in 50 male medical students without apparent heart disease. Am J Cardiol 39: 390–395

Camm AJ, Martin A, Evans KE, Arnold S, Spurrell RAJ (1978) 24-hour ambulatory monitoring. A survey of active, elderly people. ISAM 1977. Proceedings Second International Symposium on Ambulatory Monitoring, London, pp 7–12

Cats VM, Darmanata J, Durrer D (1981) Complex ventricular premature beats in healthy middle aged men during 24-hour Holter tape recording. Eur Heart J 2: 13

Clarke JM, Hamer J, Shelton JR, Taylor S, Venning GR (1976) The rhythm of the normal human heart. Lancet 2: 508–512

Djiane P, Egre A, Bory M, Savin B, Serradimigni A (1977) L'enregistrement électrocardiographique continu chez 50 sujets normaux. Proceedings Troubles du rythme et électrostimulation, Toulouse, Septembre 1977, pp 161–168

Engel UR, Burckhardt D (1975) Häufigkeit und Art von Herzrhythmusstörungen sowie EKG-Veränderungen bei jugendlichen herzgesunden Probanden. Schweiz Med Wochenschr 105: 1467–1469

Federman J, Whitford JA, Anderson ST, Pitt A (1978) Incidence of ventricular arrhythmias in first year after myocardial infarction. Br Heart J 40: 1243–1250

Goulding L (1978) Twenty-four hour ambulatory electrocardiography from normal urban and rural populations. ISAM 1977. Proceedings Second International Symposium on Ambulatory Monitoring, London, pp 13–22

Hinkle LE, Carver ST, Stevens M (1969) The frequency of asymptomatic disturbances of cardiac rhythm and conduction in middle-aged men. Am J Cardiol 24: 629–650

Kennedy HL, Caralis DG, Khan MA, Poblete PF, Pescarmona JE (1977) Ventricular arrhythmias 24 hours before and after treadmill testing. Am Heart J 94: 718–724

Kleiger RE, Senior RM (1974) Longterm electrocardiographic monitoring of ambulatory patients with chronic airway obstruction. Chest 65: 483–487

Kostis JB, Moreyra AE, Natarajan N, Gotzoyannis S, Hosler M, McCrone K, Kuo PT (1979) Ambulatory electrocardiography: What is normal? Am J Cardiol 43: 420

Leitner E-R, Andresen D, Reinhardt M, Tietze U, Schröder R (1979) Langzeit-EKG-Untersuchungen von herzgesunden Normalpersonen mit rechnercompatiblem Analysesystem. Intensivmedizin 16: 184–188

Lown B, Wolf M (1971) Approaches to sudden death from coronary heart disease. Circulation 44: 130–142

Møller M, Thayssen P (1980) Ventricular arrhythmias during exercise testing and 24 hour ecg tape recording in patients with ischaemic heart disease and in normal individuals. Acta Med Scand 208: 65–68

Orth-Gomér K (1980) Ventricular arrhythmias and risk indicators of ischemic heart disease. Acta Med Scand 207: 283–289

Raftery EB, Cashman PMM (1976) Long-term recording of the electrocardiogram in a normal population. Postgrad Med J [Suppl 7] 52: 32–38

Simonson E (ed) (1961) Differentiation between normal and abnormal in electrocardiography. Mosby, St Louis

Sobotka PA, Mayer JH, Bauernfeind RA, Kanakis C, Rosen KM (1981) Arrhythmias documented by 24-hour continuous ambulatory electrocardiographic monitoring in young women without apparent heart disease. Am Heart J 101: 753–759

Verbaan CJ, Pool J, Wanrooy JV (1978) Incidence of cardiac arrhythmias in a presumed healthy population. ISAM 1977. Proceedings Second International Symposium on Ambulatory Monitoring, London, pp 1–5

Identification of the Patient at High Risk of Sudden Cardiac Death

J. Morganroth

Introduction

Coronary artery disease, which continues to be the primary cause of death and morbidity in the western world, has a variety of potential clinical presentations. The fortunate patient is one who presents with symptoms of left ventricular dysfunction (congestive heart failure) or ischemia (angina pectoris). The presentation of the clinical syndrome of acute myocardial infarction carries with it the immediate loss of myocardial tissue and a high rate of peri-infarction death. Unfortunately, the most common presentation in the industrialized world is sudden cardiac death, which affects at least one individual per minute in the United States (Lown 1979).

Sudden cardiac death occurs prematurely, usually without precipitating cause, and is unexpected. Only about 20% of individuals affected have acute myocardial infarction, though over three-quarters have coronary artery disease. The cause of sudden cardiac death is usually a ventricular tachyarrhythmia resulting in ventricular fibrillation. Such an arrhythmia usually causes death instantaneously or within 1 h; thus, the importance of identifying the high-risk individual for this malady becomes apparent. Prevention of the occurrence of sudden cardiac death is the only logical means of stemming this epidemic problem, since therapy at its onset will not be a universally practical or a satisfying solution.

Ventricular Ectopy: The Marker for Subsequent Ventricular Tachyarrhythmia

In the 1960s the widespread use of coronary care units showed ventricular ectopy to be frequently associated with fatal ventricular arrhythmias. In such cases death could frequently be prevented by intravenous antiarrhythmic therapy (Bigger et al. 1977). Thus, the presence of ventricular premature complexes on the monitor became an important marker of fatal ventricular tachyarrhythmias over 20 years ago. Unfortunately, the degree of ventricular ectopy during the coronary-care-unit phase of acute myocardial infarction is an unreliable predictor of which patients will experience ventricular ectopy after hospital discharge (Moss et al. 1971). Epidemiologic studies conducted during the 1970s clearly identified ventricular premature complexes as important predictors of sudden cardiac death. The epidemiologic program sponsored by the National Heart Institute known as the Coronary Drug Project (Coronary Project Research Group 1973) found that the presence of even one ventricular premature beat on an electrocardiogram was associated with an increased risk of sudden death during the next 2–5-year period. Several studies in the mid-1970s (using ambulatory Holter monitoring in post-myocardial infarction patients) concluded that 50%–70% of such patients will have ventricular ectopy at or after discharge, and at least 25% of these will have complex ventricular ectopy. For patients with complex ventricular ectopy, the risk of sudden cardiac death over the next 1–3 years increased three to fourfold (Kotler et al. 1973; Vismara et al. 1975; Rehnqvist and Siogren 1977; Moss et al. 1979). In these studies ventricular ectopy was evaluated as a univariate factor.

Schulze et al. (1977b) found the presence of complex ventricular ectopy with reduced left ventricular function (as measured by radionuclide ejection fraction) in 100% of patients who died suddenly during the 6-month follow-up period. The same group (Schulze et al. 1977b) also found that the more extensive the coronary artery disease and the greater the left ventricular dysfunction at cardiac catheterization, the more likely one was to suffer sudden cardiac death, particularly in the presence of ventricular ectopy.

Davis et al. (1979) reported on the prospective evaluation of 940 patients who survived acute myocardial infarction, followed up for 12–60 months, and demonstrated that the 1-year mortality of this group without any complications was 2%, whereas those patients with electrical, ischemic, or mechanical abnormalities were noted to have more than a five fold increase in risk of sudden death. This study demonstrated that the combination of anterior wall myocardial infarction with left ventricular dysfunction in the presence of ventricular ectopy, especially if complex (ventricular couplets or ventricular tachycardia), identified a high-risk subset for sudden cardiac death that constituted 15% of the myocardial infarction population with a 6-month mortality of 15% and a 3-year mortality of 30%. In this study a low-risk subgroup was identified without these factors, constituting 2.4% of the population which had a 3-year mortality of only 6%. Using multiregression statistical analysis, this study has demonstrated that patients with complex and even simple ventricular premature complexes have an increased risk of sudden cardiac death.

A study by Ruberman et al. (1981) of 1739 male survivors of myocardial infarction clearly identified complex ventricular arrhythmias as independent and possibly unique markers of sudden cardiac death in the post-myocardial infarction population. They also demonstrated that the coexistence of underlying structural heart disease with manifest congestive heart failure was an important independent influence on the risk of death. In this particular study, simple premature ventricular contractions seen during a 1-hour monitoring period were not as predictive as in other studies which used longer monitoring periods (Davis et al. 1979). Recent studies by Bigger and Weld (1981) have demonstrated that a quantitative approach is a more predictive method than a classification system such as that used by Lown in defining prognostic significance of ventricular arrhythmias, and that the best cut-point for relating ventricular ectopic frequency to mortality appears to be $\geqslant$ 10 PVCs/h/24 h. In a series of 500 patients followed up for 1 year, mortality of this group was 25%. Bigger et al. (1981) found an incidence of ventricular tachycardia (triplets or greater) of 11.6% in 430 patients after myocardial infarction. Only 50% of these individuals had a single episode of ventricular tachycardia, and in one-third of the group the longest run was only three beats. R-on-T phenomenon was rare and the highest incidence of ventricular tachycardia occurred in patients with prior myocardial infarction, left ventricular failure, and atrial fibrillation. Patients with ventricular tachycardia had a 38% mortality at 1 year, compared with 11.6% in those without; the 36-month mortality was 54% compared with 19%.

Regarding the combination of ventricular ectopy and underlying structural heart disease manifesting as left ventricular failure, the presence of both congestive heart failure and complex arrhythmias presented a risk ratio of 6.1 compared with 1.9 with congestive heart failure alone and 3.3 with complex ventricular premature beats alone (Ruberman et al. 1981).

It is obvious that patients with underlying structural heart disease, with left ventricular dysfunction not due to coronary artery-induced myocardial infarction, might also have a high risk of sudden cardiac death in the presence of ventricular ectopy. We have shown that among patients with underlying idiopathic congestive cardiomyopathy, sudden cardiac death occurred in 47% of those who also manifested complex ventricular arrhythmias, but in only 6% of those who did not (Follansbee et al. 1980). Similar increased risk of sudden cardiac death has been suggested in patients with underlying hypertrophic cardiomyopathy concomitant with underlying ventricular irritability (Savage et al. 1979).

Profile of the Patient with the Highest Risk of Sudden Cardiac Death

When patients who have suffered out-of-hospital cardiac arrest are resuscitated, a profile of the patient who is most likely to suffer sudden cardiac death can be drawn. The studies of Myerburg et al. (1980) and Goldstein et al. (1981) define a group in which more than three-quarters of the patients have underlying coronary artery disease and the remaining patients have cardiomyopathies, severe valvular lesions, and unusual conditions such as long QT syndromes, severe hypokalemia, and preexcitation syndrome. Survivors with apparently normal hearts are a rarity, representing less than 2% of this population. Males comprise approximately 80% of the group, and the primary mechanism of sudden cardiac death is ventricular tachyarrhythmia. Two-thirds of individuals have abnormal indices of left ventricular function and use digitalis compounds frequently. In addition, patients who have had an elevation of blood urea nitrogen or pulmonary congestion during their myocardial infarction appear to be a particularly high-risk group for sudden cardiac death (Table 1).

Table 1. High risk patients for sudden cardiac death

1. Survivors of sudden cardiac death attack
2. Unstable coronary artery disease and ventricular ectopy
3. Post-myocardial infarction with ventricular dysfunction and ventricular ectopy, especially if complex
4. Structural heart disease (e.g., cardiomyopathy, valvular heart (disease) and ventricular ectopy
5. Long-QT syndrome and ventricular ectopy

Measures of Antiarrhythmic Efficacy

Ambulatory Holter monitoring has been clearly established as the most sensitive and specific means of detecting ventricular ectopy, even when compared with other noninvasive methods, such as exercise testing (Winkle 1980). Exercise testing will, however, identify arrhythmias induced by physiologic stress which is more pronounced than that which the patient spontaneously experiences during ambulatory monitoring. Thus, the two tests are essentially complementary.

The definition of antiarrhythmic drug efficacy must take into account the contexts in which ventricular premature complexes occur, of which two are important. The first is in patients in which the premature ventricular ectopy produces no significant hemodynamic embarrassment. The patient may be symptomatic in terms of occasional palpitations or dizziness but does not have syncope or advanced manifestations of hemodynamic compromise. The true measure of antiarrhythmic drug efficacy in such patients is the prevention of sudden cardiac death, since it is believed (as noted earlier) that underlying structural heart disease concomitant with ventricular ectopy places such an individual at high risk of death. Thus, antiarrhythmic suppressive therapy appears warranted if such therapy can be claimed to prevent sudden cardiac death. Unfortunately, prior antiarrhythmic drug trials aimed (for example in the post-myocardial infarction patient) at reducing sudden cardiac death (May et al. 1982) have failed to produce a statistically significant reduction, owing, probably in large part, to incorrect drug selection, inadequate sample size, or inappropriate choice of patients. It is, of course, possible that antiarrhythmic therapy does not impact upon mortality, but to be certain, a properly controlled trial is necessary. Thus, if new antiarrhythmic drugs are tested on patients with nonhemodynamically significant ventricular ectopy, the antiarrhythmic efficacy in such individuals will have to be defined as "drug effect." In such patients placebo periods are possible, prolonged outpatient studies are feasible, and Holter monitoring is the most logical method of testing.

The second important clinical setting for ventricular ectopy is when it produces hemodynamically significant ventricular arrhythmias, usually paroxysmal ventricular tachycardia and/or fibrillation, with immediate serious symptoms for which suppressive therapy is mandatory. In this context placebo periods are often not possible, inpatient studies are usually required, and invasive electrophysiologic testing is quite reasonable. The definition of antiarrhythmic efficacy in such a setting may simply be the lack of prior symptoms which, of course, would correlate with the suppression of frequent ventricular tachyarrhythmias. Another measure of efficacy would be prolongation of life.

Definition of Antiarrhythmic "Drug Effect" Based on Statistical Considerations

The establishment of antiarrhythmic drug effect is based on comparing the incidence of ventricular arrhythmias determined during a placebo-control baseline with that found over a similar environmentally controlled period during which an active antiarrhythmic agent was prescribed. The quantitative definition of such a drug effect cannot be based on anecdotal judgment as in the past but must be determined using the quantitative data obtained by long-term Holter monitoring with the appropriate use of biostatistics.

We believe that in analyzing such data it is important that one not pool treated, with controlled ventricular ectopic frequencies, for this practice will mask the percentage of individual patients who have an adverse reaction (increase in arrhythmia frequency) as well as the marked differences between individuals. Thus, individual patient drug and placebo-controlled data should be evaluated to determine the percentage of individual patients who show drug efficacy. The percentage of individual patients in a particular study who respond to a particular drug with either a reduction or an increase in the frequency of ventricular ectopy will be the most useful index of an antiarrhythmic agent's efficacy (Morganroth, 1981).

It was only a short time ago that the high frequency of spontaneous variability in the quantitation of ventricular premature beats was documented in clinically stable patients (Morganroth et al. 1978). The number of 24-h Holter monitoring sessions required to define antiarrhythmic drug efficacy and to eliminate the potential of spontaneous variability of ventricular ectopy causing an apparent change has been well established by recent studies (Morganroth et al. 1981); they suggest that two or more 24-h Holter monitoring periods be recorded during an initial placebo phase to define the degree of spontaneous variability in individual subjects under consideration. This baseline is then used as a reference for establishing the degree of suppression of ventricular arrhythmias during antiarrhythmic drug treatment. Preferably, two Holter monitoring periods should be performed during each treatment phase depending on the pharmacokinetics of the agent being tested and cost considerations. Studies should be conducted over a relatively short term (days to weeks) to determine efficacy, whereas long-term studies (over months and years) need to be performed in order that drug safety can be judged. New antiarrhythmic agents should be tested first against placebo and then against standard agents to determine comparative efficacy.

The basic measure of efficacy in individual patients will be a suppression of approximately 75% in the frequency of ventricular ectopy on drug compared with placebo (Table 2). An alternate measure would be that 100% of complex ventricular arrhythmias be abolished and a minimum of 75%–90% of ventricular unifocal ectopy be suppressed, depending on the initial inclusion criteria. If a patient is included with a mean of at least 30 ventricular ectopic beats/h/24 h, a 75% reduction would be appropriate. Patients included who have ten or more premature ventricular beats/h/24 h will require at least 90%–100% suppression to be statistically certain of a drug effect.

Table 2. Percentage of suppression required to define antiarrhythmic efficacy, comparing treatment with baseline monitoring sessions

No. days monitored		Suppression required (%)		
Before drug	On drug	VPCs	VC	VT
1	1	80	75	65
2	2	75	65	55
3	3	65	55	45

VPCs, premature ventricular contractions; VC, ventricular complexes; VT, ventricular tachycardia

Table 3. Indications for treatment of ventricular ectopy

Definite
Ventricular arrhythmias with hemodynamically induced symptoms or debilitating palpitations
Probable (Hope of preventing sudden death)
Presence of structural heart disease and
1. VPCs > 10–30/h/24 h
2. complex VPCs (VC and/or VT)
Not clear
Lack of structural heart disease and ventricular ectopy unless sustained VT is present

PVCs, premature ventricular contractions; VC, ventricular couplets; VT, ventricular tachycardia

However, until the completion of a successful, well-controlled study establishing whether or not suppression of ventricular ectopy does, in fact, prevent sudden cardiac death, we must keep an open mind as to the actual definition of antiarrhythmic drug efficacy. For example, it has been suggested (Myerburg et al. 1979) that perhaps it is not ventricular ectopic suppression through which antiarrhythmic agents protect against cardiac death, but that they may change the underlying electrophysiologic parameters and be measured according to adequate levels in the blood.

Table 3 lists the criteria we currently recommend for selecting which patients with ventricular ectopy should be treated, until such time as these important questions are answered by controlled clinical trials.

References

Bigger JT, Weld FM (1981) Analysis of prognostic significance of ventricular arrhythmias after myocardial infarction: shortcomings of Lown grading system. Br Heart J 45: 717

Bigger JT, Dresdale RJ, Heissenbuttel RH, et al. (1977) Ventricular arrhythmias in ischemic heart disease: mechanism, prevalence, significance and management. Prog Cardiovasc Dis 19: 255

Bigger JT, Weld FM, Rolnitzky LM (1981) Prevalent characteristics and significance of ventricular tachycardia detected with ambulatory electrocardiographic recording in the late hospital phase of acute myocardial infarction. Am J Cardiol 48: 815

Coronary Drug Project Research Group (1973) Prognostic importance of premature beats following myocardial infarction. JAMA 223: 116

Davis HT, DeCamilla J, Bayer LW, et al. (1979) Survivorship patterns in the posthospital phase of myocardial infarction. Circulation 60: 1252

Follansbee WP, Michelson EL, Morganroth J (1980) Nonsustained ventricular tachycardia in ambulatory patients: characteristics and association with sudden cardiac death. Ann Intern Med 92: 741

Goldstein S, Landis JR, Leighton R (1981) Characteristics of the resuscitated out-of-hospital cardiac arrest victim with coronary heart disease. Circulation 64: 977

Kotler M, Tabaygnik B, Mower M, et al. (1973) Prognostic significance of ventricular ectopic beats with respect to sudden death in the late post-infarction period. Circulation 47: 959

Lown B (1979) Sudden cardiac death: The major challenge confronting contemporary cardiology. Am J Cardiol 43: 313

May GS, Eberlein KA, Furburg CD (1982) Second degree prevalence after myocardial infarction: a review of long-term trials. Prog Cardiovasc Dis 24: 331

Morganroth J (1981) Long-term ambulatory ECG recording in the determination of efficacy of new antiarrhythmic agents. In: Morganroth J, et al. (eds) The evaluation of new antiarrhythmic drugs. Nijhoff, The Hague

Morganroth J, Horowitz LN, Josephson ME, et al. (1978) Limitations of infrequent Holter monitoring in assessing antiarrhythmic efficacy. Circulation 58: 408

Moss AJ, Schnitzler R, Green R, et al. (1971) Ventricular arrhythmia three weeks after acute myocardial infarction. Ann Intern Med 75: 837

Moss AJ, Davis HT, DeCamilla J (1979) Ventricular ectopic beats and their relation to sudden and non-sudden cardiac death after myocardial infarction. Circulation 60: 998

Myerburg RJ, Conde CA, Sheps DS, et al. (1979) Antiarrhythmic drug therapy in survivors of prehospial cardiac arrest: comparison of effects on chronic ventricular arrhythmias and recurrent cardiac arrest. Circulation 59: 855

Myerburg RJ, Conde CA, Sung RJ, et al. (1980) Clinical electrophysiologic and hemodynamic profile of patients resuscitated from prehospital cardiac arrest. Am J Med 68: 568

Rehnqvist N, Siogren A (1977) Ventricular arrhythmias prior to discharge and one year after acute myocardial infarction. Am J Cardiol 5: 425

Ruberman W, Weinblatt E, Goldberg JD, et al. (1981) Ventricular premature complexes and sudden death after myocardial infarction. Circulation 64: 297

Savage DD, Seides SF, Maron BJ (1979) Prevalence of arrhythmias during 24-hour ECG monitoring and exercise testing in patients with obstructive and non-obstructive hypertrophic cardiomyopathy. Circulation 59: 866

Schulze RA, Humphries JO, Griffith LS (1977 a) Left ventricular and coronary angiographic anatomy. Relationship to ventricular irritability in the late phase of acute myocardial infarction. N Engl J Med 55: 839

Schulze RA, Strauss HW, Pitt B (1977 b) Sudden death in the year following myocardial infarction. Relation to ventricular premature contractions in the late phase and left ventricular ejection fraction. Am J Med 61: 192

Vismara LA, Anderson EA, Mason DT (1975) Relation of ventricular arrhythmias in the late hospital phase of acute myocardial infarction to sudden death after hospital discharge. Am J Med 59: 6

Winkle RA (1980) Ambulatory ECG and the diagnosis, evaluation and treatment of chronic ventricular arrhythmias. Prog Cardiovasc Dis 23: 99

Efficacy of Oral Propafenone in Supraventricular and Ventricular Arrhythmias: Experience with 47 Cases

P. Coumel and J.-F. Leclercq

Our experience with propafenone (P) extends over a 2½-year period; we initially designed a double-blind crossover study comparing P with quinidine, but in fact, P quickly appeared as such an interesting, particular, and powerful drug that the problem was not really to prove its efficacy, but to detail all the aspects of its activity and hence, its indications according to arrhythmia mechanism and resistance to conventional therapies. This is why the standard mode of experiment was abandoned. It was replaced by an open study, carried out in symptomatic patients whose arrhythmias were often severe and poorly tolerated, and who could not deal with the drawbacks of strictly randomized treatments including placebo periods. Generally speaking, our experience is that this situation is encountered with every new compound that is really original, really active, and constitutes actual progress in antiarrhythmic therapy.

Material and Methods

We studied 47 patients, 28 males and 19 females, with a total of 50 tachyarrhythmias (21 supraventricular, 29 ventricular). The mean age was 52.4 years (extremes 7 and 78). The total duration of treatment was 237 months (mean = 5): in 21 cases it was less than 1 month, in ten cases 1–3 months, in five cases 3–12 months, and in 11 cases 12–20 months. The doses used were rather high, according to the severity of the arrhythmias: 450 mg in one child, 600 mg in 12 cases including another child, 900 mg in 29 cases, and 1 200 mg in five cases.

As most patients were symptomatic, the evaluation took into account the clinical data, except of those which were included in the initial part of the experiment. In addition to the standard electrocardiographic data, a total of 238 Holter recordings were made, 134 as control tracings and 104 in the patients treated with P. However, these numbers are far from reflecting the amount of data which were taken into account, as many patients had been followed up for years, treated beforehand with various therapies, and routinely checked by ambulatory electrocardiography.

To make the evaluation of the large variety of arrhythmias homogeneous and to make possible the comparison of the results in the whole spectrum of rhythm disturbances, we used a grading system from 1 (no effect) to 5 (complete control). It is clear that the parameters which were taken into account varied from patient to patient, or more accurately, from arrhythmia to arrhythmia. A weekly symptomatic vagal atrial fibrillation cannot be evaluated in the same way as asymptomatic ventricular premature beats. Depending on the case, either the heart rate trend or the R-R interval histogram pattern of control and treated periods was the more convenient and reliable parameter of evaluation. We must always be aware that comparing apparently identical parameters only on the basis of their number may be very misleading (Coumel et al. 1981).

Results

Tables 1 and 2 provide the detailed diagnostic data and the results of the various treatments in supraventricular and ventricular arrhythmias respectively.

Supraventricular Tachycardias

We have classified our 21 cases according to the arrhythmia mechanism present, and particularly according to the role of the autonomic nervous system, because the effect of P is closely related to it.

Table 1. Results of single therapies and combined treatment in supraventricular arrhythmias

Diagnosis	Case no.	Name	Sex	Age	Single therapies				Combined therapies			
									AM +		BBL +	
					P	MST	BBL	AM	P	MST	P	MST
ST	1	Gar	F	54	3	2	3	–	–	–	–	–
APB	2	Alm	M	57	3	3	–	–	–	–	–	–
APB	3	Bou	M	74	1	1	–	–	–	–	–	–
AT	4	Car	M	74	5	2	1	3	–	–	–	–
AT	5	Des	M	42	4	2	3	–	–	–	–	–
AT	6	Ber	M	56	1	1	1	2	–	–	–	–
JT	7	Dom	F	47	3	1	2	4	–	–	–	–
VAA	8	Gen	M	62	3	4	1	1	5	–	–	–
VAA	9	Del	M	56	1	3	2	3	–	5	–	–
VAA	10	Kov	M	57	2	1	1	3	–	5	–	–
VAA	11	Pet	M	37	1	2	1	2	–	–	–	–
VAA	12	Tch	M	64	1	2	1	2	–	–	–	–
VAA	13	Dum	M	56	1	2	1	3	–	4	–	–
VAA	14	Lec	M	57	1	1	1	2	–	2	–	–
AAA	15	Elh	M	36	5	1	–	3	–	–	–	–
AAA	16	Gau	F	69	1	1	3	5	–	–	–	–
AAA	17	Buv	M	67	5	2	2	2	–	3	–	–
AAA	18	Car	F	58	4	1	3	3	–	–	5	–
AAA	19	Sch	M	66	5	5	5	–	–	–	–	–
AAA	20	Pel	F	55	3	1	3	–	–	–	5	4
AAA	21	Rob	F	60	5	1	3	5	–	–	–	4

ST, sinus tachycardia; APB, atrial premature beats; AT, ectopic atrial tachycardia; JT, paroxysmal junctional tachycardia; VAA, vagal atrial arrhythmia; AAA, adrenergic atrial arrhythmia; P, propafenone; MST, membrane stabilizer; BBL, beta-blocker; AM, amiodarone

Table 2. Results of single therapies and combined treatment in ventricular arrhythmias

Diagnosis	Case no.	Name	Sex	Age	Single therapies				Combined therapies			
									AM	+	BBL	+
					P	MST	BBL	M	P	MST	P	MST
IB-VPB	19	Sch	M	66	5	5	–	–	–	–	–	–
IB-VPB	22	Dem	F	65	4	4	–	–	–	–	–	–
IB-VPB	23	Rob	M	45	5	4	1	5	–	–	–	–
IB-VPB	24	Tau	M	78	4	3	–	–	–	–	–	–
IB-VPB	25	Pet	F	33	5	3	2	5	–	–	–	–
IB-VPB	26	Cau	M	50	4	3	–	–	–	–	–	–
IB-VT	27	Nor	F	18	4	2	2	–	–	–	4	–
IB-VT	28	Leb	F	35	4	3	2	5	–	–	–	4
IB-VT	29	Des	M	43	4	3	2	5	–	–	–	5
IB-VT	30	Gar	M	26	4	3	3	5	–	–	5	4
IB-VT	31	Flo	M	23	5	2	2	5	–	–	–	3
IB-VT	32	God	F	52	4	2	2	3	–	4	–	3
CVT	4	Car	M	74	5	3	1	3	–	–	–	–
CVT	33	Rou	M	58	4	3	–	5	–	–	–	–
CVT	34	Gia	F	57	5	5	–	–	–	–	–	–
MVPVT	35	Glo	F	60	4	1	2	2	–	–	–	2
MVPVT	36	Lec	M	57	4	1	1	3	5	3	–	–
MVPVT	37	Fou	F	62	4	2	2	3	4	2	–	2
MVPVT	38	Mac	F	32	3	2	3	4	–	–	4	3
IS-VT	13	Dum	M	56	1	2	1	3	–	4	–	–
IS-VT	39	Gue	M	7	5	2	2	5	–	–	–	2
IS-VT	40	Leb	F	9	4	2	2	4	–	–	–	3
IS-VT	41	Sei	F	68	3	2	2	4	5	5	–	–
PMI-VT	42	Gai	M	57	2	1	–	5	–	–	–	–
PMI-VT	43	Bra	F	69	4	2	–	3	3	4	–	–
PMI-VT	44	Deb	M	57	5	3	3	–	–	4	–	–
PMI-VT	45	Fra	M	61	5	3	–	3	–	4	–	–
PMI-VT	46	Pet	M	64	1	1	–	1	–	1	–	–
TP	47	Sai	F	72	5	1	–	–	–	–	–	–

IB-VPB, idiopathic benign ventricular premature beats; IB-VT, idiopathic benign ventricular tachycardia; CVT, cardiomyopathy with ventricular tachycardia; MVPVT, mitral valve prolapse with ventricular tachycardia; IS-VT, idiopathic severe ventricular tachycardia; PMI-VT, post-myocardial infarction ventricular tachycardia; TP, *torsades de pointes;* P, propafenone; MST, membrane stabilizer; BBL, beta-blocker; AM, amiodarone

Miscellaneous Supraventricular Arrhythmias: In a group of seven patients there was one with sinus tachycardia, two with atrial premature beats, three with ectopic atrial tachycardia, and one with paroxysmal junctional tachycardia. The mean effect (1.7) of treatment with membrane stabilizers (in practice always quinidine, plus others in numerous cases) indicates that the arrhythmias were rather resistant: in comparison, the P effect (2.9) is satisfactory, though not perfect. The following two categories of arrhythmias are in fact more interesting for an understanding of the mode of effect of P.

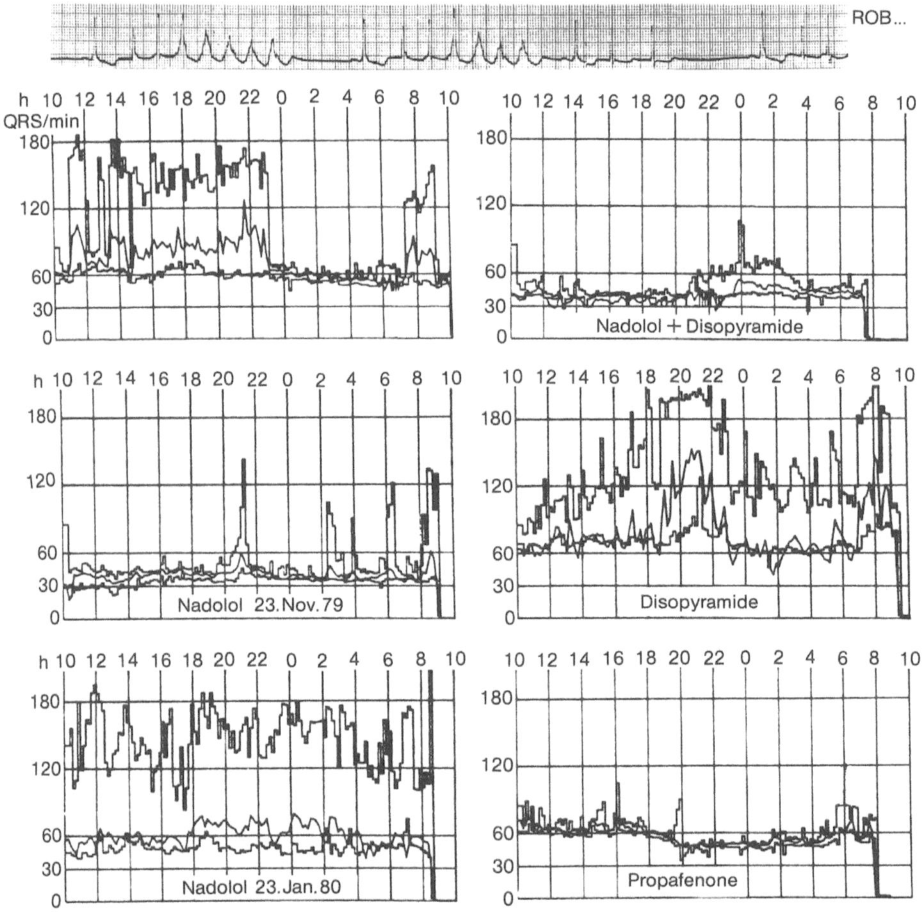

Fig. 1. Adrenergic atrial arrhythmia (case no. 21). Frequent bursts of ectopic atrial tachycardia (*top tracing*) are responsible for runs of tachycardia with an intermittent maximal preexcitation pattern. The particularity of this intractable tachyarrhythmia is to occur only during the day. The computerized analysis of the control 24-h ambulatory recording (*upper left panel*) clearly illustrates the fact in the large difference between the trends of maximal and minimal frequency which encompass the mean heart rate curve. Nadolol alone controls the arrhythmia (*middle left panel*) but an escape phenomenon appears after 2 months (*lower left panel*). Then the combination of nadolol and disopyramide again controls the arrhythmia (*upper right panel*), and nadolol remains necessary, as shown by the arrhythmia recurrence when disopyramide is given alone (*middle right panel*). The good long-term result obtained by propafenone (*lower right panel*) is probably related to both the membrane-stabilizing and beta-adrenergic inhibitory effects of the drug

Vagal Atrial Arrhythmias: Seven patients had particularly resistant forms of vagal-induced atrial flutter and fibrillation, a syndrome observed predominantly in males (all of these seven were men) and characterized by frequent paroxysmal attacks, occurring usually at night, or during the resting periods following lunch or dinner (Coumel et al. 1978). The onset of arrhythmia is usually preceded by a progressive and relative bradycardia at a rate of 55–60/min which reflects the increased vagotonic drive. It can be reproduced by vagal maneuvers and its mechanism is clearly the same as that of experimental acetylcholine-induced atrial fibrillations.

Our therapeutic experience with this syndrome is wide and uniform. These patients are resistant to, and usually aggravated by beta-blockers (mean effect = 1.1). Quinidine is only partially effective, and the seven cases presently under discussion were selected for their resistance to membrance stabilizers, the mean efficacy of which was graded 2.1. Amiodarone is usually effective in about half the cases, reflected here by a mean efficacy of 2.4. The combination of amiodarone and quinidine usually gives better results: 4.0 in the four cases where it was used.

P was ineffective in this syndrome (1.4). To be exact, not only did most of them not improve, but their arrhythmias became more frequent (for example from weekly to daily attacks of longer duration). This result is, in fact, unsurprising if the beta-inhibitory effect of P is taken into account, and the effect of the drug on sinus frequency confirms it.

Adrenergic Atrial Arrhythmias: The situation is opposite in the following seven patients, whose arrhythmia was characterized essentially by its predominance during the day, and the clear triggering effect of effort or emotion (Coumel et al. 1982). These patients were chosen for the characteristic pattern of their arrhythmia, and the difficulty of, if not always the resistance to treatment. Beta-blocking therapy is indeed effective in this situation, if strong doses of powerful drugs like nadolol are used, but has the limitation of an escape phenomenon frequently observed after 1–2 months (Fig. 1). In our seven patients the average effect of beta-blockers was 2.7, a better result than in the miscellaneous group, and opposite to that of the vagal arrhythmias. Type I antiarrhythmic agents were

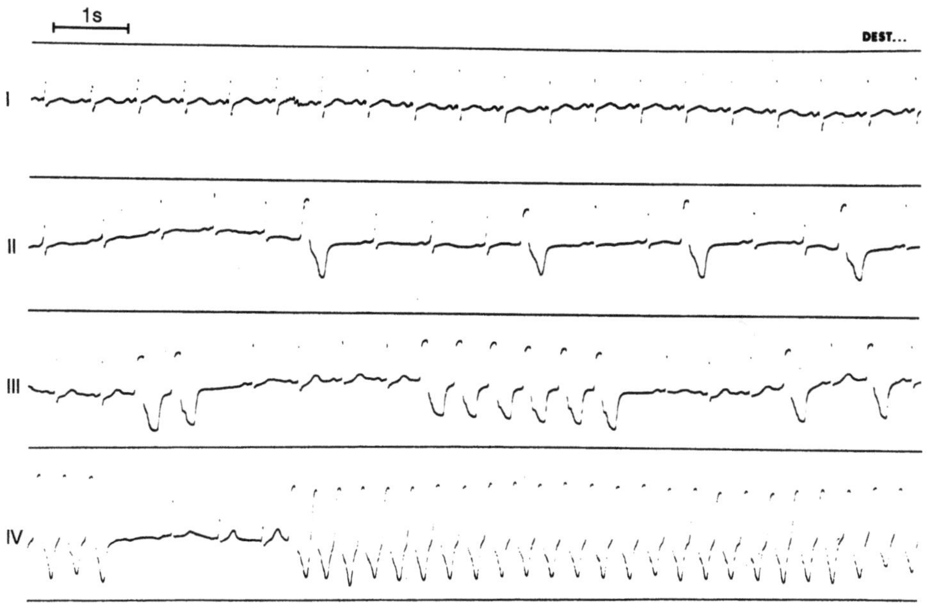

Fig. 2. Idiopathic benign ventricular tachycardia (case no. 29). Sinus rate, isolated ventricular premature beats, salvos, or runs of sustained ventricular tachycardia are observed in this patient. As he was perfectly able to define the various states and to classify them into four classes of feeling (*I to IV*), his history was of great help in following the effects of therapy on a long-term basis (see Fig. 3)

not effective (1.7), but amiodarone was (3.6), and the combination of quinidine agents and beta-blockers as well.

The efficacy of P by far exceeded that of the previous agents: the mean result was 4.0, and in two patients combining P and beta-blocker achieved complete control.

Ventricular Arrhythmias

A total of 29 cases covered the entire spectrum of either common or rare ventricular tachyarrhythmias, which can be separated into categories (Table 2).

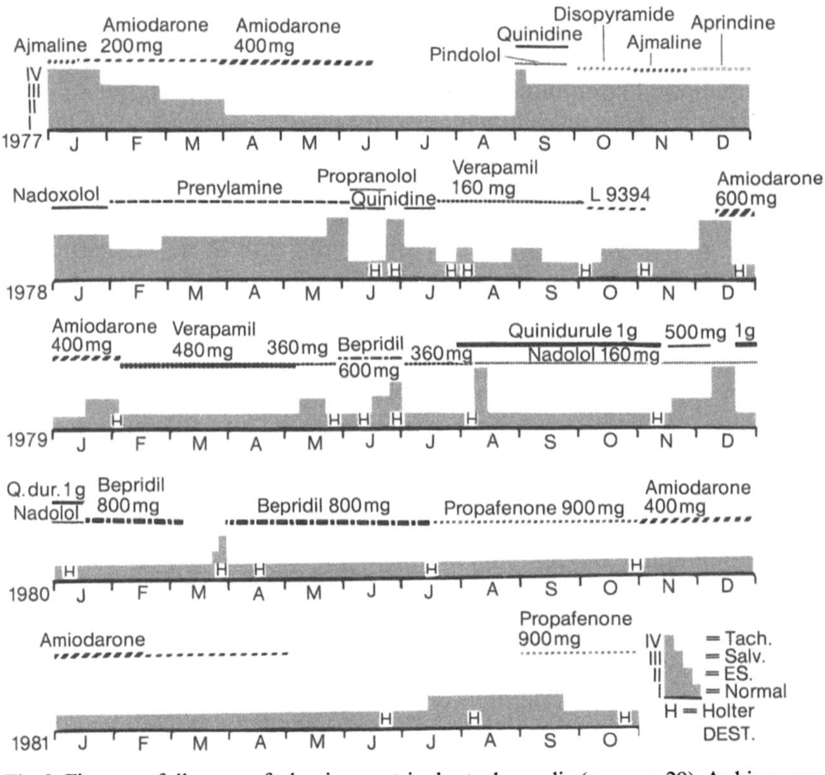

Fig. 3. Five-year follow-up of a benign ventricular tachycardia (case no. 29). As his perception of the various classes (*I*, sinus rhythm; *II*, isolated premature beats; *III*, salvos; *IV*, sustained ventricular tachycardia) was reliable, and repeatedly verified by ambulatory recordings (*H*), a number of open therapeutical trials were carried out with this very cooperative patient. Amiodarone was used first, from January to June 1977, and remained efficacious for 2½ months after it was discontinued. From September 1977 to Mai 1978, various type I antiarrhythmics were ineffective when given alone, and quinidine was effective (June 1978) only when given with propranolol. After various trials with Ca-blockers (verapamil, bepridil), and with amiodarone and its equivalent L9394, over a 1-year period (July 1978–July 1979), the necessity of combining quinidine with beta-blockers (nadolol) was again verified over a 6-month period. Propafenone has been tested twice (first July–October 1980 and again starting in September 1981) and has proven equal in effect to the above combination

Idiopathic Benign Ventricular Premature Beats: This is the most widely used model for experimenting with new antiarrhythmic drugs. Actually we started with these patients in a strictly-defined protocol. As stated in the introduction, P quickly proved effective (4.5), but quinidine did as well (3.7), so that this was not the best model for pointing up the difference between the two drugs.

Idiopathic Benign Ventricular Tachycardia: When this arrhythmia occurs in doublets, in salvos, or in runs of ventricular tachycardia, it is possibly not more severe but certainly more troublesome (Fig. 2) and the chronic arrhythmia can be followed on a long-term basis by both subjective and objective methods (Fig. 3). The arrhythmia is usually more

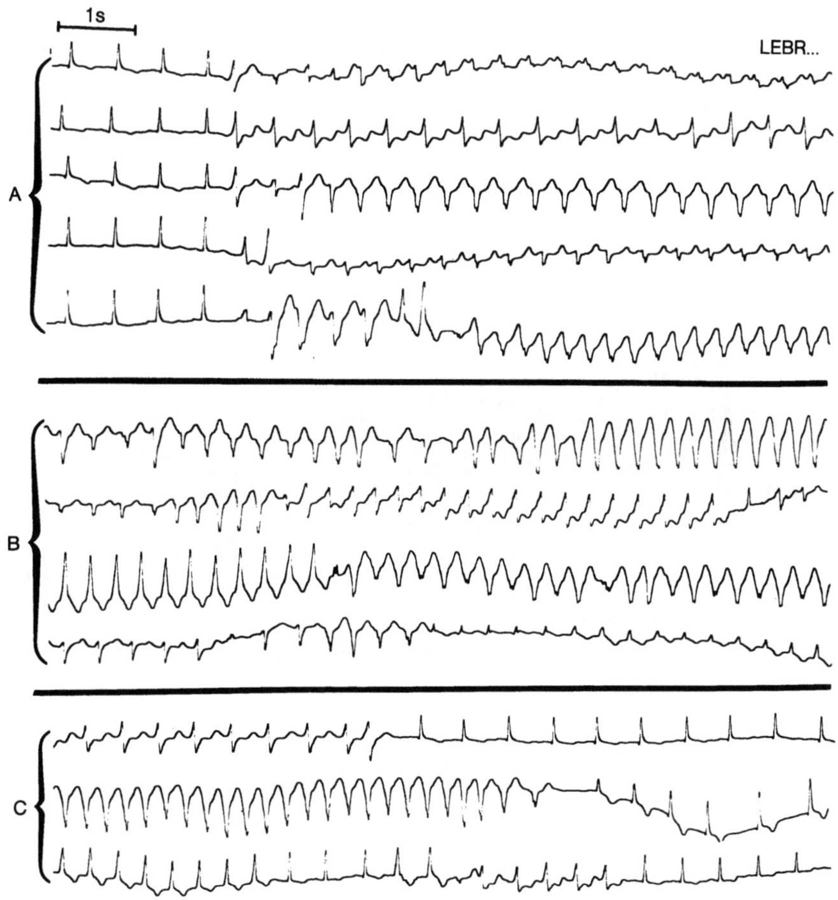

Fig. 4 A–C. Severe, polymorphic, idiopathic ventricular tachycardia in a child (case no. 40). The panels show the impressive variety of ventricular activity starting **A**, changing **B**, and terminating spontaneously **C** during a single Holter recording in this 9-year-old child. This arrhythmia proved resistant to all type I antiarrhythmics, whether given alone or in combination with beta-blockers. Amiodarone, which was efficient, had to be discontinued after 2 years because of bluish skin discoloration (See also Fig. 5)

resistant than isolated premature beats to quinidine (2.5 instead of 3.7), and not sensitive to beta-blockers (2.2), but combining both drugs is useful (3.8 in five cases). Of course, amiodarone is effective in most cases (4.5), but P is not far from this level of efficacy, with an average result of 4.2.

Cardiomyopathies and Mitral Valve Prolapse: Three cases of cardiomyopathy and four of mitral valve prolapse were studied with severe, polymorphic runs of irregular ventricular tachycardia occurring mainly during exercise or stress. The severity of these arrhythmias is demonstrated by the poor effect of single therapies with quinidine (2.4), beta-blockers (1.8), or even amiodarone (3.3); and in comparison the positive P effect (4.1) deserves to be emphasized.

Idiopathic Severe Ventricular Tachycardia: Four cases of severe, resistant ventricular tachycardia, resembling the preceding ones in many respects but without evidence of any heart disease, were treated with P. Two patients were children (Figs. 4 and 5), and although the tachycardia could be controlled by amiodarone (4.0), the continuation of treatment with this drug on a long-term basis is a problem. Quinidine and a number of other type I antiarrhythmics were quite insufficient (2.0), and beta-blockers were even

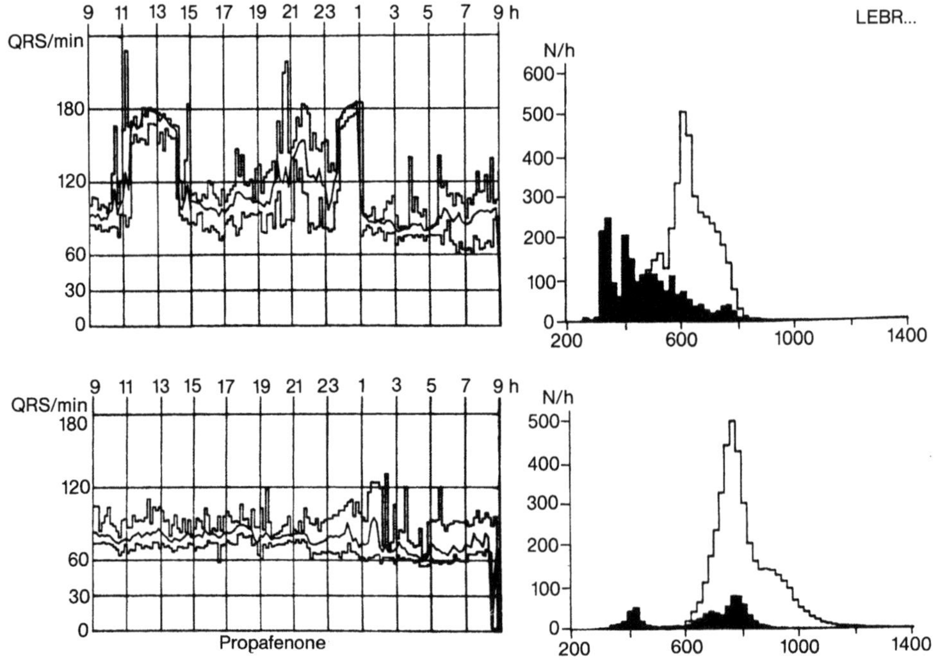

Fig. 5. Propafenone efficacy in a severe ventricular tachycardia (case no. 40, tracings in Fig. 4). The upper panels show the computerized analysis of a 24-h control tracing, in terms of cardiac rate (maximal, minimal and mean frequency) and R-R interval histograms which differentiate the enlarged (*solid*) and narrow (*open*) QRSs. The lower panels show the effect of propafenone, which was positive but incomplete: the daily dosage was limited to 450 mg in this 9-year-old child because of the presence of a sinus bradycardia at night

less effective (1.8). The P results was again in sharp contrast (3.3), though less favorable than that of amiodarone.

Post-myocardial Infarction Ventricular Tachycardia: Propafenone was given in five cases of recurrent paroxysmal ventricular tachycardia in the chronic phase of myocardial infarction. In most cases it was given on a long-term basis after quinidine (2.0) or amiodarone (3.0) had proven insufficient, or when they had to be combined for better efficacy. The P effect was graded 3.4 in these difficult patients, and in three cases it was actually the only possible treatment if the problems of congestive heart failure and long-term tolerance were taken into account. Figure 6 shows the case of patient no. 45, who died after his frequently recurring ventricular tachycardia had been controlled for almost 2 years. The terminal ECG is that of an electromechanical dissociation largely explained by the myocardial damage, the persistant angina – spontaneous and during exercise, and the concomitant Ca-blocking treatment: however, the point is that P did control the ventricular tachycardia.

Torsades de Pointes (WHO/ISFC Task Force, 1978): We had two cases of *torsades de pointes,* one in the context of ionic disorders, quinidine treatment, and chronic AV block

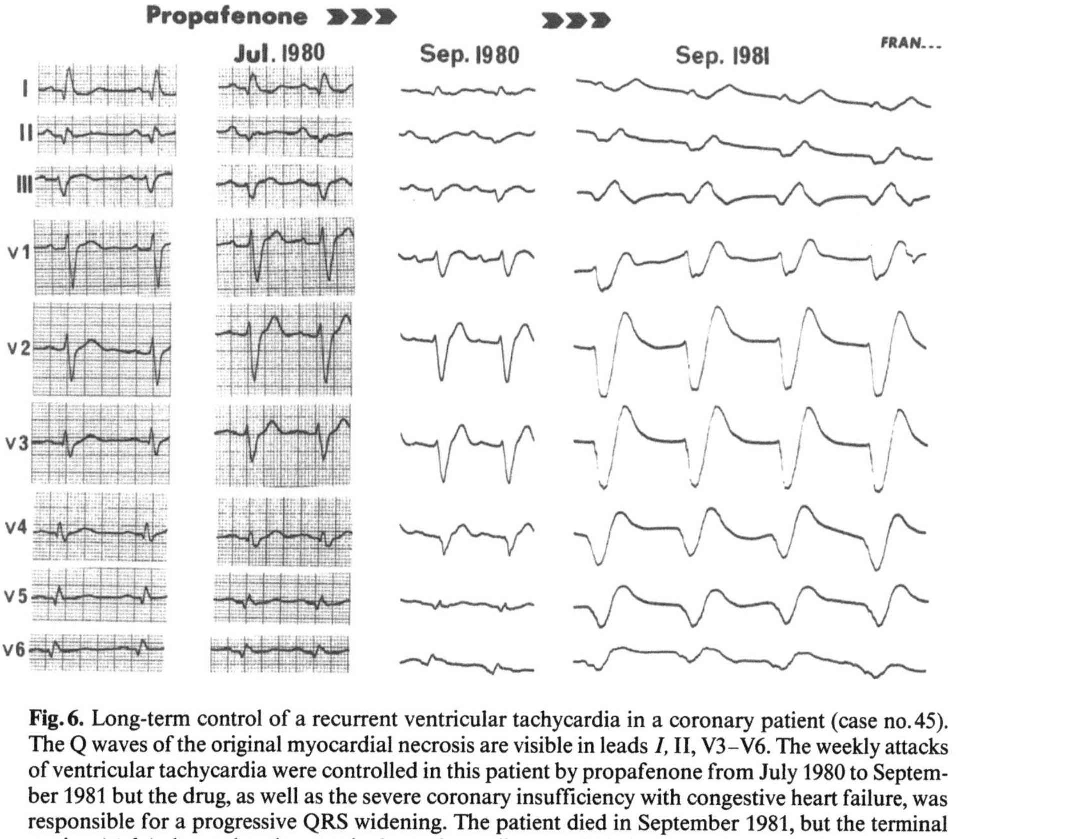

Fig. 6. Long-term control of a recurrent ventricular tachycardia in a coronary patient (case no. 45). The Q waves of the original myocardial necrosis are visible in leads *I*, II, V3–V6. The weekly attacks of ventricular tachycardia were controlled in this patient by propafenone from July 1980 to September 1981 but the drug, as well as the severe coronary insufficiency with congestive heart failure, was responsible for a progressive QRS widening. The patient died in September 1981, but the terminal tracing (*right*) shows that the ventricular tachycardia was still being controlled at that time

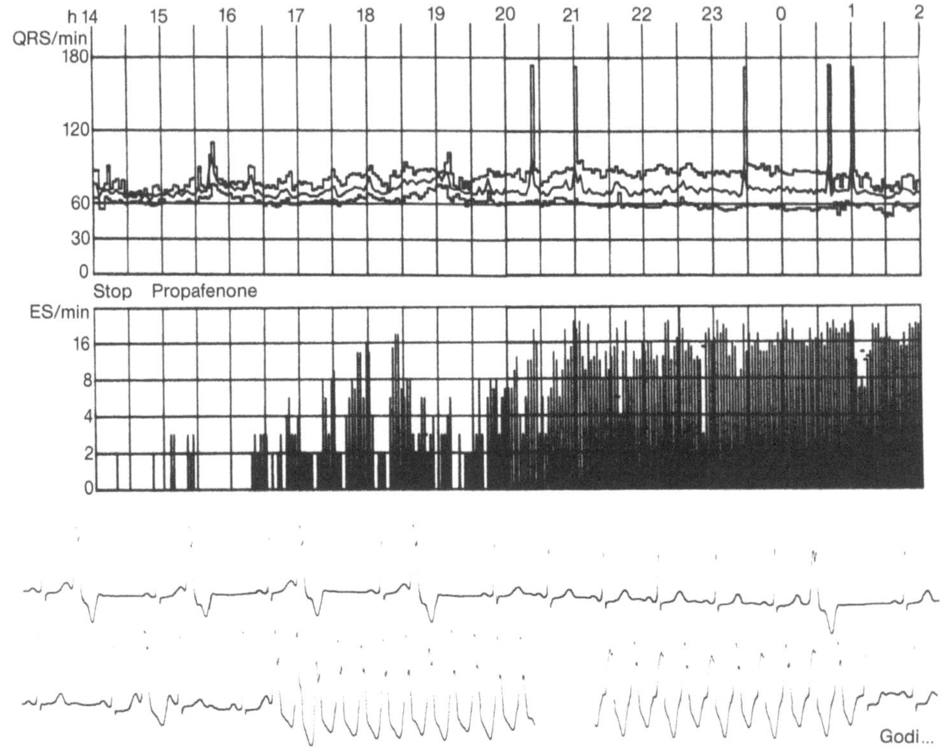

Fig. 7. Duration of action of propafenone (case no. 32). The last uptake of 300 mg propafenone is at 1 p.m. in this relatively resistant ventricular tachycardia. The number of ventricular premature beats increases progressively during the following hours, but they are isolated (*upper tracing*) until 8:30 p.m., at which time the first run of ventricular tachycardia (*lower tracing*) is detected from the maximal heart rate curve. This was observed after a treatment of 24-h duration. After a longer impregnation (several weeks), the duration of action was also longer: it took 8 h after the last uptake before the first isolated premature beats were observed

in a 72-year-old woman (no. 47). Although *torsades de pointes* persisted after the pacemaker implantation, P helped to control them. In case no. 34, where quinidine treatment was indeed effective but had been complicated by *torsades de pointes,* P could be given without observing this known toxic effect of type I anti-arrhythmic drugs (Fig. 8).

Sinus Rate, PR Interval and QRS Width

The sinus frequency could be studied over a 24-h period, with and without P treatment, in only ten patients (nos. 2, 8, 19, 22, 23, 25, 26, 32, 33, 35 and 45). The arrhythmias in the untreated patients were so frequent and so severe that accurate evaluation of the basic sinus rate on a statistical basis was not possible from the Holter recordings. In these ten patients (Table 3), with a mean age of 54, the basic 24-h mean heart rate was 74.7/min, and P slowed it by 13% ($P < 0.01$). The daytime frequency, evaluated over an 8-h period was slowed from 81.3/min to 72.4/min ($p < 0.02$) while the night frequency evaluated

Table 3. Comparison of sinus frequency with and without propafenone treatment, studied over a 24-h period

Sinus rate ($n = 10$, mean age = 54)				
Sinus frequency	Basal (mean min ± SD)	Propafenone (mean/min ± SD)	%	*P*
Over 24 h	74.7 ± 12.2	66.2 ± 11.5	−13%	< 0.01
Day (11 a.m.–7 p.m.)	81.3 ± 14.5	72.4 ± 13	−12%	< 0.02
Night (1 a.m.–5 a.m.)	63.7 ± 8.5	57.9 ± 11.8	−10%	< 0.05
Day/night ratio	1.27 ± 0.1	1.27 ± 0.2	0	NS

over a 4-h period was slowed by only 10% ($P < 0.05$). Yet the day-to-night ratio of the mean heart rate, which is a meaningful biological constant (1.27 + 0.1), was absolutely unchanged by P, confirming that the beta-inhibitory effect of the drug is comparable to that of amiodarone, but quite different from that of beta-blockers (Leclercq et al. 1980). The PR interval was almost constantly prolonged (from a mean value of 180 ms to 194 ms), as was the QRS width (from 103 ms to 117 ms).

Timing and Duration of Action

Propafenone acts rapidly by the oral route, and its first effects are visible within 1 h of uptake. It is also rapidly eliminated, and many patients with permanent arrhythmias describe the recurrence of their symptoms 6–8 h after the last uptake very precisely. This is well illustrated in Fig. 8 where the isolated premature beats reappear before the salvos. This may indicate a difference between the two aspects of P activity (membrane-stabilizing and beta-adrenergic inhibitory effect). In addition, the more sensitive the arrhythmia, the longer the drug effect, which indicates that duration of action is also a matter of threshold of activity. Finally, the antiarrhythmic effect takes longer to wear off after several weeks of impregnation than after a few days: in the subject of Fig. 8 the reappearance took 9 h after a prolonged treatment, instead of about 5.

Adverse Side Effects

Some degree of digestive intolerance was observed: a bitter taste in the mouth for eight patients, with nausea in four, and vomiting in two. Dizziness was noted in eight cases, and fatigue in six. These tolerance problems diminished as the doses used were decreased, and in only six patients was the treatment discontinued: it must be pointed out that in four cases the treatment was discontinued because of the ineffectiveness of P on the arrhythmia (nos. 10–12 and 16), and in two because although it was effective, it could be replaced by another drug (nos. 22 and 23). The other patients tolerated these side effects in exchange for freedom from arrhythmia.

Adverse cardiac side effects were observed on 12 occasions. A left bundle-branch block appeared in patients no. 11 and no. 44: the treatment was continued in the latter without further conduction disturbance. A marked sinus bradycardia or a definite sinoatrial block was noted in eight cases (Fig. 7), and, curiously, all were women. In three

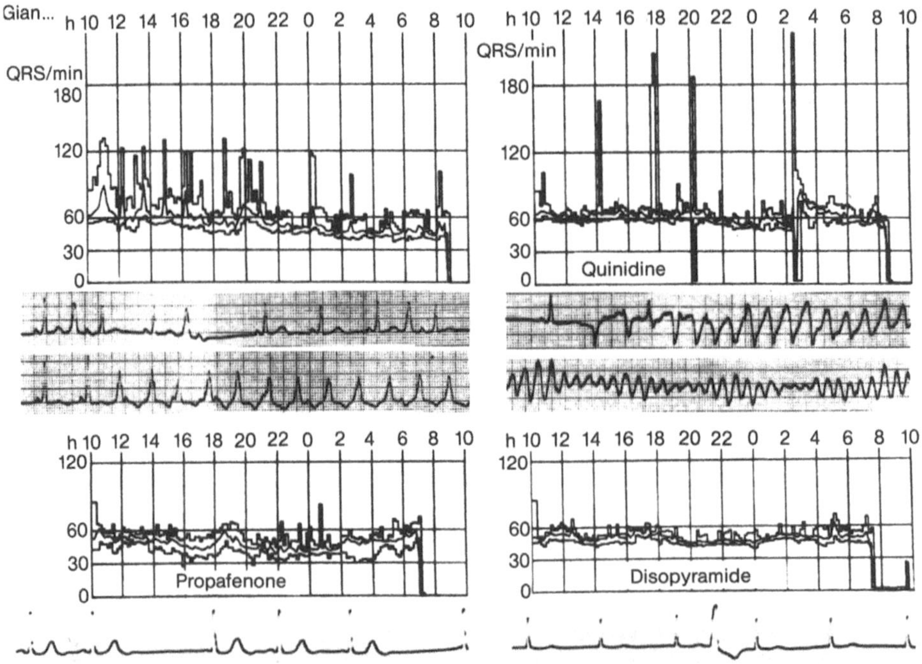

Fig. 8. Cardiac tolerance to quinidine, propafenone, and disopyramide (case no. 34). The *left upper panel* shows the runs of ventricular tachycardia in a 57-year-old patient with a congestive cardiomyopathy. Quinidine treatment (*right uper upper panel*) is indeed effective in suppressing the arrhythmia but induces four attacks of *torsades de pointes* in the 24-h period, two of which degenerate into ventricular fibrillation requiring electrical countershock. Propafenone does not have this toxicity at the ventricular level but induces a sinoatrial block (*left lower panel*). While on disopyramide (*right lower panel*) the patient had repeated isolated extrasystoles but no adverse cardiac side effects

(nos. 7, 34, 43) the treatment was discontinued for this reason; in four (nos. 21, 34, 37, 41) the bradycardia was well tolerated and P was maintained without further complication, and in one it was continued with the protection of an implanted pacemaker (no. 40). In two cases (nos. 23 and 29) of ventricular arrhythmias, a typical vagal atrial fibrillation was documented while patients were under treatment, and it should probably be attributed to P, as it was never again observed before or after in these patients, who were followed up on a long-term basis. Finally, we did not observe any particular depressive effect on the myocardial function, even in patients with enlarged hearts.

Discussion

The two main electrophysiological properties (membrane-stabilizing and beta-inhibitory effect) of the drug are well illustrated in these 47 patients who cover a very large range, if not the entire spectrum of rhythm disturbances. Abandoning the classical mode of a double-blind, randomized, control experiment very early in the study allowed us to use in a comprehensive way patients with severe, poorly tolerated supraventricular and ventricular arrhythmias. Standardized experiments are, almost by definition, carried out in asymptomatic patients: this applies only to a dozen cases of the present series, most of them having benign atrial or ventricular premature beats. It is certain that very objective, precise quantitative evaluations, with complete and indisputable statistical analysis are possible with such patients: the problem is that such a study is more effective in eliminating unworthy drugs than in detecting the outstanding ones. This general reflection applies to amiodarone as well as to propafenone.

A consideration of the global results shows that the type I antiarrhythmic effect of P is very marked, and surpasses that of the more conventional drugs, particularly quinidine: the mean efficacy of P is 2.8 in supraventricular and 4.0 in ventricular arrhythmias, and the corresponding values are 1.9 and 2.7 for quinidine. Of course, it must be emphasized that the patients were often chosen precisely for their relative or definite resistance to quinidine, and in any case these values do not express the specificity of P.

Propafenone in Supraventricular Arrhythmias

The particular indications for P in supraventricular tachyarrhythmias are well shown by the two groups of seven patients each whose arrhythmias are closely dependent on the vagosympathetic balance. P is of no value in vagal-induced atrial flutter and fibrillation, and this is confirmed by the two cases in which this arrhythmia occurred as a complication of the treatment. This is in keeping with the beta-adrenergic inhibitory effect also evidenced by the modifications of the sinus frequency. Amiodarone has the same effect, yet it is effective in this arrhythmia because its main electrophysiological property of lengthening the action potential partially counterbalances the otherwise deleterious bradycardia. This is not the case with P.

On the other hand, every time an increased sympathetic tone is implicated in the arrhythmia mechanism, as happened in the last group of seven patients, P is as effective as amiodarone, and its better tolerance on a long-term basis makes it very useful.

Propafenone in Ventricular Arrhythmias

At the ventricular level, the two effects of P are useful whenever an adrenergic factor is present. This is not the case for idiopathic ventricular premature beats when they are isolated, but doublets, salvos, and runs of ventricular tachycardia are mostly present during the day or after exercise. In general, this applies to any complex ventricular arrhythmia occurring in the context of a myocardial disease, or whenever the characteristics of the ventricular arrhythmia are distinctive because of their occurrence during effort, the left ventricular origin of the extrasystoles, or the irregularity and the polymorphism of the tachycardias (Coumel et al. 1982). This is why it is not realistic to compare P with quinidine, except in idiopathic, isolated ventricular premature beats.

In fact, it is more meaningful to compare P with amiodarone, or with the quinidine–beta-blocker or quinidine–amiodarone combination. This was done using two groups of our patients, and the results are shown in Fig. 9. The first group was formed of

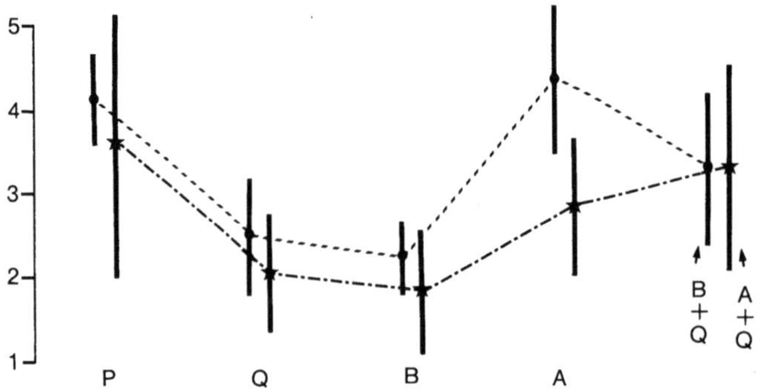

Fig. 9. Effects of single and combined therapies in ventricular tachycardias. Propafenone (*P*), quinidine (*Q*), beta-blockers (*B*) and amiodarone (*A*) were given alone in two groups of ten and nine patients respectively, followed by the combination of Q and B, or A and Q according to the resistance shown to single therapies. The mean results ± SD were graded from 1 (no effect) to 5 (complete control). It is clear that propafenone results more or less surpass those of the other treatments, in patients who have been chosen specifically because of the resistance of their tachyarrhythmias

ten patients (nos. 28–32, 35, 37–40) who received P, quinidine, beta-blockers and amiodarone as single therapies, and quinidine + beta-blockers as combined therapy. The second group was formed of nine patients (nos. 32, 36, 37, 13, 41, 43–46) who received the single therapies, and quinidine + amiodarone as combined therapy. Patients no. 32 and 37 received both types of combined therapies (Table 2). It is clear from the figure that the groups were not identical in terms of severity and resistance of their ventricular arrhythmias. This is not surprising as the combined treatment was not chosen by chance or to follow any previously designed protocol, but simply for the practical purpose of controlling the arrhythmia. Patients in the second group were more severely diseased: the difference is not significant when the two groups are considered separately with P, quinidine, or beta-blocker as single therapies, but it becomes significant when they are considered together, and above all when amiodarone is taken into account.

The main point of this comparison is to show (a) that in the first group, combined quinidine–beta-blocker therapy, though less effective than P, is no longer statistically different from it, and (b) that the same applies to the second group of more severe arrhythmias when they are treated with combined amiodarone and quinidine. Finally, P and amiodarone are not incompatible, and may be combined for better efficacy. This was done successfully in four of our most severe cases (nos. 36, 37, 41, 43), and these patients are now being followed up on a long-term basis.

Conclusion

Propafenone is indeed an important contribution to the therapeutic armamentarium in severe, resistant tachyarrhythmias. Though they are essentially very different, we consider this drug as important as amiodarone in many respects. Contrary to that of amiodarone, the P metabolism is very rapid, probably too rapid, and this is an inconvenience.

But the particularly slow metabolism of amiodarone may be inconvenient as well. On the other hand, P covers part of the indications for amiodarone, except for the particular category of vagal atrial arrhythmias. This eliminates some indications for amiodarone, and thereby some of its side effects. But P does not have the protective myocardial effect of amiodarone in coronary patients. In short, for the clinician, these drugs are complementary in many difficult situations, and the relative absence of cardiac toxicity when they are administered, combined with their great efficacy, makes both of them very useful in the modern treatment of tachyarrhythmias.

References

Coumel P, Attuel P, Lavallee JP, Flammang D, Leclercq JF, Slama R (1978) Syndrome d'arrythmie auriculaire d'origine vagale. Arch Mal Coeur 71: 645–656

Coumel P, Leclercq JF, Attuel P (1981) Les limites des méthodes d'évaluation quantitative. Arch Mal Coeur 74: 37–46

Coumel P, Rosengarten MD, Leclercq JF, Attuel P (1982) Role of the sympathetic nervous system in non-ischaemic ventricular arrhythmias. Br Heart J 137–147

Coumel P, Attuel P, Leclercq JF, Friocourt P (1982) Arythmies auriculaires d'origine vagale ou catecholergique. Effets comparés du traitement beta-bloquant et phénomène d'échappement. Arch Mal Coeur 75: 373–387

Leclercq JF, Rosengarten MD, Attuel P, Kural S, Milosevic D, Coumel P (1980) Les effets des antiarrythmiques sur le rythme sinusal. Appréciation gràce aux enregistrements électrocardiographiques de longue durée quantifiés par le systeme Atrec. Arch Mal Coeur 73: 903–912

WHO/ISFC Task Force (1978) Definition of terms related to cardiac rhythm. Eur T Cardiol 8: 127–144

The Possible Relevance of Late Potentials for the Identification of Patients Needing Antiarrhythmic Treatment*

G. Breithardt, M. Borggrefe, U. Karbenn, K. Haerten, J. Ostermeyer and L. Seipel

A large proportion of patients with coronary artery disease succumb to sudden cardiac death [1]. Complex ventricular arrhythmias have been shown to be a harbinger of sudden cardiac death in these patients, mainly in those with underlying abnormalities of left ventricular function [2–9]. The large spontaneous variability of ventricular ectopic beats and above all of complex forms such as pairs, salvos, and runs of ventricular tachycardia [10–13], requires extended periods of Holter monitoring. However, the accuracy of Holter monitoring in correctly identifying those patients at risk has recently been questioned [14]. Therefore, other parameters that could serve as indicators of increased ventricular vulnerability would be useful. The ideal parameter would be one that can easily be detected by noninvasive methods, that shows no spontaneous variability, and that is as closely linked to the inherent mechanism of ventricular tachyarrhythmias as possible.

Recently, ventricular late potentials that probably result from regional slow ventricular activation [15–21] have emerged as a new noninvasive parameter [22–32]. Whether these late potentials as recorded from the body surface are a better indicator of an increased risk of ventricular tachycardia or ventricular fibrillation in coronary patients than Holter monitoring has not yet been settled. Thus, the purpose of this paper is to review our present experience [25, 26, 33–42] with the use of the signal-averaging technique for the noninvasive detection of late ventricular potentials, and to discuss their possible relevance for the identification of patients in need of antiarrhythmic treatment.

Patients and Methods

A total of 402 patients were studied. Group I were apparently healthy controls ($n = 27$); group II were patients in whom ventricular tachycardia or ventricular fibrillation had already been documented, thus representing a retrospective sample ($n = 69$); groups III and IV were patients studied prospectively after recent myocardial infarction ($n = 160$) and with stable coronary artery disease ($n = 146$) respectively.

Registration of late potentials from the body surface using high-gain amplification and the digital signal-averaging technique was performed as recently described [25, 26]. The rate was 10000 samples/s. Single-pole analog filters were used (6 db/octave). The jitter for QRS triggering was 1.5 ms. In all cases, the reproducibility of the recordings was tested by repeating the averaging process with the electrodes in the same positions. Duration and amplitude of late potentials were defined as previously reported [35].

---

* Supported by the Johann A. Wülfing-Stiftung and the Sonderforschungsbereich 30 (Kardiologie) of the Deutsche Forschungsgemeinschaft/Bonn

In 179 patients (69 group-II patients and 110 of group IV), electrophysiological studies were performed as previously described [43]. The patients were in the postabsorptive and nonsedated state. All antiarrhythmic drugs if any were withheld for at least 4–5 half-lives. Digitalis was discontinued 5 days before the study. The stimulation protocol included the introduction of single and double ventricular extrastimuli during sinus rhythm and a paced ventricular rhythm at rates of 120, 140, 160, and 180 bpm. After every eighth beat, one premature stimulus was introduced beginning in late diastole, and then progressively earlier until ventricular refractoriness was reached. Then the coupling interval of the premature stimulus (S_2) was prolonged again until effective capture of the ventricles was achieved. The second premature stimulus (S_3) was then introduced beginning at a coupling interval that was about 150 ms longer than S_1–S_2 and decreased in decrements of 10 ms. A repetitive ventricular response was considered to be present if one or more nonstimulated premature ventricular depolarizations occurred after single or double premature stimulation. Sustained ventricular tachycardia was defined as tachycardia lasting more than 30 s, or requiring termination before that time because of hemodynamic deterioration. In those patients who did not have documented ventricular tachyarrhythmias (group IV), programmed ventricular stimulation was stopped as soon as four or more consecutive ventricular echo beats or ventricular tachycardia (defined as 10 or more consecutive echo beats) were induced.

Results

Prevalence of Late Potentials in Various Groups of Patients (Table 1)

In 27 "normal" subjects (12 medical students or physicians of the hospital, 15 patients with no evidence of coronary artery disease or left ventricular dysfunction during heart catheterization), no late potentials were detected. In all cases there was a smooth transition from the QRS complex to the ST segment in the high-amplitude recording (Fig. 1).

In group II, 69 patients with previously documented ventricular tachycardia and/or ventricular fibrillation in whom these arrhythmias could be reproducibly initiated by programmed ventricular stimulation were studied. One patient had normal coronary arteries and normal left ventricular function, nine had dilative cardiomyopathy, in four pa-

Table 1. Prevalence of late potentials in various groups of patients

Group		*n*	Late potentials (%)	Mean duration (ms)
I	Controls	27	–	–
II	Patients with VT/VF	69	74	51 ± 31.4
III	Patients after recent myocardial infarction	160	51	27 ± 15.5
IV	Patients without VT/VF	146	34	31 ± 15.3
	Total	402		

VT/VF, ventricular tachycardia and/or fibrillation

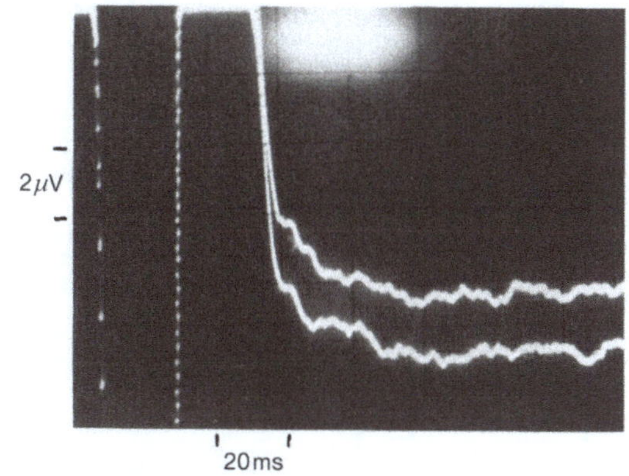

Fig. 1. Averaged high-gain amplified and filtered (100–300 Hz, 6 db/octave) recording of the terminal portion of the QRS complex and the onset of the ST segment in a normal subject. There was a smooth transition from the QRS complex into the ST segment. To demonstrate the reproducibility two consecutive recordings were performed

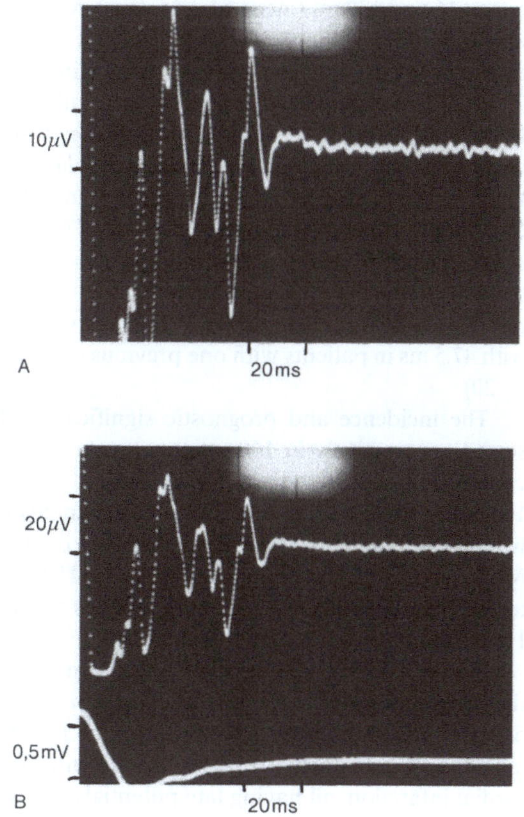

Fig. 2 A, B. Averaged recording in a patient with ventricular tachycardia. A multiphasic potential is recorded that extends from the terminal portion of the QRS complex into the ST segment. The tracing in **A** and the upper tracing in **B** show highly amplified recordings; in the *lower tracing* in **B**, the end of the QRS complex and the ST segment are shown at low amplification

tients coronary artery and valvular heart disease coexisted, and in 51 patients coronary artery disease was documented. The remaining patients were not studied angiographically.

The overall incidence of late potentials was 74% (51 of 69 patients). Typical examples are shown in Figs. 2 and 3. The mean duration of these late potentials ranged be-

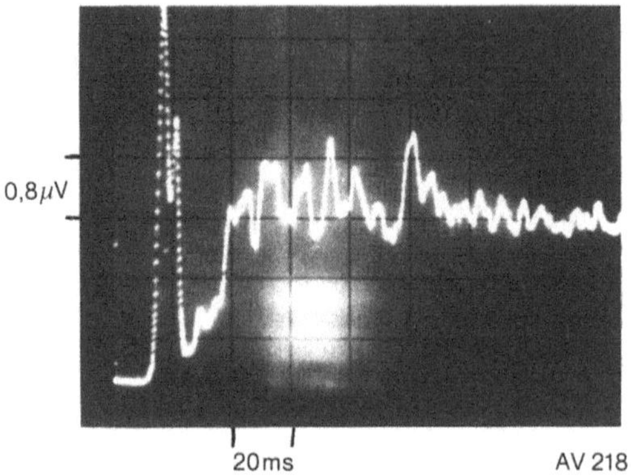

Fig. 3. Averaged recording in a patient with ventricular tachycardia showing a signal of very low amplitude of about 70-ms duration

tween 16 and 180 ms (mean 51 ± 31.4 ms). Mean amplitude was 9.0 ± 9.6 μV. The degree and extent of coronary artery involvement did not influence the prevalence of late potentials. However, these were associated with left ventricular contraction abnormalities. Three of five patients with a normal ventricular angiogram, nine of 15 (60%) with diffuse hypokinesia, and 35 of 41 (85%) with akinesia or aneurysm had late potentials. Neither of two patients with right ventricular dysplasia had late potentials. The remaining patients were not studied angiographically. In patients with ventricular tachycardia (n = 57), the prevalence of late potentials was 77%, as compared with 58.3% in those with a single episode of ventricular fibrillation ($n = 12$). Mean duration of late potentials in patients with one previous episode of ventricular fibrillation was 16.5 ms ($n = 12$), as compared with 40 ms in patients with recurrent ventricular tachycardia ($p < 0.05$); ($n = 37$) or with 47.5 ms in patients with one previous episode of ventricular tachycardia ($p < 0.05$; $n = 20$).

The incidence and prognostic significance of late ventricular potentials were assessed prospectively in 160 patients (mean age 56 ± 8.3 years) shortly after acute myocardial infarction (median day of study 25.5). Late potentials were recorded in 81 of 160 patients (50.6%); a duration of less than 20 ms was observed in 33 patients (20.6%), whereas late potentials of 20 ms duration or more were present in 48 patients (30%). Mean duration of late potentials was 27 ± 15.5 ms. There was no significant correlation to the frequency and type of spontaneous ventricular arrhythmias during 10- to 24-h Holter monitoring.

During a follow-up period of 7.5 ± 3.2 months (mean ± SD; maximum 15.8 months), the course after discharge was uneventful in 136 patients (85%). Sudden cardiac death occurred in seven patients (4.4%) after 3.7 ± 3.4 months (range 0.7 to 8.3 months). Sustained ventricular tachycardia was documented in four cases 2.9 ± 1.3 months after myocardial infarction, all having late potentials (Fig. 4). The overall incidence of ventricular tachycardia in patients with late potentials of 20 ms duration and more was 4 in 48 patients (8.3%), increasing to 16.6% (3/18 patients) when only patients with late potentials greater than 40 ms were considered. Sudden cardiac death occurred in three of 79 patients (3.8%) without late potentials. In patients with late potentials of less than 40-ms duration, the incidence of sudden death was 3.2% (2 of 63 patients), but it increased to 11.1% (2 of 18 patients) with late potentials of 40 ms duration of more. Ventricular tachycardia or sudden death occurred in 21.7% of patients with late potentials and anterior

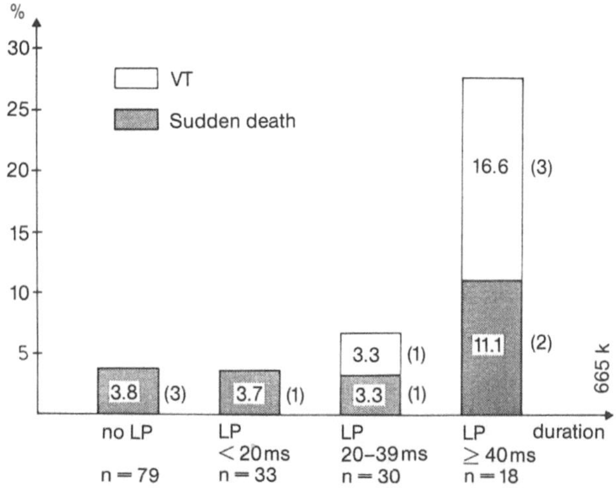

Fig. 4. Prognostic significance of late potentials in 160 patients studied shortly after myocardial infarction. The incidence of ventricular tachycardia (VT) and sudden death (< 1 h) is indicated in relation to the absence or presence of late potentials and their respective duration. *LP*, late potential

wall infarction, compared with 5.5% in patients with late potentials and inferior wall infarction ($P < 0.05$). Only one of 79 patients (1.3%) without late potentials died of a nonsudden cardiac cause (reinfarction), compared with three of 81 patients (3.7%) with late potentials irrespective of duration.

In a subset of 21 patients (eight with anterior wall infarction and 13 with inferior wall infarction) with late potentials during their first examination, a second examination was done after a mean follow-up time of 13 months (range 4.8–21.3 months); in six of eight patients with anterior wall infarction and in four of 13 with inferior wall infarction, late potentials were no longer present at the follow-up. In the remaining patients, late potentials were still present with no significant change in duration.

In 146 patients without previously documented ventricular tachycardia and/or fibrillation and without a history of syncope (group IV), coronary angiography and ventriculography were clinically indicated in order to establish or exclude the diagnosis of coronary heart disease. Of these 146 patients, 23 had no coronary heart disease, 34 had one-vessel disease, 40 two-vessel disease, and 49 three-vessel disease. Regional contraction abnormalities without significant (greater than 50%) stenosis of at least one vessel were found in 14 patients. In group IV, 49 patients (33.6%) demonstrated late potentials. Mean duration was 31 ± 15.3 ms (median 25 ms; range 10–68 ms), being 40 ms or more in 16 patients (32.6%). In 9 patients (18.4%) exhibiting late potentials the duration was less than 20 ms, whereas in the remaining 24 (49%) the duration was between 20 and 39 ms. Mean amplitude of late potentials was 16.5 ± 22.4 µV.

There was a close correlation between the detection of late potentials and left ventricular function. In 32 cases with an angiographically normal contraction pattern of the left ventricle (15 normals and 17 patients with coronary artery disease) without ventricular tachycardia, only three patients (9.4%) exhibited late potentials, which were of short duration (18, 26, and 28 ms). Six out of 24 patients with diffuse hypokinesia, patients had late potentials. In patients with regional contraction abnormalities, the prevalence of late potentials was higher in those with akinesia (14 of 26 patients, 53.8%) or with left ventricular aneurysm (18 of 43 patients, 41.9%) than in those with hypokinesia (8 of 36 patients, 22.2%). On the other hand, the degree and extent of coronary artery involvement did not influence the prevalence of late potentials. Thus, the main factor associated with the occurrence of late potentials was the presence of left ventricular wall motion abnormalities.

Correlation Between Late Potentials and Spontaneous Ventricular Arrhythmias

In 73 patients without previously documented ventricular tachycardia or syncope, the results of 24-h Holter monitoring (Reynolds Pathfinder) was correlated to spontaneous ventricular arrhythmias. In 45 patients without late potentials, the average number of ventricular ectopic beats p/h was 37 ± 91.7 (mean ± SD); 14 of 45 patients (31.1%) had sporadic ventricular couplets or triplets. In the remaining 28 patients with late potentials the average number of ventricular ectopic beats was 41 ± 97.6 p/h; eight patients (28.6%) had sporadic couplets or triplets.

Correlation Between Late Potentials and the Repetitive Ventricular Response

In 70 patients in whom no late potentials could be detected from the body surface, four or more ventricular echo beats were induced less frequently than in 40 patients with late potentials.

More precisely, the repetitive response was absent in two patients without late potentials, but all patients with late potentials demonstrated a repetitive ventricular response. Four or more ventricular echo beats, considered an endpoint for stimulation, were induced in 20 of 70 patients (28.6%) without, and in 24 of 40 patients (60%) with late potentials. In the latter group, the incidence of abnormal responses (four or more ventricular echo beats or ventricular tachycardia) increased in relation to the increased duration of late potentials (Fig. 5). Ventricular fibrillation was not induced in any patient of either group. In patients in whom four or more echo beats were induced, the rate (mean ± SD) of the induced responses decreased from 267 ± 33.0 bpm in those without late potentials to 258 ± 37.0 bpm in those with late potentials of less than 20-ms duration, to 254 ± 54.5 bpm with a duration between 20 and 39 ms, and finally to 242 ± 37.6 bpm in those with late potentials equal to or greater than 40 ms. The proportion of patients with late potentials in whom four or more echo beats were induced was higher in those with akinesia or aneurysm compared with those without (Fig. 6).

Effect of Antiarrhythmic Drugs on Late Potentials

The effect of various antiarrhythmic drugs on late potentials was compared with the inducibility of ventricular tachycardia in 11 patients, all of whom had had previously documented sustained ventricular tachycardia.

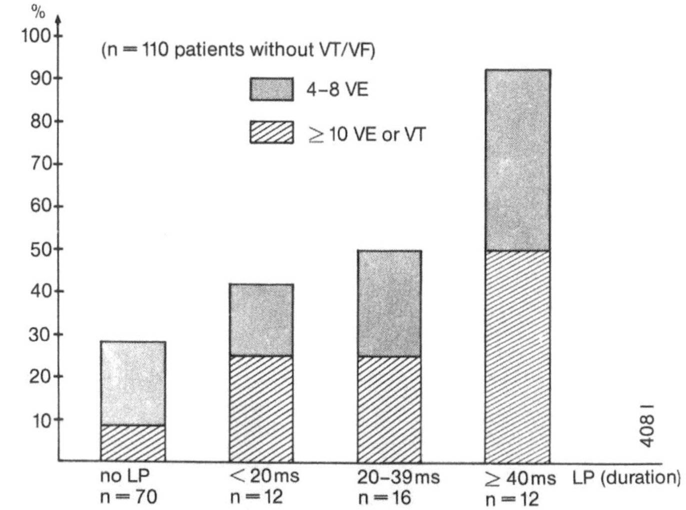

Fig. 5. Relationship between presence or absence of late potentials and the results of programmed ventricular stimulation in 110 patients. With increasing duration of late potentials, the percentage of inducible ventricular arrhythmias (4–9 ventricular echo beats [*VE*] or ⩾10 VE or ventricular tachycardia [*VT*] increases to a maximum of 92% in patients with late potentials of duration ⩾40 ms. *VT/VF*, ventricular tachycardia and/or fibrillation

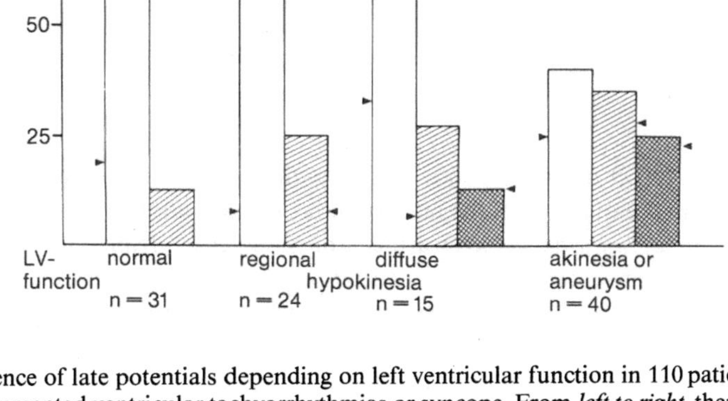

Fig. 6. Presence or absence of late potentials depending on left ventricular function in 110 patients without previously documented ventricular tachyarrhythmias or syncope. From *left to right*, there is an increasing proportion of patients with late potentials of short (< 40 ms) or long (⩾40 ms) duration. An "abnormal" response to programmed ventricular stimulation (defined as ⩾4 consecutive ventricular echo beats, marked by small *arrows* was highest in patients with akinesia or aneurysm

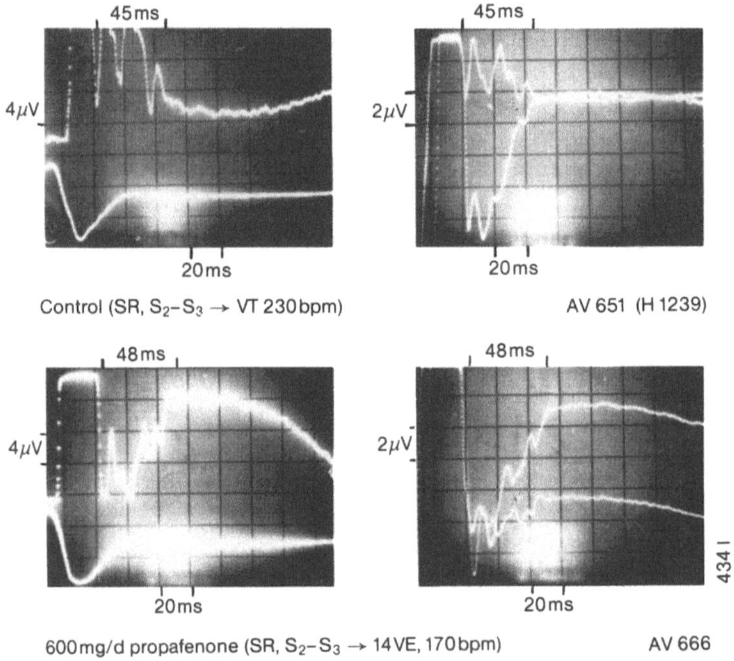

Fig. 7. Effect of propafenone (600 mg/day) on duration of late potentials in a patient with ventricular tachycardia. Despite a decrease in the rate of induced tachycardia, there was no signficant change in the duration of the late potential

Table 2. Lack of effect of various class I antiarrhythmic drugs on the duration of late potentials in patients with ventricular tachycardia (VT)

Change in inducibility	Duration of late potentials (ms)	
	Controls	Under therapy
None	34 ± 30	34 ± 27
↑	37 ± 55	35 ± 43
↑↑	17 ± 7	20 ± 7
↑↑↑ or no longer inducible	46 ± 50	40 ± 40

Black arrows denote changes in inducibility of VT using a step-like stimulation program

The effect of propafenone in one patient is shown in Fig. 7. There was a slight increase in the duration of the late potential, concomitant with a change of the inducibility and rate of ventricular tachycardia, which decreased from 230 bpm to 170 bpm. During control, ventricular tachycardia could be induced by two premature beats during sinus rhythm; after propafenone (600 mg/day), nonsustained ventricular tachycardia could still be initiated.

On the whole, in contrast to what was expected, there was no significant correlation between changes in the duration of late potentials and the mode of initiation or the abolition of ventricular tachycardia in 11 patients studied while on various antiarrhythmic drugs (Table 2).

Effect on Map-guided Surgery in Patients with Ventricular Tachycardia

The response of late potentials to surgical intervention in patients with documented ventricular tachycardia and coronary artery disease can be used to study their pathophysiological significance. Therefore we studied 19 patients pre- and postoperatively, 16 with previously documented sustained ventricular tachycardia (VT) and three with only inducible VT (one of whom had recurrent syncope), due to previous myocardial infarction. Mean age was 53 ± 6 years, 16 were male, three female. In all but one, VT could be induced preoperatively by programmed right ventricular stimulation. Indication for surgery was either intractable VT or need for bypass grafting and/or aneurysmectomy. Preoperatively, mean duration of late potentials was 54 ± 37.7 ms and mean amplitude was 12 ± 14.0 μV. Surgery was guided by epi- and endocardial mapping. In 14 cases endomyocardial encircling ventriculotomy was the main procedure, whereas in five patients only aneurysmectomy and bypass grafting were performed. Postoperatively, late potentials were no longer detectable in 12 cases, whereas in six of seven cases there was a decrease in duration, but no essential change in amplitude. A postoperative electrophysiological study was performed in 18 cases. In those 12 patients in whom late potentials were abolished, the maximal number of inducible ventricular echo beats using an extended stimulation program from three right ventricular sites ranged between one and five in 9 cases and between 10 and 11 in 2 cases, while VT was induced in only one case. Of six patients in whom late potentials were still detectable, ventricular tachycardia could still be induced in two cases and a maximal response of ten echo beats was observed in another.

Discussion

Among coronary patients, mainly those who have survived an episode of acute myocardial infarction are at high risk of subsequent sudden cardiac death after hospital discharge. Identification of these patients is still one of the major problems of clinical cardiology [1]. There seems to be sufficient evidence that most episodes of sudden cardiac death are due to ventricular fibrillation [44]. Multivariate statistical techniques have provided evidence that frequent, and above all complex, ventricular arrhythmias detected by long-term ECG recording [2–9] independently contribute to prognosis; they are thus considered precursors of sudden death. However, some doubt has recently been shed on the usefulness of the long-term ECG for the identification of individual patients at risk of sudden death [14]. Furthermore, the usefulness of spontaneous ventricular arrhythmias may be limited by their great spontaneous variability [10–13]. In addition, though noninvasive, long-term recording of the ECG over 24 h is time-consuming with regard to both recording and evaluation even if semiautomatic or automatic arrhythmia detection devices are used. In contrast to the spontaneous variability of ventricular arrhythmias, recording of late potentials does not have the disadvantage of spontaneous variability, as they seem to be stable for many months (unpublished results).

Ventricular late potentials are a new electrocardiographic parameter, which is based on experimental studies [15–19, 45, 46] and clinical observations [21, 47, 50]. These have consistently shown the presence of delayed fractionated activity during diastole in regions of old experimental infarctions and in patients with ventricular tachycardia due to left ventricular aneurysms. This diastolic activity resulting from regional slow activation represents one of the prerequisites for reentry, i.e., slow conduction; the other two prerequisites are unidirectional block and recovery of the tissue ahead of the wave front of excitation [51]. Delayed fractionated potentials have also been observed during intraoperative epicardial [23, 49, 50, 52] and endocardial catheter mapping [20, 21] in patients with ventricular tachycardia. The amplitude of these signals which occur in localized areas may be in the order of several millivolts if bipolar recordings are used. Using conventional methods of ECG recording these signals can be recovered from the body surface only in very rare cases [48]. However, Berbari et al. [22], in the experimental animal, and Fontaine et al. [23], in patients with idiopathic ventricular tachycardia, were the first who reported that these signals can be recorded from the body surface by the use of high-gain amplification and computer averaging techniques. This has been confirmed by some recent studies in the experimental animal [16, 53] and in man [24–31].

In the present study, the averaging technique was used as a totally noninvasive method to detect regional delayed activation of the ventricles. Late potentials were in the range of some microvolts at the filter settings used. These data are in agreement with those obtained in experimental myocardial infarction [16, 22, 53]. Therefore, high-gain amplification was necessary to record the low-magnitude precordial signals. In order to reduce the amount of noise as much as possible, a high-gain preamplifier was selected on the basis of its very high signal-to-noise ratio. Signal filtering and averaging were used to eliminate remaining random noise. With increasing repetitions of the averaging process the signal-to-noise ratio increased. Generally, 200 repetitions were sufficient to obtain a stable signal, with no further improvement by prolonged averaging.

To date only a few reports on the prevalence of late potentials in small groups of patients exist [24–31]. Some differences in prevalence in the various reports may be due to differences in the equipment used and the methods of selecting patients. The data presented in this paper show that ventricular late potentials can be found in patients both without and with ventricular tachycardia (Table 1). Thus, the presence of late potentials is neither highly sensitive nor specific for patients with clinically evident ventricular tachyarrhythmias. In addition, there is a large overlap in the duration of late potentials among patients with ventricular tachycardia or fibrillation and patients without a history of these arrhythmias. The longer duration of late potentials in patients with ventricular tachycardia may indicate that in these cases regional activation is more fragmented and possibly slower than in those without previously documented ventricular tachycardia.

Our results of noninvasive recording of late potentials are in agreement with recent invasive studies by Klein et al. [50] and Spielman et al. [54] who studied patients during open heart surgery by epi- and endocardial mapping or during endocardial catheter mapping. These groups found a greater incidence and extent of delayed and fragmented ventricular activity in patients with documented ventricular tachyarrhythmias compared to those without. These data and the greater prevalence of late potentials in our patients with regional or diffuse ventricular contraction abnormalities suggest that the anatomic precondition for late potentials is diseased tissue. Obviously, a transmural infarction may show no abnormal activation pattern because such tissue is "electrically" silent. On the other hand, tissue immediately adjacent to the infarction contains viable myocardium interspersed with fibrotic tissue [15]. Such tissue may result in fragmentation of the propagating electromotive surface with the consequent development of high-frequency components [55–57]. It was possible to identify the border zone of old myocardial infarcts as the site of origin for delayed ventricular potentials by comparing precordial recordings using the averaging technique and intraoperative mapping techniques (own observation; 58). The fact that late potentials were abolished [33, 34] by subendocardial partial or complete encircling ventriculotomy [59] in patients with documented ventricular tachycardia is an important argument in favor of the hypothesis that these late potentials are related to the propensity to ventricular tachycardia, and that they probably originate in the border zone between myocardial scars and normal myocardium.

The question arises as to why late potentials cannot be detected in all patients with documented ventricular tachycardia and/or fibrillation. There are several reasons. First, instable triggering may prevent the recording of late potentials which are canceled by the always changing timing. This seems to be of minor importance, as the jitter for triggering was relatively small in our system. Second, these signals may have amplitudes too low to be differentiated from noise. Third, fragmented activation of a certain area of the myocardium may occur so early that it is still covered within the QRS complex; therefore, it need not always outlast normal ventricular activation. Fourth, the signals may be too small and may occur immediately at the end of QRS at a time when filter ringing occurs. Fifth, in some patients a "stress" such as premature excitation by ectopic beats or artificially by premature stimuli may be necessary to slow conduction to a sufficient degree to evoke reentry [19]. Lastly, in some patients with inducible ventricular tachycardia, the functional basis for tachycardia may not be reentry but triggered automaticity [60]. This, however, remains speculative, as triggered automaticity as a mechanism for ventricular tachycardia has not yet been proven in man.

In those patients without documented ventricular tachycardia or fibrillation, the presence of late potentials has to be considered an indicator of abnormally conducting tissue which may set the stage for reentrant tachycardia. However, slow conduction is only one of the prerequisites for reentry. Some limited follow-up data suggest that some of these patients may later develop ventricular tachycardia or sudden death [26]. The differences in duration of late potentials in patients with and without ventricular tachycardia suggest that a critically prolonged regional conduction delay may favor the occurrence of reentry. Nevertheless, in none of the cases with or without ventricular tachycardia was conduction delay sufficiently long to reach beyond ventricular refractoriness, which would make reexcitation of normal tissue possible. Thus, it has to be assumed that some "stress" is necessary to prolong regional conduction delay to a critical value. Similar responses of regional fragmented activity to premature beats have been observed in experimental myocardial infarction [19].

Late potentials as could be shown in the present prospective pilot study are a frequent finding after recent myocardial infarction. Half the patients exhibited late potentials of varying duration at the end of or after the QRS complex. This study is the first to show that averaging might be able to predict the subsequent occurrence of sustained ventricular tachycardia in patients after recent myocardial infarction. All four patients who developed sustained ventricular tachycardia, three of whom had to be resuscitated, exhibited late potentials. In contrast, no patient without late potentials had an episode of documented symptomatic ventricular tachycardia.

There was a higher incidence of sudden death in those with late potentials of duration $\geqslant$40 ms. However, these differences were not significant. The incidence of sudden death or ventricular tachycardia was significantly less (3.6%) in patients without late potentials or with late potentials of less than 20-ms duration compared to those with late potentials longer than or equal to 20 ms (14.6%; $P < 0.01$). None of the patients who died suddenly or had ventricular tachycardia had conduction abnormalities in their discharge ECG. Thus, it seems justified to assume that the cause of sudden death in these patients was ventricular fibrillation. Whether the occurrence of sudden death in those patients with late potentials was related to primary reentrant arrhythmias remains unsettled. In contrast, sudden death in those without late potentials might be due to a new ischemic event leading to ventricular fibrillation. Though this hypothesis seems attractive, there is presently no way to determine the cause of death in the individual case.

Clinical Implications

Recording of late potentials from the body surface is a new and promising technique which may help to identify patients at risk of ventricular tachycardia or sudden death after myocardial infarction. Further studies are necessary to prove their predictive value in patients with recent myocardial infarction in conjunction with other parameters such as 24-h, long-term ECG recording. In the mean time no premature conclusions should be drawn as to the indication for antiarrhythmic therapy of patients with late potentials. Before definite proof of their prognostic signficance has been obtained, this could expose such patients to an unnecessary risk of potential side effects without sufficient evidence of benefit. Another question still to be answered concerns the significance of late potentials in patients long after myocardial infarction. The same attitude is mandatory toward drug intervention as toward patients after recent myocardial infarction to avoid premature conclusions. The high incidence of inducible ventricular tachycardia in those patients with late potentials of 40 ms duration or more (92%) suggests that these potentials are indeed an expression of increased ventricular vulnerability.

Whether late potentials will prove to be a better indicator for future development of ventricular tachycardia than for sudden death is a crucial question. First, there was a tendency to shorter late potentials in those patients who survived an episode of ventricular fibrillation compared with those with sustained ventricular tachycardia. Second, there was an inverse relationship between duration of late potentials and rate of ventricular tachycardia. Third, all patients who developed ventricular tachycardia after recent myocardial infarction (group III) had had late potentials whereas those who died suddenly did not all have late potentials. It is an attractive hypothesis that those who died suddenly and who did not have late potentials died from a new ischemic event, whereas those who had late potentials died of chronic electrophysiological abnormalities. This hypothesis needs further elucidation.

The lack of any significant effects of antiarrhythmic drugs on the duration of late potentials, at least as far as pooled patient data are concerned, is unexpected. Similar results have recently been reported by others [61, 62]. One would expect a prolongation of late potentials above all with antiarrhythmic drugs that slow conduction. The reasons for the lack of observed effect remain obscure. A possibility is that late potentials recorded by the averaging technique represent the sum of many cardiac cycles. Thus, dynamic changes that might occur on alternate beats might be canceled out during the averaging process. Another reason might be that the effect of antiarrhythmic drugs on electrophysiologic parameters is less during sinus rhythm than during premature discharges.

For the evaluation of the success of surgery in patients with ventricular tachycardia and previous myocardial infarction, signal averaging represents a new noninvasive approach, whereby patients can be identified for whom surgery might not be successful in ablating the site of origin of ventricular tachycardia. Abolition of late potentials by surgery suggests that the surgical procedure has been successful in removing electrophysiologically abnormal tissue. However, even when late potentials are still present after surgery, the propensity to ventricular tachycardia may have been abolished.

References

1. Lown B (1979) Sudden cardiac death: The major challenge confronting contemporary cardiology. Am J Cardiol 43: 313–328
2. Kotler MN, Tabatznik B, Mower MM, Tominaga S (1973) Prognostic significance of ventricular ectopic beats with respect to sudden death in the late postinfarction period. Circulation 47: 959
3. Moss AJ, DeCamilla JJ, Davis HP, Bayer L (1977) Clinical significance of ventricular ectopic beats in the early posthospital phase of myocardial infarction. Am J Cardiol 39: 635
4. Moss AJ, Davis HT, DeCamilla J, Bayer LW (1979) Ventricular ectopic beats and their relation to sudden and nonsudden cardiac death after myocardial infarction. Circulation 60: 998
5. Geltman EM, Ehsani AA, Campbell MK, Schechtman K, Roberts R, Sobel BE (1979) The influence of location and extent of myocardial infarction on long-term ventricular dysrhythmia and mortality. Circulation 60: 805
6. Ruberman W, Weinblatt E, Goldberg JD, Frank CW, Shapiro S,(S, Chaudhary BS (1980) Ventricular premature complexes in prognosis of angina. Circulation 61: 1172–1178
7. Moss AJ (1980) Clinical significance of ventricular arrhythmias in patients with and without coronary artery disease. Prog Cardiovasc Dis 23: 33–52
8. Califf RM, Wagner GS, Rosati RA (1981) Prognostic value of ventricular arrhythmias. Am J Cardiol 47: 397
9. Schulze RA Jr, O'Neal Humphries J, Griffith LSC et al. (1977) Left ventricular and coronary angiographic anatomy. Relationship to ventricular irritability in the late hospital phase of acute myocardial infarction. Circulation 55: 839–843
10. Morganroth J, Michelson EL, Horowitz LN, Josephson ME, Pearlman AS, Dunkman WB (1978) Limitations of routine long-term ambulatory electrocardiographic monitoring to assess ventricular ectopic frequency. Circulation 58: 408–414
11. Winkle RA (1978) Antiarrhythmic drug effect mimicked by spontaneous variability of ventricular ectopy. Circulation 57: 1116–1121
12. Michelson EL, Morganroth J (1980) Spontaneous variability of complex ventricular arrhythmias detected by long-term electrocardiographic recording. Circulation 61: 690–695
13. Andresen D, Leitner E-R v, Wegscheider K, Schröder R (1982) Nachweis komplexer tachykarder ventrikulärer Rhythmusstörungen im Langzeit-EKG. Dtsch Med Wochenschr 107: 571–574
14. Cats VM, Lie KI, Capelle FJL van, Durrer D (1979) Limitations of 24 hour ambulatory electrocardiographic recording in predicting coronary events after acute myocardial infarction. Am J Cardiol 44: 1257–1262
15. Daniel T, Boineau J, Sabiston D (1971) Comparison of human ventricular activation with canine model in chronic myocardial infarction. Circulation 44: 74–89
16. Simson MB, Euler DE, Michelson EL, Falcone R, Spear JF, Moore N (1981) Confirmation of a new technique for detecting slow ventricular activation on the body surface. Am J Cardiol 47: 488

17. El-Sherif N, Scherlag BJ, Lazzara R, Hope RR (1977) Reentrant ventricular arrhythmias in the late myocardial infarction period. I. Conduction characteristics in the infarction zone. Circulation 55: 686–702
18. El-Sherif N, Scherlag BJ, Lazzara R, Hope RR (1977) Reentrant ventricular arrhythmias in the late myocardial infarction period. II. Patterns of initiation and termination of reentry. Circulation 55: 702–719
19. El-Sherif N, Lazzara R, Hope RR, Scherlag BJ (1977) Reentrant arrhythmias in the late myocardial infarction period. III. Manifest and concealed extra-systolic grouping. Circulation 56: 225–234
20. Klein H, Werner P, Frank G, Bethge KP, Lichtlen PR (1981) Value of left ventricular endocardial catheter mapping in patients with ventricular arrhythmias. Eur Heart J [Suppl A] 2: 42
21. Josephson ME, Horowitz LN, Farshidi A (1978) Continuous local electrical activity: A mechanism of recurrent ventricular tachycardia. Circulation 57: 569–665
22. Berbari EJ, Scherlag BJ, Hope RR, Lazzara R (1978) Recording from the body surface of arrhythmogenic ventricular activity during the ST segment. Am J Cardiol 41: 697–702
23. Fontaine G, Frank R, Gallais Hamonno F, Allali I, Phan-Thuc H, Grosgogeat Y (1978) Electrocardiographie des potentiels tardifs du syndrome de post-excitation. Arch Mal Coeur 71: 854–864
24. Uther JB, Dennett CJ, Tan A (1978) The detection of delayed activation signals of low amplitude in the vectorcardiogram of patients with recurrent ventricular tachycardia by signal averaging. In: Sandoe E, Julian DG, Bell JW (eds) Management of ventricular tachycardia – Role of Mexiletine. Excerpta Medica, Amsterdam Oxford, p 80–82
25. Breithardt G, Becker R, Seipel L (1980) Non-invasive recording of late ventricular activation in man. Circulation [Suppl III] 62: 320
26. Breithardt G, Becker R, Seipel L, Abendroth R-R, Ostermeyer J (1981) Non-invasive detection of late potentials in man – A new marker for ventricular tachycardia. Eur Heart J 2: 1–11
27. Hombach V, Höpp H-W, Braun V, Behrenbeck DW, Tauchert M, Hilger HH (1980) Die Bedeutung von Nachpotentialen innerhalb des ST-Segmentes im Oberflächen-EKG bei Patienten mit koronarer Herzkrankheit. Dtsch Med Wochenschr 105: 1457–1462
28. Simson M, Horowitz L, Josephson M, Moore EN, Kastor J (1980) A marker for ventricular tachycardia after myocardial infarction. Circulation [Suppl III] 62: 262
29. Oeff M, Leitner E-R v, Brüggemann T, Andresen D, Sthapit R, Schröder R (1982) Methodische Probleme bei der Registrierung ventrikulärer Spätpotentiale. Z Kardiol 71: 204
30. Rozanski JJ, Mortara D, Myerburg RJ, Castellanos A (1981) Body surface detection of delayed depolarizations in patients with recurrent ventricular tachycardia and left ventricular aneurysm. Circulation 63: 1172–1178
31. Simson MB (1981) Use of signals in the terminal QRS complex to identify patients with ventricular tachycardia after myocardial infarction. Circulation 64: 235–242
32. Höpp H-W, Hombach V, Braun V, Behrenbeck DW, Tauchert M, Hilger HH (1981) Kammerarrhythmien und ventrikuläre Spätdepolarisationen bei akutem Myokardinfarkt. Z Kardiol 70: 319
33. Breithardt G, Seipel L, Karbenn U, Abendroth R-R, Ostermeyer J, Borggrefe M, Yeh HL (1981) Verhalten ventrikulärer Spätpotentiale nach operativer Therapie ventrikulärer Tachykardien. Z Kardiol 70: 612
34. Breithardt G, Seipel L, Ostermeyer J, Karbenn U, Abendroth R-R, Yeh HL, Bircks W (1982) Effect of surgery on late ventricular potentials recorded by precordial signal averaging in patients with ventricular tachycardia. Am Heart J 104: 996–1003
35. Breithardt G, Borggrefe M, Karbenn U, Abendroth R-R, Yeh HL, Seipel L (1982) Prevalence of late potentials in patients with and without ventricular tachycardia – Correlation to angiographic findings. Am J Cardiol 49: 1932–37
36. Breithardt G, Schwarzmeier J, Haerten K, Seipel L (1981) Häufigkeit ventrikulärer Spätpotentiale in der Postinfarktphase. Z Kardiol 70: 332
37. Breithardt G, Schwarzmaier J, Abendroth R-R, Borggrefe M, Seipel L (1981) Prospective study on the incidence of late potentials in postmyocardial infarction patients. Circulation [Suppl IV] 64: 328
38. Breithardt G, Schwarzmeier J, Borggrefe M, Haerten K, Seipel L (in press) Prognostic significance of late ventricular potentials after acute myocardial infarction. Eur Heart J

39. Breithardt G, Abendroth R-R, Borggrefe M, Karbenn U, Seipel L (1982) Ventrikuläre Vulnerabilität und Nachweis ventrikulärer Spätpotentiale bei Patienten ohne dokumentierte ventrikuläre Tachykardien. Z Kardiol 71: 206
40. Borggrefe M, Breithardt G, Karbenn U, Seipel L (1981) Incidence of late ventricular activation in patients without previously documented ventricular tachycardia. Circulation [Suppl IV] 64: 172
41. Borggrefe M, Breithardt G, Seipel L (1981) Häufigkeit ventrikulärer Spätpotentiale bei Patienten mit ventrikulären Tachykardien oder Kammerflimmern. Z Kardiol 70: 612
42. Haerten K, Borggrefe M, Weyers FJ, Breithardt G (1982) Langzeitverhalten ventrikulärer Spätpotentiale bei Patienten nach Infarkt. Z Kardiol 71: 205
43. Breithardt G, Seipel L, Abendroth RR, Loogen F (1980) Serial electrophysiological testing of antiarrhythmic drug efficacy in patients with recurrent ventricular tachycardia. Eur Heart J 1: 11–24
44. Iseri L, Humphrey SB, Siner EJ (1978) Prehospital brady-asystolic cardiac arrest. Ann Intern Med 88: 741–745
45. Waldo AL, Kaiser SGA (1973) A study of ventricular arrhythmias associated with acute myocardial infarction in the canine heart. Circulation 43: 1222
46. Williams DO, Scherlag BJ, Hope RR, El-Sherif N, Lazzara R (1974) The pathophysiology of malignant ventricular arrhythmias during acute myocardial ischemia. Circulation 50: 1163–1172
47. Josephson ME, Horowitz LN, Farshidi A, Spielman SR, Michelson EL, Greenspan AM (1978) Sustained ventricular tachycardia: Evidence for protected localized re-entry. Am J Cardiol 42: 416
48. Fontaine G, Guiraudon G, Frank R, Vedel J, Grosgogeat Y, Cabrol C, Facquet J (1977) Stimulation studies and epicardial mapping in ventricular tachycardia: Study of mechanisms and selection for surgery. In: Kulbertus HE (ed) Re-entrant arrhythmias, mechanisms and treatment. MTP Press, Lancaster, p 333–350
49. Ostermeyer J, Breithardt G, Kolvenbach R, Körfer R, Seipel L, Schulte HD, Bircks W (1979) Intraoperative electrophysiologic mapping during cardiac surgery. Thorac Cardiovasc Surg 27: 260–270
50. Klein H, Karp RB, Kouchoukos NT, James TN, Waldo AL (1979) Ventricular mapping of abnormal myocardium in patients with and without arrhythmias. Circulation [Suppl II] 60: 24
51. Zipes DP (1975) Electrophysiological mechanisms involved in ventricular fibrillation. Circulation [Suppl III] 52: 120–130
52. Fontaine G, Guiraudon G, Frank R (1978) Intramyocardial conduction defects in patients prone to ventricular tachycardia, III. The post-excitation syndrome in ventricular tachycardia. In: Sandoe E, Julian DG, Bell JW (eds) Management of ventricular tachycardia – role of Mexiletine. Excerpta Medica, Amsterdam Oxford, p 67–69
53. Simson MB, Euler D, Michelson EL, Falcone RA, Spear JF, Moore EN (1981) Detection of delayed ventricular activation on the body surface in dogs. Am J Physiol 241: 363–369
54. Spielman SR, Untereker WJ, Horowitz LN, Greenspan AM, Simson MB, Kastor JA, Josephson ME (1981) Fragmented electrical activity – relationship to ventricular tachycardia. Am J Cardiol 47: 448
55. Langner PH Jr, Geselowitz DB, Briller SA (1973) Wide band recording of the electrocardiogram and coronary heart disease. Am Heart J 86: 308–317
56. Flowers NC, Horan LG, Thomas JR, Tolleson WJ (1969) The anatomic basis for high frequency components in the electrocardiogram. Circulation 39: 531–539
57. Reynolds EW, Muller BF, Anderson GJ, Muller BT (1967) High frequency components in the electrocardiogram. A comparative study of normals and patients with myocardial disease. Circulation 35: 195–206
58. Simson M, Spielman S, Horowitz L, Josephson M, Harken A, Kastor J (1981) Slow ventricular activation detected on the body surface in patients with ventricular tachycardia after myocardial infarction. Am J Cardiol 47: 498
59. Guiraudon G, Fontaine G, Frank R, Escande R, Etievent P (1978) Encircling endocardial ventriculotomy. A new surgical treatment for lifethreatening ventricular tachycardias resistant to medical treatment following myocardial infarction. Ann Thorac Surg 26: 438–444
60. Wyndham CRC, Arnsdorf MF, Levitsky S, Smith TC, Dhingra RC, Denes P, Rosen KM (1980)

Succesful surgical excision of focal paroxysmal atrial tachycardia. Observations in Vivo and in Vitro. Circulation 62: 1365–1372
61. Höpp HW, Deutsch H, Hombach V, Braun V, Hilger HH. Medikamentöse Beeinflußbarkeit ventrikulärer Spätpotentiale. Z Kardiol 71: 206
62. Simson MB, Spielman SR, Horowitz LN, Waxman HL, Falcone RA, Marcus NH, Josephson ME (1982) Effects of antiarrhythmic drugs on body surface late potentials in patients with ventricular tachycardia. Am J Cardiol 49: 1030

Simulation Studies for the Interpretation of Delayed Potentials

R. Frank, G. Fontaine, M. Pierfitte* and Y. Grosgogeat

Introduction

Delayed potentials, defined as ventricular activity recorded after the end of the surface QRS complex, have been related in some selected cases to the occurrence of ventricular tachycardia [1]. We described these potentials after recording them with close bipolar electrodes (1-mm) during epicardial mapping in patients with ventricular tachycardia not related to coronary artery disease [2]. We then found them by 1-cm wide bipolar endocardial recording during electrophysiological studies [3] and by surface ECG after high amplification and averaging techniques in similar cases [4]. These potentials have been interpreted as the consequence of very slow conduction in a localized zone of diseased myocardium, thus showing one of the prerequisites for reentry mechanism.

However, the morphology of the recorded potentials changes from one technique to another:

1. Surface ECG displays multiple potentials of low amplitude, 1–10 μV, in the ST segment (Fig. 1).
2. Endocardial 1-cm bipolar potentials usually have a similar pattern, recorded in localized zones of the ventricles, with a QRS synchronous potential followed by a smaller potential (0.1 mV) occurring during the ST segment (Fig. 1).
3. There may be different patterns on 1-mm bipolar recording (Fig. 2):
   (a) Usually the first QRS synchronous potential is broad and of low amplitude and is followed, after an isoelectric line, by a second potential, sharp and of high amplitude.
   (b) That potential may be followed by another, of similar morphology but with different orientation.
   (c) In some cases, the QRS synchronous potential is followed by multiple fragmented potentials of low amplitude.

Recording of these potentials in patients with ventricular tachycardia seemed to differ from one pathology to another. In right ventricular dysplasia, delayed activation was constantly recorded from the epicardium with 1-mm spaced electrodes [1], whereas preoperative endocavitary studies could only record it in approximately half the cases with 1-cm spaced bipolar electrodes. In contrast, epicardial mapping in old myocardial infarction could seldom record a fragmented activation following the QRS synchronous potential [5].

---

* Ingenieur de l'Ecole Nationale Supérieure des Télécommunications de Paris. This work was realized with the material assistance of La Caisse Régionale d'Assurances Maladie de Paris (C.R.A.M.P.) and L'Association de Recherche et d'Entraide Cardiologique et Angéiologique (A.R.E.C.A.)

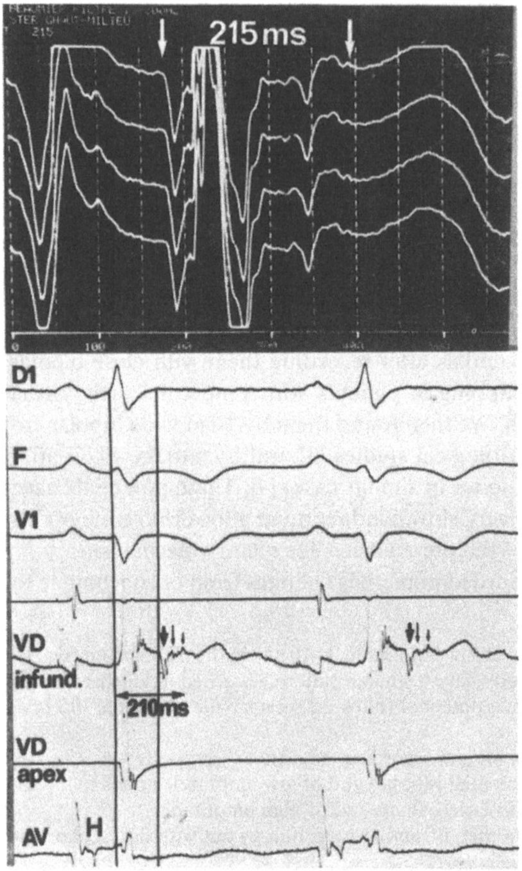

Fig. 1. *Top.* four successive averaged cycles of 100 ECG beats in a patient with right ventricular dysplasia, showing delayed activation of up to 215 ms after the onset of the QRS. *Bottom.* surface ECG and endocavitary recording with delayed activation of up to 210 ms in the pulmonary infundibulum (1-cm bipolar recording)

Method

For a better understanding of the laws which may influence the recording of these potentials, we developed a computer program to simulate the potentials detected by a unipolar or bipolar electrode system when one or multiple dipoles are passing by. The purpose was to look at the conditions which could generate patterns similar to those observed in delayed activation.

Without entering into the details of the mathematical model, which has been described elsewhere [6], we consider an electrically homogeneous medium in which basic electrostatic laws may be applied. The model allows computation of the electric field produced by one or more dipoles moving at constant speed and in a straight line. Three equidistant electrodes define a surface. Dipoles may move at any angle, and at any depth from that surface. The program allows modification of the interelectrode distance, the size and orientation of the dipole, and distance from the tripolar system. The display

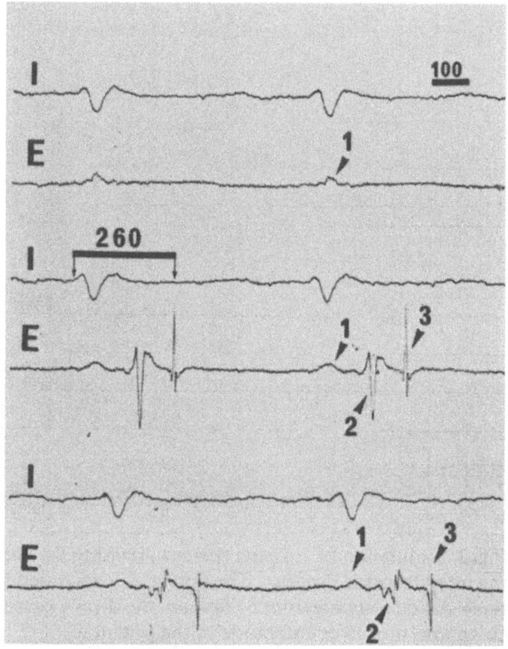

I = Lead 1 of the ECG
E = Epicardial recording

Fig. 2. Different patterns of epicardial (*E*) delayed activation (1-mm bipolar recording)

is the computerized recording from each of the three bipolar leads and three unipolar leads that can be derived from the tripolar system.

We will assume that the size of the elementary dipole generated by a myocardial fiber is in the 1-mm range. Studies by Spach et al. [7] by indirect means on Purkinje fibers indicated a value near 0.5 mm. In our simulation, the electrode size is first in the same 1-mm range as in the epicardial study. A "wide" interelectrode distance will be ten times wider than the dipole, about 10-mm, as in the endocavitary catheterization studies.

Results

The simulation procedure allows display of the basic electrostatic laws included in the program [6].

Amplitude of a unipolar potential is inversely related to the square of the dipole electrode distance. Amplitude of a bipolar potential is inversely related to the cube of the dipole electrode distance. An abnormal activation can be more precisely localized with a bipolar than a unipolar electrode, but the latter is more sensitive to distant potentials (Fig. 3).

Prolongation of the potential duration appears with the increase of the distance between the electrodes and the dipoles (Fig. 3). The potential becomes broader and its du-

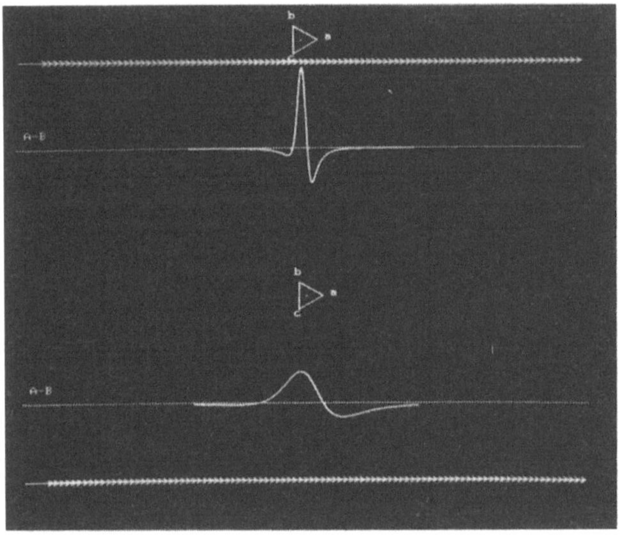

Fig. 3. Simulation of a dipole (*arrows*) passing the electrode system. The dipole size is the same as the interelectrode distance. The potential is recorded by the AB lead. *Top.* the dipole passes at 1 interelectrode distance from B. *Bottom:* the dipole passes at 6 interelectrodes from B. Note the broadening and the lower amplitude of the potential

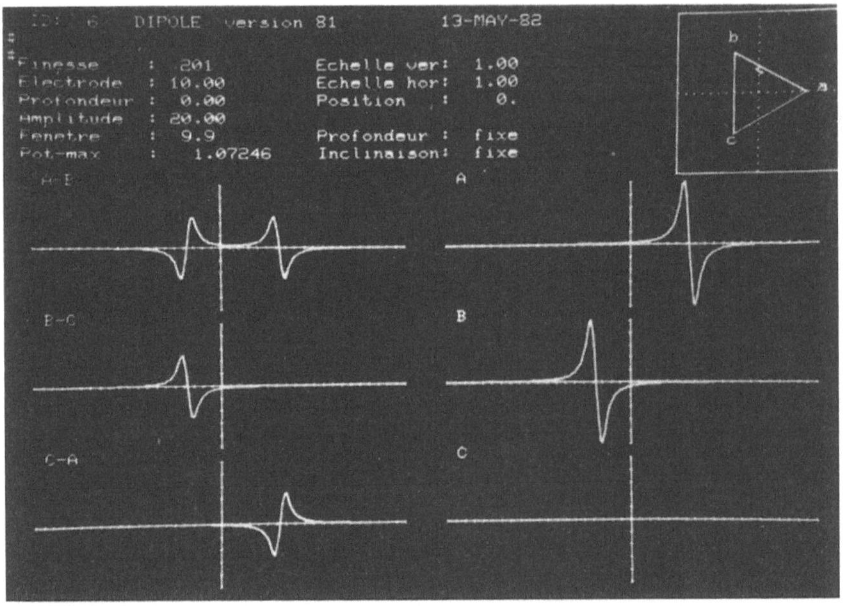

Echelle = Scale

Fig. 4. Typical display from the program. *Top left,* a small dipole, represented by an *arrow* (size 1 mm) passes parallel to a wide (10 mm) electrode pair AB at a very small distance. Recording on the bipolar AB lead displays a double potential. Note that the other bipolar (BC, CA) and the unipolar (A, B) recordings only show the earlier or the later potential

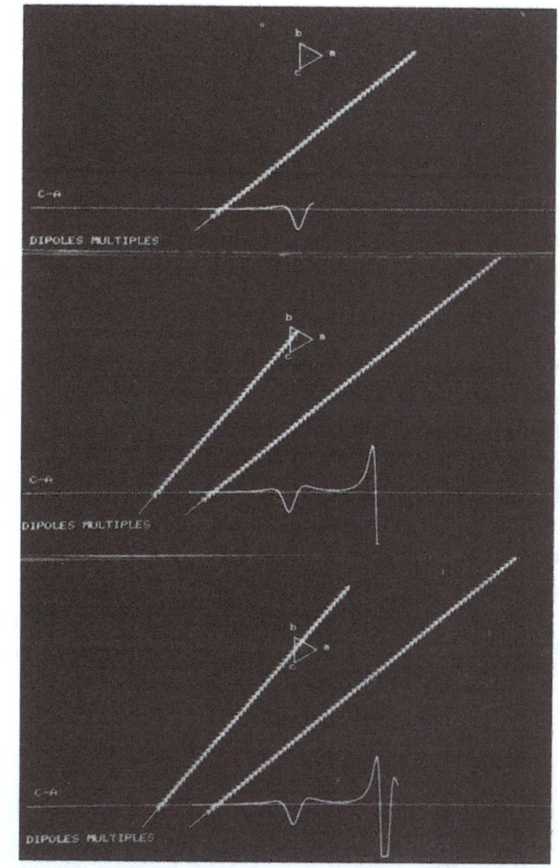

Fig. 5. Simulation of delayed activation, the interelectrode distance being the same as the dipole size. The first dipole (*top*) passes far from the CA lead and generates a low potential. The second dipole (*middle and bottom*) passes near the CA lead and generates a high potential

ration is proportional to the distance, but its amplitude decreases markedly on bipolar lead. It will also widen when that distance is too small in relation to the interelectrode width. The minimum duration is observed when the dipole passes at a distance which is about a quarter of that width. However, a broad potential should be considered as a potential passing far from the electrode. The broadening of the potential may be interpreted as the recording of the electrical phenomenon from a wider angle.

A double potential may be obtained with a single activation dipole, when the dipole is smaller than the interelectrode width (one-tenth in our example) and passes near each electrode. The bipolar system acts then as two unipolar electrodes, each one recording a deflection as the dipole passes by (Fig. 4). However, in that situation the recorded potentials have a symmetry which is not present in the actual pattern of delayed potential. Such a pattern may be compared with the "split His" recording with 10-mm spaced electrodes.

The morphology of delayed potentials is reproduced by multiple dipoles passing by the electrode; a sharp potential is due to a dipole passing near the electrode and a broad potential is due to a dipole passing at a distance. When two dipoles are generated, one early passing far from the bipolar system and one delayed passing close to the electrode, the potentials reproduce the pattern of delayed potentials recorded in arrhythmogenic right ventricular dysplasia, with 1-mm spaced electrodes: The first (QRS synchronous) potential is broad and of low amplitude, and the second is sharp whith a higher amplitude (Fig. 5).

The effect of multiple successive dipoles will be to create multiple deflections, according to their relationship with the electrode system, reproducing "fragmented" activation (Fig. 6). They will also interfere with one an other according to their timing and their special relationship, resulting in mutual cancellation or enhancement. Multiple parallel dipoles will be enhanced, simultaneous dipoles with different orientation may cancel each other out. These phenomena are well known on the ECG, where left ventricular activation usually cancels out right ventricular activation. We may then create a new simulated model (Fig. 7), with a first activation front consisting of many parallel dipoles, reproducing the "normal ventricular activation wave," and a delayed activation front with only one dipole, representing the delayed activation. With a 1-mm spaced electrode, the pattern will not change much from the previous potential simulation, the broad activation front being relatively far from the electrode pair.

All these patterns suppose that the interelectrode distance is comparable with the dipole size. Similarity between simulated potentials and the recorded ones with a 1-mm electrode may imply that the local heart "dipole" is really in the 1-mm range.

If the size of the recording system is much wider than the dipole, as with 1-cm wide bipolar electrodes (ratio 10:1), the pattern will change. If we look at the same model of

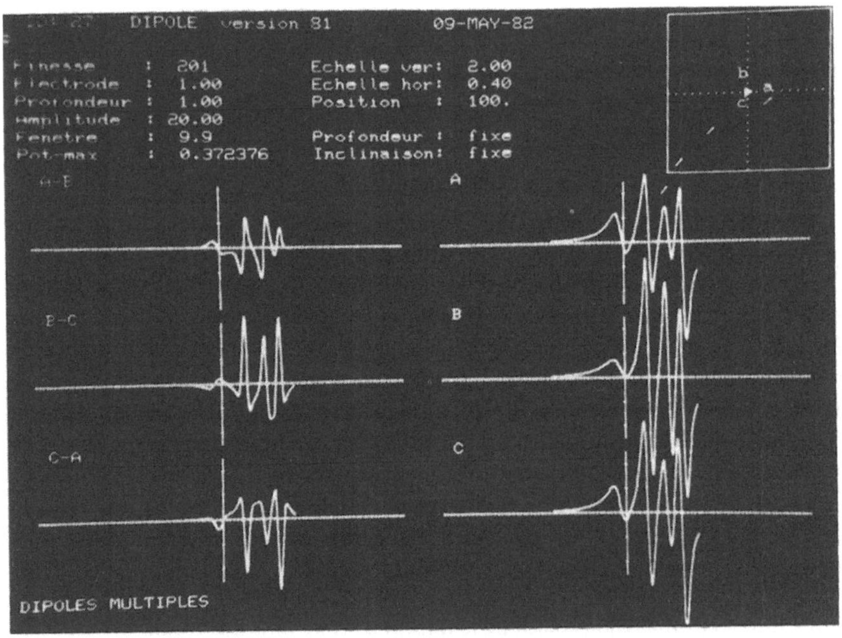

Echelle = Scale

Fig. 6. Display of multiple dipoles passing by the tripolar system one after the other, reproducing fragmentation of potentials

the first activation front, with summation of many dipoles representing the ventricular activation and a later dipole passing on one electrode representing a delayed potential (Fig. 8), the amplitude of the signal will change but not in the same way. The first activation will have a recording from the wide bipolar system with a higher amplitude, possibly explained by the fact that both electrodes are relatively nearer the whole activation front which passes in between. In contrast, the delayed activation will have a much smaller amplitude. It is in fact recorded only by one of the two electrodes, the nearest to the dipole, and is relatively very far from the other electrode. It will not be recorded by the electrode pair located remotely, either in the bipolar or the unipolar mode. Such a pattern is very similar to endocardial recordings of delayed activation and may explain some difficulties in finding these potentials when the electrode is not properly located in the abnormal zone.

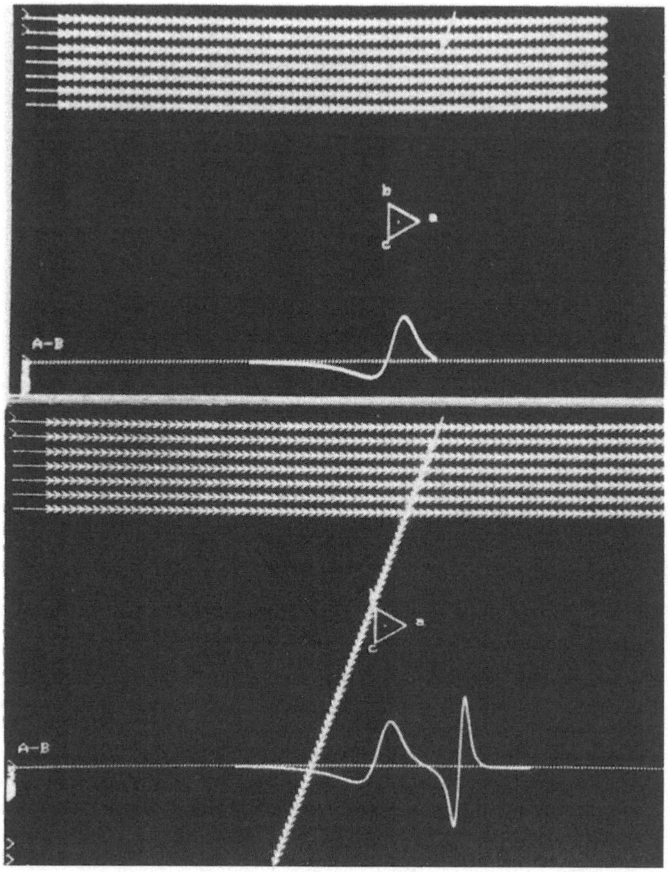

Fig. 7. Simulation of delayed activation as in Fig. 5, with a first activation front with multiple dipoles and a delayed one passing the B electrodes. Note that there is little difference from the simulation in Fig. 5

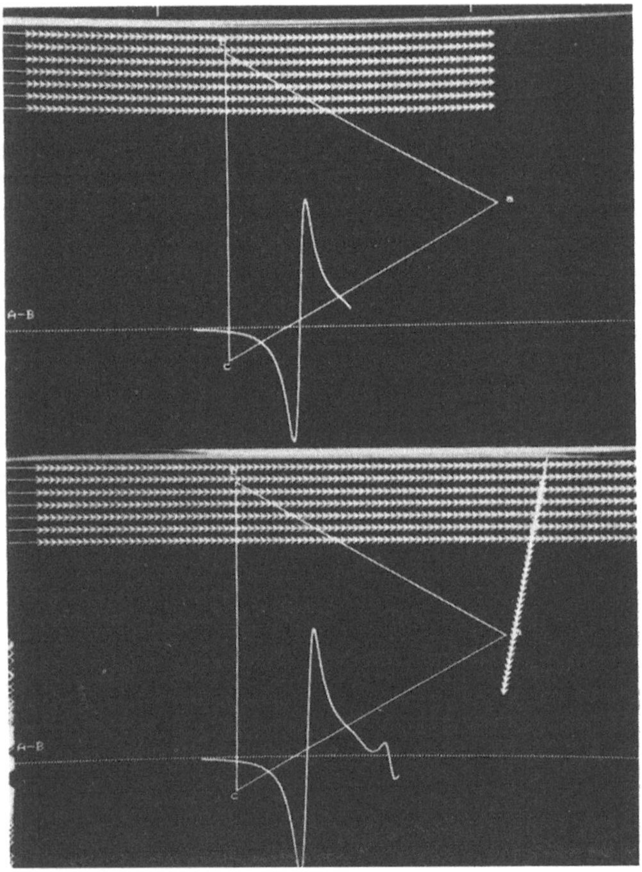

Fig. 8. Same simulation as Fig. 7, but the interelectrode distance is ten times the dipole size. The first potential is high, and the delayed activation, despite passing the A electrode, is of reduced amplitude

Consequences

These findings may explain the problems in recording delayed potentials with 1-mm spaced electrodes:

1. In myocardial infarction, most delayed potentials are subendocardial [8], in the border zone between normal and diseased myocardium. Epicardial mapping with close bipolar electrodes has a low sensitivity to distant small potentials, which explains the lack of recording of delayed potentials in comparison with that obtained with endocardial mapping.
2. In right ventricular dysplasia, histologic studies [9] showed that the anomaly started at the epicardial aspect of the right ventricle, which is infiltrated with fat, only leaving strands of living myocardium, where delayed activation may occur, when the subendocardium stays normal a longer time. Epicardial mapping with close bipolar leads will then easily record the abnormal bipolar potential, while endocardial mapping is too distant from the abnormal zone.

Differences of patterns between close bipolar and wide bipolar recordings are due to the geometry of the recording electrodes. As the widely spaced electrode pair is distant from the abnormal zone, the local potentials will be of smaller amplitude. Recording of a delayed activation with close bipolar electrodes allows precise localization of the abnormal zone.

Simulation studies favor the hypothesis that delayed potentials are related to a delayed activation of a localized ventricular zone. The various recorded patterns are due to successive or simultaneous interacting electrical dipoles passing close to the electrodes, as already suggested by Spach in earlier studies [7].

In conclusion, one should bear in mind that the model of the heart activation is just that, only a model. This means that the hypotheses formed have to be coroborated with clinical experience. Similarity of pattern does not mean that the basic phenomenon has to be the same. These data have to be considered as the reflection of how careful the electrophysiologist must be in interpreting the recorded pattern, recording being affected not only by the amplifiers and the filter setting, but also by the relationship between the recorded dipole and the bipolar interelectrode distance, the electrode position, and, as multiple dipoles are always considered with summation, phenomena which may enhance, but mostly cancel out, the potentials on the recording.

References

1. Fontaine G, Guiraudon G, Frank R (1978) Intramyocardial conduction defects in patients prone to ventricular tachycardia. I. The postexcitation syndrome in sinus rhythm. In: Sandoe E, Julian DG, Bell JW (eds) Management of ve ventricular tachycardia. Role of mexiletine. Excerpta Medica, Amsterdam, pp39–55
2. Fontaine G, Guiraudon G, Frank R, Gerbaux A, Cousteau JP, Barillon A, Gay J, Cabrol C, Facquet J (1975) La cartographie epicardique et le traitement chirurgical par simple ventriculotomie de certaines tachycardies ventriculaires rebelles par reentree. Arch Mal Coeur 68: 113–124
3. Frank R, Fontaine G, Vedel J, Mialet G, Sol C, Guiraudon G, Grosgogeat Y (1978) Electrocardiologie de quatre cas de dysplasie ventriculaire droite arythmogene. Arch Mal Coeur 71: 963–972
4. Fontaine G, Frank R, Gallais-Hamonno F, Allali I, Phan-Thuc H, Grosgogeat Y (1978) Electrocardiographie des potentiels tardifs du syndrome de post-excitation. Arch Mal Coeur 71: 854–864
5. Fontaine G, Guiraudon G, Frank R, Vedel J, Grosgogeat Y, Cabrol C, Facquet J (1977) Stimulation studies and epicardial mapping in ventricular tachycardia: study of mechanisms and selection for surgery. In: Kulbertus H (ed) Reentrant arrhythmias. MTP, Lancaster, pp334–350
6. Fontaine G, Pierfitte M, Tonet JL, Fillette F, Frank R, Grosgogeat Y (1981) Interpretation of afterpotentials registered from epicardium, endocardium and body surface in patients with chronic ventricular tachycardia. In: Hombach V, Helger HH (eds) Signal averaging technique in clinical cardiology. Schattauer, Stuttgart New York, p177
7. Spach MS, Barr RC, Johnson FA, Kootsey MY (1973) Cardiac extracellular potentials. Analysis of complex wave forms about the Purkinje network in dogs. Circ Res 38: 465
8. Wiener I, Mindich B, Pitchon R (1982) Determinants of ventricular tachycardia in patients with ventricular aneurysms: results of intraoperative epicardial and endocardial mapping. Circulation 65: 856
9. Fontaine G, Tereau Y, Frank R, Guiraudon G, Fillette F, Chomette G, Grosgogeat Y (1982) Dysplasie ventriculaire droite arythmogene et maladie de Uhl. Arch Mal Coeur 75: 361

Electrophysiologic Testing in Patients with Ventricular Tachycardia

E. N. Prystowsky, G. V. Naccarelli, J. J. Heger, and D. P. Zipes

Patients with ventricular tachycardia run a substantial risk of sudden death; therefore, therapy to prevent such arrhythmias is critical. However, noninvasive tests such as continuous electrocardiographic recordings, exercise testing, or both, often provide data insufficient for determining antiarrhythmic drug efficacy. For example, occurrences of arrhythmia may be separated widely in time, and many patients who are given drugs that seem to be effective at the time of hospital discharge die suddenly or are readmitted because of recurrent arrhythmias and/or syncope. Further, antiarrhythmic drugs are also arrhythmogenic and can result in sudden death although the arrhythmogenicity of the drug may not be apparent for weeks or months (Rinkenberger et al. 1982; Selzer and Wray 1964; Meltzer et al. 1978).

Electrophysiologic testing has recently been advocated as a procedure for evaluating drug efficacy in patients with ventricular tachycardia (Fisher et al. 1977; Mason and Winkle 1978; Horowitz et al. 1978; Naccarelli et al. 1981; Naccarelli et al. 1982) and out-of-hospital cardiac arrest (Ruskin et al. 1980). We (Naccarelli et al. 1981; Naccarelli et al. 1982) and others (Fisher et al. 1977; Mason and Winkle 1978; Horowitz et al. 1978; Ruskin et al. 1980) demonstrated that suppression of ventricular arrhythmias on electrophysiologic testing during drug therapy predicted lack of recurrence of these arrhythmias during 1–2 years of follow-up. However, we consider serial drug testing in patients who have ventricular tachycardia to be experimental and feel that many issues are unresolved, such as who requires serial electrophysiologic study, what constitutes an "acceptable" electrophysiologic response during drug therapy, and what is an adequate ventricular tachycardia pacing protocol? In this chapter we present recent data from our laboratory in an attempt to answer some of these questions.

Repetitive Ventricular Response – Not a Useful Marker for Recurrent Ventricular Tachycardia

In 1978, Greene et al. reported that induction of repetitive ventricular responses in man "identifies patients with life-threatening ventricular instability." To test for repetitive ventricular response induction electrode catheters were inserted in the heart, and during atrial pacing the ventricle was stimulated prematurely at various coupling intervals until either ventricular refractoriness was reached or repetitive ventricular responses were induced. Repetitive ventricular responses were defined as two or more premature ventricular complexes in response to a single ventricular stimulus; that is, when the ventricle was stimulated prematurely, the stimulus resulted in a paced ventricular complex followed by at least one nonpaced ventricular complex (Figs. 1 and 2). Green et al. did not

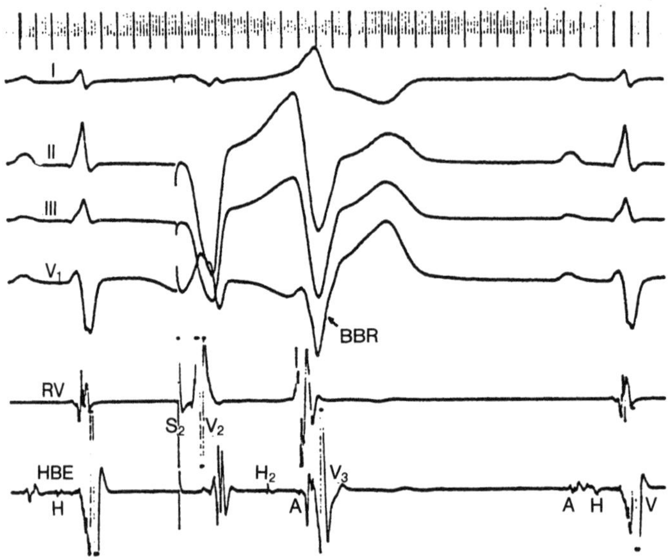

Fig. 1. Demonstration of bundle-branch reentry *(BBR)* induced during sinus rhythm following a premature ventricular stimulus (S_2). Note that the H_2V_3 interval (80 ms) exceeds the HV interval (60 ms) during sinus rhythm. *HBE,* His bundle electrogram; *RV,* right ventricular electrogram; H_2, retrograde His potential from V_2; V_2, ventricular response induced by S_2 (Reprinted with permission of the Br Heart J, Naccarelli et al. 1981)

identify the mechanism of repetitive ventricular responses induced in their patients. Further, they concluded that repetitive ventricular responses did not occur in normal patients but were present in 88% of patients with recurrent ventricular tachycardia. In post-myocardial infarction patients, the induction of a repetitive ventricular response presaged a high incidence of symptomatic ventricular tachycardia or sudden death. In another study by this same group, Schaeffer et al. (1978) showed that suppression of repetitive ventricular responses during treatment with aprindine correlated with successful antiarrhythmic therapy. These results were promising, for they suggested that a relatively simple procedure could predict patients at risk of sudden death and demonstrate effectiveness of drug therapy in preventing ventricular tachycardia.

We performed repetitive ventricular response testing in 148 electrophysiologic studies of 125 patients who were being studied for ventricular tachycardia, supraventricular tachycardia, bradyarrhythmias, and syncope of unknown origin. Specifically, we determined (a) the prevalence of repetitive ventricular responses caused by non-bundle-branch reentry and bundle-branch reentry in 47 patients with, and 50 patients without a history of ventricular tachycardia (previous reports have not distinguished patients with bundle-branch reentrant repetitive ventricular responses which appear to be physiologic); (b) the prevalence of both forms of repetitive ventricular responses using two types of electrophysiologic stimulation, namely, single premature ventricular stimulation during sinus rhythm or atrial pacing, and single premature ventricular stimulation during ventricular pacing; and (c) whether the induction of non-bundle-branch reentry could be used to identifiy those patients at risk either of subsequently developing symptomatic ventricular tachycardia or of sudden death.

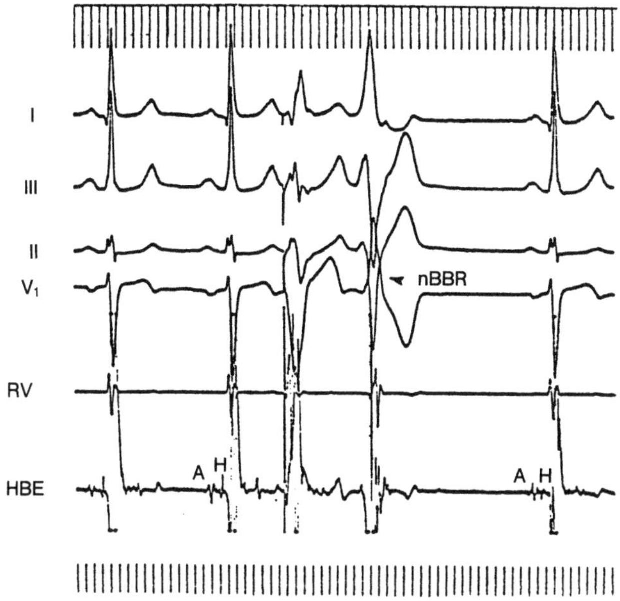

Fig. 2. Demonstration of non-bundle-branch reentry *(nBBR)* induced :uring sinus rhythm following a premature ventricular stimulus (S_2). Note that the nBBR complex has a different configuration than the paced ventricular complex (V_2) and that no His potential is recorded before the nBBR complex. *I, II, III, V_1,* scalar electrocardiographic leads; ***HBE,*** His bundle electrogram; ***RV,*** right ventricular electrogram; S_2, premature ventricular stimulus; V_2, ventricular response induced by S_2; V_3, repetitive ventricular response. (Reprinted with permission of the Br Heart J, Naccarelli et al. 1981)

To induce repetitive ventricular responses, single premature ventricular stimuli were introduced after every eighth beat, beginning in late diastole during sinus rhythm or control of the heart rate by atrial pacing and/or ventricular pacing. The premature interval was decreased by 10–20-ms steps until a repetitive ventricular response was induced or ventricular refractoriness was reached. In 93% of the studies more than one pacing cycle length, and in 81% more than one right ventricular pacing site (apex and outflow tract) were used during ventricular pacing. During atrial pacing, a second ventricular pacing site was used in 22%, and a second atrial pacing cycle length in 16% of the patients who did not have a repetitive ventricular response induced at the first ventricular site or pacing cycle length tested. Our pacing protocol used to initiate ventricular tachycardia has been published in detail (Rinkenberger et al. 1982) and consists of incremental atrial pacing, premature atrial stimulation, premature ventricular stimulation at one or more right ventricular sites using 1 and 2 extrastimuli while pacing the ventricle at $\geqslant$ two cycle lengths, and burst ventricular pacing with 3–8 complexes at cycle lenghts $\geqslant$ 250 ms.

A repetitive ventricular response was defined as two or more premature ventricular complexes produced by a single premature ventricular stimulus delivered during sinus rhythm, atrial pacing, or ventricular pacing. A repetitive ventricular response was interpreted as bundle-branch reentry only if it occurred after a critical V_2H_2 delay and had an H_2V_3 interval greater than or equal to the HV interval of the conducted supraventricular complexes (Fig. 1). The QRS morphology of the repetitive ventricular response was

Table 1. Prevalence of repetitive responses (RVR)

	VT ($n = 47$)		Non-VT ($n = 50$)	
	Ventricular pacing	Atrial pacing	Ventricular pacing	Atrial pacing
No.	47	27	50	21
RVR	38 (80.9%)	10 (37.0%)	33 (66.0%)	2 (9.5%)
nBBR	33 (70.2%)	9 (33.3%)	15 (30.0%)	1 (4.8%)
BBR	22 (46.8%)	1 (3.7%)	28 (56.0%)	2 (9.5%)

RVR, repetitive ventricular responses; BBR, bundle-branch reentry; nBBR, non-bundle-branch reentry; VT, ventricular tachycardia

usually similar to the QRS complex induced by right ventricular apical pacing. All other repetitive ventricular responses were interpreted as non-bundle-branch reentry. These repetitive ventricular responses usually had a configuration different from the complex initiated during right ventricular apical pacing, and most often no His deflection was seen or, if present, the H_2V_3 interval was shorter than the HV interval of the conducted supraventricular impulses (Fig. 2).

Ninety-seven patients, 47 with and 52 without a history of ventricular tachycardia, were tested electrophysiologically using a single premature ventricular stimulus during ventricular pacing, and in 48 of these patients one ventricular extrastimulus was induced during sinus rhythm, atrial pacing, or both (hereafter considered as the atrial pacing group).

The prevalence of repetitive ventricular responses using both stimulation techniques is shown in Table 1. In the 47 patients who had ventricular tachycardia and in the 50 without ventricular tachycardia, both non-bundle-branch reentry and bundle-branch reentry occurred more often during ventricular pacing than during atrial pacing. Non-bundle-branch reentry was induced more often ($P < 0.001$) by both pacing methods in patients who had ventricular tachycardia than in those patients who did not. In addition to the 97 studies performed in the control state, 51 studies were performed in patients taking antiarrhythmic drugs. The prevalence of repetitive ventricular responses was not statistically different between these patients and those who were not taking drugs.

To determine if induced non-bundle-branch reentry could identify patients at risk of developing future symptomatic ventricular tachycardia or sudden death, 59 patients receiving antiarrhythmic therapy to suppress ventricular tachycardia had an electrophysiology study just before discharge and were followed up for an average of 10.9 months. Predictive accuracy was determined using the formula:

$$\frac{\text{True positive and True negative}}{\text{Total number of patients}}$$

True positive was defined as non-bundle-branch reentrant repetitive ventricular responses present on discharge study with recurrence of ventricular tachycardia during follow-up. True negative was defined as non-bundle-branch reentrant repetitive ventricular responses not induced and no occurrence of arrhythmia during follow-up. We found that non-bundle-branch reentry induced during ventricular and atrial pacing had a predictive accuracy of 59% and 64% respectively. Thus, neither technique yields a predictive accuracy sufficiently high to make the test clinically useful.

One additional observation deserves comment. The predictive accuracy of non-bundle-branch reentrant repetitive ventricular responses induced during atrial pacing appeared to be greater in patients who also had ventricular tachycardia initiated during the same electrophysiologic study. For example, 16 patients who had ventricular tachycardia induced at their discharge study also had repetitive ventricular response testing during atrial pacing. Eight patients had non-bundle-branch reentry induced in addition to the induced ventricular tachycardia and seven of these had recurrent arrhythmias or died suddenly. In contrast, only two of eight without induced non-bundle-branch reentry had ventricular tachycardia during follow-up. Further investigations are necessary to determine predictive accuracy using multiple electrophysiologic variables.

Electrophysiologic Testing in Patients With Ventricular Tachycardia but Without Coronary Artery Disease

In contrast to repetitive ventricular response testing, serial electrophysiologic testing appears to be worthwhile if the ability to induce ventricular tachycardia is the end point used to judge the success of drug therapy (Fisher et al. 1977; Mason and Winkle 1978; Horowitz et al. 1978; Naccarelli et al. 1981, 1982; Ruskin et al. 1980; Prystowsky et al. 1982). Thus, patients who have ventricular tachycardia induced before but not after drug therapy usually have no recurrence of ventricular tachycardia if they continue the dosage of the antiarrhythmic drug that prevented induction of ventricular tachycardia at the time of electrophysiologic study (Fisher et al. 1977; Mason and Winkle 1978; Horowitz et al. 1978; Naccarelli et al. 1981, 1982; Ruskin et al. 1980; Prystowsky et al. 1982).

One obvious prerequisite for serial electrophysiologic testing is the ability to induce ventricular tachycardia at the pre-drug control study. Previous investigations (Fisher et al. 1977; Mason and Winkle 1978; Josephson et al. 1978; Vandepol et al. 1980) demonstrated that ventricular tachycardia could be initiated reproducibly by programmed electrical stimulation in more than 80% of patients who had a history of sustained ventricular tachycardia. Other studies (Wellens et al. 1976; Denes et al. 1976) have reported induction of ventricular tachycardia in a substantially smaller percentage of patients. Although different pacing protocols may partly explain the variability of ventricular tachycardia induction in the above reports, differences in the populations of patients and types of ventricular tachycardia studied may also be important, as the latter groups (Wellens et al. 1976; Denes et al. 1976) had a higher percentage of patients who did not have coronary artery disease.

We performed electrophysiologic studies prospectively on 161 consecutive patients referred for evaluation of ventricular tachycardia to determine whether the presence and type of heart disease, or the duration of spontaneous ventricular tachycardia, or both, affected the frequency of induction of ventricular tachycardia. Seventy-eight patients had coronary artery disease and 83 had either no identifiable heart disease (primary electrical disease), or heart disease other than coronary artery disease. No patient was taking an antiarrhythmic drug other than digitalis at the time of his or her electrophysiologic test. All patients underwent the same pacing protocol (Rinkenberger et al. 1982; vide supra) in an attempt to induce ventricular tachycardia.

Patients without coronary artery disease were subclassified into the following groups: (a) cardiomyopathy – patients diagnosed as having congestive cardiomyopathy, if cardiomegaly and diminished left ventricular contractility were documented by left ventriculogram and/or echocardiogram, or as having hypertrophic myopathy if asymmetric or concentric left ventricular hypertrophy was documented by echocardiogram; (b) primary electrical disease – patients who had arrhythmias but no evidence of structural heart disease noted by physical examination, echocardiogram (seven patients), or cardiac catheterization (21 patients); and (c) mitral valve prolapse documented by echocardiography. Induced ventricular tachycardia was classified as sustained if it lasted ≥ 30 s or required termination prior to this time due to hemodynamic compromise. Nonsustained ventricular tachycardia was tachycardia that terminated spontaneously within 30 s.

Ventricular Tachycardia Induction in Patients Without Coronary Artery Disease

Thirty-seven patients had cardiomyopathy: 30 congestive, four hypertrophic without outflow obstruction, and three congestive cardiomyopathy secondary to valvular heart disease. Twenty-eight patients had primary electrical disease and 18 had mitral valve prolapse. There were 44 men and 39 women with a mean age of 44.2 ± 17.1 years; 39 patients had a history of syncope, 28 had presyncope or dizziness, seven had only palpitations, and six were asymptomatic. Each of the 34 patients who had histories of sustained ventricular tachycardia had at least one prior cardioversion because of his or her arrhythmia.

We initiated 4.2 ± 1.2 episodes of ventricular tachycardia per patient in those in whom ventricular tachycardia could be induced. The presence and type of heart disease affected the initiation of ventricular tachycardia in the laboratory. Among those who had a history of sustained ventricular tachycardia, induction of ventricular tachycardia occurred in 13 of 25 patients (52%) with cardiomyopathy, in all nine of those who had primary electrical disease, and in all five with mitral valve prolapse. In patients with a history of nonsustained ventricular tachycardia, initiation of ventricular tachycardia was successful in four of 12 (33%) who had cardiomyopathy, six of 19 (32%) with primary electrical disease, and five of 13 (39%) with mitral valve prolapse. Combining all groups, ventricular tachycardia was induced in 69% of patients who had a history of sustained ventricular tachycardia and in 34% of patients who had a history of nonsustained ventricular tachycardia ($P < 0.05$). It should be noted that in patients with a history of nonsustained ventricular tachycardia, none had sustained ventricular tachycardia induced.

An interesting subgroup of nine patients were those with "repetitive nonsustained ventricular tachycardia" (Parkinson and Papp 1947; Rahilly et al. 1982). Of these nine patients, six had primary electrical disease and three had mitral valve prolapse; two had ventricular tachycardia induced in the laboratory.

Nine patients had left ventricular programmed stimulation in addition to stimulation of the right ventricle. Ventricular tachycardia was induced in three of nine patients from both ventricles, in two of nine from the right ventricle only, and in one of nine from the left ventricle only. Ventricular tachycardia was not induced from either ventricle in three patients.

Ventricular Tachycardia Induction in Patients with Coronary Artery Disease

Fifty-six of 59 patients (95%) who had a history of sustained ventricular tachycardia and 15 of 19 patients (79%) with a history of nonsustained ventricular tachycardia had initiation of ventricular tachycardia in the laboratory. Ventricular tachycardia was induced more frequently in the patients who had coronary artery desease than in those who did not. This difference was significant for patients who had a history of sustained ventricular tachycardia ($P < 0.01$) and for patients who had a history of nonsustained ventricular tachycardia ($P < 0.05$).

In conclusion, it is clear that initiation of ventricular tachycardia in the electrophysiology laboratory depends on many factors, some of which are the presence and type of heart disease, and the type of ventricular tachycardia being investigated. The frequency of ventricular tachycardia induction in patients with repetitive nonsustained ventricular tachycardia is so low that we no longer recommend electrophysiologic testing for these patients.

Acknowledgements: This study was supported in part by the Herman C. Krannert Fund; by Grants HL-06308, HL-07182, and HL-18795 from the National Heart, Lung and Blood Institute of the National Institutes of Health, Bethesda, Maryland; and by the American Heart Association, Indiana Affiliate, Inc.

References

Denes P, Wu D, Dhingra RC, Amat-Y-Leon F, Wyndham C, Mautner RK, Rosen KM (1976) Electrophysiologic studies in patients with chronic recurrent ventricular tachycardia. Circulation 54: 229–236

Fisher JD, Cohen HL, Mehra R, Altschuler H, Escher DJW, Furman S (1977) Cardiac pacing and pacemakers. II. Serial electrophysiologic-pharmacologic testing for control of recurrent tachyarrhythmias. Am Heart J 93: 658–668

Greene HL, Reid PR, Schaeffer AH (1978) The repetitive ventricular response in man. A predictor of sudden death. N Engl J Med 299: 729–734

Horowitz LN, Josephson ME, Farshidi A, Spielman SR, Michelson EL, Greenspan AM (1978) Recurrent sustained ventricular tachycardia. 3. Role of the electrophysiologic study in selection of antiarrhythmic regimens. Circulation 58: 986–997

Josephson ME, Horowitz LN, Farshidi A, Kastor JA (1978) Recurrent sustained ventricular tachycardia. 1. Mechanisms. Circulation 57:431–440

Mason JW, Winkle RA (1978) Electrode-catheter arrhythmia induction in the selection and assessment of antiarrhythmic drug therapy for recurrent ventricular tachycardia. Circulation 58: 971–985

Meltzer RS, Robert EW, McMorrow M, Martin RP (1978) Atypical ventricular tachycardia as a manifestation of disopyramide toxicity. Am J Cardiol 42: 1049–1053

Naccarelli GV, Prystowsky EN, Jackman WM, Heger JJ, Rinkenberger RL, Zipes DP (1981) The repetitive ventricular response. Prevalence and prognostic significance. Br Heart J 46: 152–158

Naccarelli GV, Prystowsky EN, Jackman WM, Heger JJ, Rahilly GT, Zipes DP (1982) Role of electrophysiologic testing in managing patients who have ventricular tachycardia unrelated to coronary artery disease. Am J Cardiol 50: 165–171

Parkinson J, Papp C (1947) Repetitive paroxysmal tachycardia. Br Heart J 9: 241–262

Prystowsky EN, Heger JJ, Zipes DP (1982) The recognition and treatment of patients at risk for sudden Death. In: Eliot RS (ed) Cardiac emergencies. Futura, Mount Kisco/New York, 353–384

Rahilly GT, Prystowsky EN, Zipes DP, Naccarelli GV, Jackman WM, Heger JJ (1982) Clinical and electrophysiologic findings in patients with repetitive monomorphic ventriculartachycardia and otherwise normal electrocardiogram. Am J Cardiol 50: 459–468

Rinkenberger RL, Prystowsky EN, Jackman WM, Naccarelli GV, Heger JJ, Zipes DP (1982) Drug conversion of nonsustained ventricular tachycardia to sustained ventricular tachycardia during serial electrophysiologic studies: Identification of drugs that exacerbate tachycardia and potential mechanisms. Am Heart J 103: 117–184

Ruskin JN, DiMarco JP, Garan H (1980) Out-of-hospital cardiac arrest: electrophysiologic observations and selection of long-term antiarrhythmic drug therapy. N Engl J Med 303: 607–613

Schaeffer AH, Greene HL, Reid PR (1978) Suppression of the repetitive ventricular response: an index of long-term antiarrhythmic effectiveness of aprindine for ventricular tachycardia in man. Am J Cardiol 42: 1007–1012

Selzer A, Wray HW (1964) Quinidine syncope. Paroxysmal ventricular fibrillation occurring during treatment of chronic atrial arrhythmias. Circulation 30: 17–26

Vandepol CJ, Farshidi A, Spielman SR, Greenspan AM, Horowitz LN, Josephson ME (1980) Incidence and clinical significance of induced ventricular tachycardia. Am J Cardiol 45: 725–731

Wellens HJJ, Duren DR, Lie KI (1976) Observations on mechanisms of ventricular tachycardia in man. Circulation 54: 237–244

Results of Invasive Methods

H. J. Wellens

If one wants to discuss the value of programmed stimulation of the heart to study mechanisms and treatment of tachycardias, it is helpful to divide the patient population into three groups:

1. Patients with electrocardiographically documented tachycardias
2. Patients with a history but no documentation of tachycardia
3. Patients at high risk of death from an arrhythmia

Our methods of programmed stimulation and recording in patients have been published elsewhere and will not be discussed here (1).

Patients with Electrocardiographically Documented Tachycardias

As can be seen from Tables 1 and 2, in most patients suffering from electrocardiographically documented long-lasting tachycardias the same arrhythmia can be initiated during the stimulation study. Sufficient electrocardiographic recordings should be made during the stimulation study to prove that the arrhythmia initiated is identical to the one occurring clinically. We have commented previously upon the importance of using different stimulation sites, basic pacing rates, and numbers of extrastimuli to obtain the greatest possible amount of information (2). Briefly, in all our patients at least three different basic cycle lengths and up to four premature stimuli are used.

Table 1. Results of programmed electrical stimulation in 442 Patients with documented Supraventricular Tachycardia

		n	Initiation	Termination
Atrial tachycardia		55	33 (60)	37 (67)
Atrial flutter		59	4 (7)	55 (93)
AV junction tachycardia	Intranodal	105	105 (100)	105 (100)
	Conc. acc. p.	56	56 (100)	56 (100)
	Pathway unknown	4	4 (100)	4 (100)
	Digitalis	5	0	0
SVT of unknown origin		6	0	
WPW		152	152 (100)	152 (100)
Total		442		

Values in parentheses are percentages

Abbreviations: Conc. acc. p., concealed accessory pathway; SVT, supraventricular tachycardia; WPW, Wolff-Parkinson-White syndrome

Table 2. Results of programmed electrical stimulation in 165 patients with documented ventricular Tachycardia

	n	Initiation	Termination
VT of short duration	23	2 (9)	2 (9)
Exercise-induced VT	6	3 (50)	1 (17)
Long QT syndrome	14	3 (21)	0
Sustained VT			
MI < 24 h	8	0	2 (25)
MI 24 h–5 weeks	5	2 (40)	4 (80)
MI > 5 weeks	65	59 (90)	63 (97)
Idiopathic	30	27 (90)	27 (90)
Other	14	7 (50)	5 (35)
Total	165		

Values in parentheses are percentages
Abbreviations: VT, ventricular tachycardia; MI, myocardial infarction

Table 3. Considerations in studying drug effects by programmed electrical stimulation of the Heart

1. Mode of drug administration: acute intravenous vs. chronic oral
2. Timing of measurements after drug administration
3. Importance of predrug electrophysiological values
4. Differences in effect on anterograde and retrograde conduction
5. Stability of electrophysiological properties

The ability to initiate the clinically occurring tachycardia reproducibly in the catheterization laboratory gives us the opportunity to study the effect of intravenous and oral medications on the arrhythmia. The pitfalls and limitations of this approach should, however, be realized (Table 3). We want to stress that while prevention of tachycardia initiation suggests at least short-term efficacy of the drug, inability to prevent reinitiation of tachycardia following administration does not exclude clinical effectiveness. Amiodarone is an example of a drug falling in the latter category.

Patients with a History of Tachycardia but no Electrocardiographic Documentation

As shown in Table 4 a sustained tachycardia could be initiated during programmed stimulation of the heart in 53 of 80 patients with a history of tachycardia but no previous electrocardiographic documentation. In 8 of the 19 patients in whom an AV nodal tachycardia could be initiated, this was only possible after atropine administration. All these patients showed dual AV nodal pathway curves before atropine, suggesting that the electrophysiologic substrate for AV nodal reentry was available. It is of interest that

Table 4. Results of programmed electrical stimulation in 80 patients with a history but no documentation of Tachycardia

	Tachycardia type	*n*
WPW	CMT	15
Other	Conc. acc. p.	5
	AV nodal	19
	Atrial	6
	Atrial flutter	2
	Ventricular	6
	None	27

Abbreviations: WPW, Wolff-Parkinson-White syndrome; CMT, circus movement tachycardia; Conc. acc. p., concealed accessory pathway

in all Wolff-Parkinson-White syndrome patients with a history of tachycardia, a circus movement tachycardia could be initiated using the AV node-His pathway and the accessory atrioventricular connection.

Identification of High-Risk Patients

Correct identification of the patients with coronary heart disease, Wolff-Parkinson-White syndrome, and cardiomyopathy who are at high risk of sudden life-threatening arrhythmias would be of obvious clinical importance. What role can be played by programmed stimulation of the heart?

It is important to realize that nonsustained polymorphic ventricular tachycardia can be initiated during programmed stimulation in many hearts where no cardiac abnormalities can be identified. Table 5 lists every ventricular arrhythmia that could be induced during programmed stimulation in 32 patients without a history of cardiac arrhythmia. In 29 Patients concomitant cardiac disease was absent; two patients had a cardiomyopathy, one an old myocardiac infarction. The average number of ventricular premature beats required to initiate those arrhythmias was three. Table 5 indicates that we have to be very careful before attaching significance to induction of nonsustained polymorphic

Table 5. Ventricular arrhythmias initiated during programmed electrical stimulation in 32 patients with no documentation of ventricular arrhythmias

Repetitive responses ($\leq$3 beats)	30
Nonsustained polymorphic VT ($\geq$6 beats)	15
Nonsustained monomorphic VT (16 beats)	1
VF → CMP	1
VF → Normal heart	1
Ventricular flutter	1

Abbreviations: VT, ventricular tachycardia; VF, ventricular fibrillation; CMP, cardiomyopathy

ventricular tachycardia as a marker of high risk. The importance of the number of premature stimuli required to initiate these polymorphic ventricular tachycardias deserves further study.

Of interest in this regard is a recently completed investigation by Richards et al. (3). In survivors of acute myocardial infarction, they observed a high first-year mortality (35%) in patients in whom electrical instability like ventricular fibrillation, sustained ventricular tachycardia, or polymorphic ventricular tachycardia lasting at least 10 s could be initiated during programmed stimulation. The heart was paced just above the sinus rate. No more than two ventricular premature beats at two right ventricular sites were given, with a stimulus strength of twice diastolic threshold and 20 mA. Patients who were comparable in site and size of infarction and number of coronary arteries involved but not showing this electrical instability during programmed stimulation had a first-year mortality of only 9%.

It has been shown that in patients with the Wolff-Parkinson-White syndrome, the presence of a short anterograde refractory period of the accessory pathway indicates risk for high ventricular rates if atrial fibrillation supervenes (4).

The value of programmed stimulation of the heart in identifying cardiomyopathy patients at risk is not known at the present time. One of the problems in assessing the value of programmed stimulation of the heart to identify patients at high risk of sudden death is the use of different stimulation protocols in different centers. We believe that worldwide agreement on stimulation protocols is essential in order to ascertain the true value of programmed stimulation of the heart as soon as possible.

References

1. Ross DL, Farré J, Bär FW, Vanagt EJ, Dassen WR, Wiener I, Wellens HJJ (1980) Comprehensive clinical electrophysiological studies in the investigation of documented or suspected tachycardias: time, staff, problems and costs. Circulation 61: 1010
2. Wellens HJ (1978) Value and limitations of programmed electrical stimulation of the heart in the study and treatment of tachycardias. Circulation 57: 845
3. Richards DA, Cody DV, Denniss AR, Russell PA, Uther JB, Young AA (1982) Ventricular electrical instability during the first year following myocardial infarction. Am J Cardiol 49: 929
3. Wellens HJ, Bär FW, Farré J, Ross D, Vanagt EJ (1979) Sudden death in the Wolff-Parkinson-White syndrome. In: Kulbertus H, Wellens HJJ (eds) Sudden death. Nijhoff, The Hague, p 392

Specific Antiarrhythmic Drugs for Specific Arrhythmias

R. W. F. Campbell

Arrhythmia diagnosis and selection of appropriate therapy are important facets of cardiological practice. It seems not unreasonable to expect that for each specific arrhythmia there would be a specific treatment, but in clinical reality such situations are rare. This may reflect inaccurate arrhythmia diagnosis, inadequate drug therapy, or an inability to recognize specificity.

Specificity

The word "specific", first used in a medical context in 1677, implies of a medication that it is "exclusively efficacious for, or acting upon, a particular ailment" (Onions 1973). In medical practice, specific medications for specific conditions are uncommon, but include hormone replacement for deficiency states, and desferrioxamine in the management of hemochromatosis and iron poisoning.

Drug specificity when treating cardiac arrhythmias might be reflected by the reliable termination of an arrhythmia, by a single intravenous administration of a drug, and in other situations by the successful long-term prophylaxis of an arrhythmia by oral administration of a drug. In the former context, clinical specificity approaches that which might be determined by in vitro experiments, but in the latter case, specificity may be obscured by pharmacodynamic problems and by toxicity. Most clinical trials of antiarrhythmic therapy are reported on an "intention to treat" principle – an entirely laudable stance which examines the practical implications of recommending a drug regimen for a selected patient population. Specificity of an antiarrhythmic drug would be better identified by considering its effect in those patients who continue therapy and in whom acceptable plasma levels of the drug are maintained. The results might have little eventual clinical relevance, as for example specificity identified for an extremely toxic drug which would be tolerated by only a minority of individuals.

The Importance of Specificity in Arrhythmia Management

The success of clinical arrhythmia management is often constrained by unacceptable drug interference with sinus node function, AV nodal conduction, His-Purkinje conduction, and enhanced automatic activity. The precision of antiarrhythmic action implied by specificity might minimize these unwanted electrophysiological effects, although, as discussed, general adverse effects are a separate issue. Specificity is also associated with efficacy. These considerations identify a specific drug as one which is effective and selective. Specific drugs, if available, would reduce trial and error in clinical arrhythmia management.

Specific Drugs for Specific Arrhythmias – General Considerations

Specificity is more likely to be observed in simple conditions of arrhythmogenesis. Theoretically, arrhythmias might be caused by an abnormality of automatic behavior in a single cell (Wit and Rosen 1981 a). The electrophysiological derangement in that cell might be relatively simple and easily modified. If this arrhythmogenic basis could be identified in other clinical contexts, the same treatment could be employed with the expectation of success. Arrhythmias are usually more complex, however, and depend upon the geometry and characteristics of many cells, some normal and some abnormal (Wit and Rosen 1981 b; Arnsdorf 1977; Corr and Sobel 1979). Rarely will such complex individual factors be repeated and it is clinically impossible to distinguish the important characteristics of each arrhythmia substrate. Furthermore, the arrhythmia substrate may be acted upon by outside influences, such as the modulation of a ventricular parasystolic focus by the sinus node (Moe et al. 1977), the activation of a reentry pathway by an ectopic beat (Wellens 1977), and the alteration of artrioventricular conduction by autonomic tone (Lichtman et al. 1973). The many factors involved in clinical arrhythmogenesis confound easy identification of specific therapy but do offer a number of possibilities for therapeutic action, explaining how an antiarrhythmic drug can be effective against diverse arrhythmias (e. g., quinidine used for the control of reciprocating tachycardia in the Wolff-Parkinson-White (WPW) syndrome and for the management of ventricular tachyarrhythmias).

Development of a specific drug for a specific arrhythmia requires detailed knowledge of both. Knowledge of the action of drugs in vitro and in vivo is improving, but relatively little is known about drug effects in diseased tissues. Moreover, it is difficult to separate direct and indirect effects of drugs, for example when a drug (e. g., beta-blockers, digitalis, disopyramide) alters the rate of sinus node discharge or alters autonomic tone. Tissue bath and intact animal investigations of drug actions provide valuable information, but some aspects such as ventricular fibrillation threshold aeterations are difficult to relate to clinical practice (Arnsdorf 1977). Most drugs have a variety of electrophysiological effects although one effect is usually sufficiently predominant to place the compound in a classification system such as that described by Vaughan Williams (1978). These classifications are useful for appreciating general principles of antiarrhythmic action, but none is of major clinical relevance for the selection of therapy for an individual arrhythmia. Part of the problem is that the electrophysiological features by which a drug is classified may have been determined in normally oxygenated cells bathed by a balanced perfusate containing standard electrolyte concentrations – rare circumstances for the genesis of clinical arrhythmias.

As important as detailed knowledge of antiarrhythmic actions are precise definitions of arrhythmias. Current arrhythmia definitions are based on standard surface electrocardiograms and are, by necessity, crude. Ventricular ectopic complexes which result from altered automaticity, reentry, or triggered activity (Wit and Rosen 1981 a, b) are indistinguishable, and ideal therapy is likely to differ for each mechanism. There is considerable need for a system which identifies and separates clinically important arrhythmia variations (Campbell 1981). Torsades de pointes (Zilcher et al. 1980; Editorial 1980) is a well-discussed example of a variant ventricular tachyarrhythmia but its definition remains imprecise, being largely dependent on subjective interpretation of the QRS vector. Invasive electrophysiological testing has permitted better characterization of a variety of arrhythmias and can separate, relatively reliably, superficially identical narrow QRS tachycardias of atrial origin, of AV nodal reentry, and of the preexcitation syndrome. The technique can also provide information on the relative efficacy of individual antiarrhythmic agents in patients with ventricular tachycardia (Kaster et al. 1981). If reliably initiated and terminated by programmed stimulation, ventricular tachycardia is probably due to reentry or triggered activity, while that which is uninfluenced by stimulation either is automatic or has a stimulation site remote from the origin of the arrhythmia (Josephson et al. 1978). The complex and time-consuming nature of invasive electrophysiology precludes its general use, but information from this source may eventually be correlated with the 12-lead electrocardiogram to improve arrhythmia classification by noninvasive methods.

Practical Situations of General Specificity

Cardiac arrhythmias occurring in individual patients may be so unique that each requires a specific drug for control. However there are certain specific drug effects generally observed in clinical situations.

Verapamil

Verapamil, a Vaughan Williams class IV antiarrhythmic drug, inhibits the membrane transport of calcium and has a marked action on calcium-dependent cells which are concentrated in the sinoatrial and atrioventricular nodes. Reentry tachycardia, which can occur within these structures, is very effectively treated by verapamil (Singh et al. 1978; Tonkin et al. 1980). Other supraventricular tachycardias also respond to verapamil administration, particularly if the atrioventricular node is part of a reentry pathway as is the case in the reciprocating tachycardia of the WPW syndrome. Success rates for arrhythmia termination approach 96% for AV nodal tachycardia and 92% for reciprocating tachycardia. This specificity is marred by occasionally dramatic hypotension and by unstable plasma levels during oral administration.

Lignocaine

Lignocaine, a Vaughan Williams class I antiarrhythmic drug, depresses the maximal rate of depolarization of the action potential. Conduction in myocardial cells may be slowed, converting unidirectional conduction to complete block (El-Sherif et al. 1977). This action would be expected to be beneficial in the treatment of reentrant arrhythmias, the most important example of which is ventricular fibrillation; the electrical abnormality probably comprising multiple interlacing wavelets of reentrant excitation. Lignocaine is the only drug shown to be effective for the prophylaxis of ventricular fibrillation in acute myocardial infarction (Lie et al. 1974). It is unlikely that its electrophysiological action is truly specific, but the pharmacokinetic properties of lignocaine permit rapid safe attainment of therapeutic levels by intravenous dosing. Unfortunately, a significant first pass effect precludes the oral use of lignocaine, and analogues which can be given by mouth have not yet been shown to be effective for ventricular fibrillation prophylaxis (Campbell et al. 1979, 1981).

Digoxin

Digoxin, which slows conduction in the AV node by a vagal action, is unclassified in the Vaughan Williams system. Its use as a first-line drug in the management of atrial fibrillation and other rapid atrial arrhythmias is to reduce the attendant fast ventricular response rate rather than to correct the basic arrhythmia. In over 90% of treated patients, satisfactory control of the ventricular rate can be achieved. The impressive long-term safety of digoxin and its relative freedom from adverse effects make it an important antiarrhythmic agent, and while it cannot be accurately described as specific, there is no other single medication which offers its spectrum of action.

Bretylium

The electrophysiological effects of bretylium are imprecisely understood and there is controversy as to its classification in the Vaughan Williams system. Bretylium has been recommended as a unique complement to DC shock in the management of drug-resistant ventricular tachycardia and repetitive ventricular fibrillation (Kumana and Hamer 1979), but there is insufficient controlled evidence to assess the value of this strategy.

Propafenone

Propafenone is a Vaughan Williams class I antiarrhythmic agent with additional sympatholytic properties (Seipel and Breithardt 1980). It is highly effective for many types of arrhythmias, whether supraventricular or ventricular, but appears especially active both in the termination and the prophylaxis of tachycardias associated with the WPW syndrome (Rudolph et al. 1979; Waleffe et al. 1981).

Amiodarone

Amiodarone is a Vaughan Williams class III antiarrhythmic agent which prolongs refractoriness in all cardiac tissues. Numerous reports of its high level of efficacy against a wide variety of arrhythmias have been published (Heger et al. 1981; Rosenbaum et al.

1976; Kaski et al. 1981). Unlike most other potent antiarrhythmic agents, it possesses little, if any, negative inotropic property and has a specific indication in the management of serious ventricular arrhythmias in patients with severely depressed ventricular function, as occurs, for example, in cardiomyopathies. A further specific indication is the prophylaxis of paroxysmal atrial fibrillation and flutter – an arrhythmic situation which is poorly controlled by other available drugs. Amiodarone may also play a unique role in the long-term oral prophylaxis of ventricular fibrillation. There are no controlled studies to support this indication, but numerous case reports suggest benefit (Nademanee et al. 1981).

Beta-Adrenoreceptor-Blocking Drugs

Beta-adrenoreceptor-blocking drugs constitute the class II of Vaughan Williams. They are specific for the treatment of exercise dependent arrhythmias whether occurring during or following exertion (Coumel et al. 1978). High dose beta-adrenoreceptor blocking drugs are the most useful medical management for patients with the long QT syndrome (Schwartz et al. 1975). In selected patients following myocardial infarction, beta-adrenoreceptor blocking therapy used prophylactically, has reduced mortality (Editorial 1982) but it is unclear whether this effect is mediated by an antiarrhythmic or an anti-ischaemic action.

Atropine

Atropine, a vagolytic agent, is not classified in the Vaughan Williams system. It is specifically indicated for arrhythmias related to transient vagotonia – a situation most frequently encountered in acute myocardial infarction where ventricular arrhythmias may complicate marked sinus bradycardia and hypotension (Scheinmann et al. 1975)

Conclusions

Arrhythmias and antiarrhythmic drugs are extremely complex. At present it remains unlikely that detailed information regarding the mechanism of any given arrhythmia will be obtained from the surface electrocardiogram, but better characterization and description of arrhythmias should prove of therapeutic benefit. Knowledge of antiarrhythmic drug action in diseased as well as normal tissues is crucial to the understanding of a drug's effect on a given arrhythmia.

Few specific drugs are recognized for specific arrhythmias but for many arrhythmias there is a clear first-line drug choice. These agents are not truly specific, but represent a clinical compromise of anticipated efficacy, tolerance, and toxicity, as antiarrhythmic drug selection takes into account not only the arrhythmia requiring control but also the patient's myocardial performance, underlying pathological process, and concurrent disease.

This should not encourage continued empiric approaches to antiarrhythmic treatment. Hopefully, antiarrhythmic drug selection can be improved as diagnoses become more accurate and better drugs become available. Yet even today, important information may be neglected. For instance, in the event of failure of a chosen drug, any modification of the arrhythmia by that drug is not systematically used in the selection of the next best alternative. If drugs with a highly selective antiarrhythmic action were developed, it might be possible to characterize an arrhythmia by its serial response to a battery of trial agents.

However, the most important cardiac arrhythmias are those which threaten life. For these, treatment must be rapid and effective. Identification of specific therapies is mandatory, and the indication for their use should be based on a simple, fast, noninvasive test, preferably the 12-lead electrocardiogram.

Prognostically important arrhythmias are controversial, as their suppression does not necessarily alter prognosis. Until the mechanism by which these arrhythmias are related to prognosis is understood it is unlikely that specific therapy will be defined.

Finally, patients with symptomatic arrhythmias require treatment. Therapy should relieve symptoms and cause no unwanted effects. The latter requirement may preclude identification of general specific therapy, as each patient must be treated as an individual. In an electrophysiological sense, specific drugs for specific arrhythmias may already exist, but in clinical practice specificity is modified by many other factors and is difficult to recognize. Long-term specificity is particularly subject to these external influences. Short-term specificity primarily concerns the arrhythmia and the electrophysiological action of the drug and should be most easily recognized in situations where rapid drug administration terminates an established arrhythmia. Thus, verapamil for AV nodal reentrant tachycardia is the best clinical example of a specific drug for a specific arrhythmia.

Acknowledgments: I should like to thank Mrs. D. Naisby, Miss S. Atkinson and Mr. R. Jordan for their invaluable assistance in the preparation of this manuscript.

References

Arnsdorf MF (1977) Membrane factors in arrhythmogenesis: concepts and definitions. Prog Cardiovasc Dis 19: 413–429

Campbell RWF (1981) Evaluation of antiarrhythmic drugs. Should the Lown classification be used as a measure of efficacy? In: Morganroth J, Moore EN, Dreifus LS, Michelson EL (eds) The evaluation of new antiarrhythmic drugs. Nijhoff, The Hague pp 113–121

Campbell RWF, Achuff SC, Pottage A, Murray A, Prescott LF, Julian DG (1979) Mexiletine in the prophylaxis of ventricular arrhythmias during acute myocaridal infarction. J Cardio Pharm 1: 43–52

Campbell RWF, Bryson LG, Bailey BJ, Murray A, Julian DG (1981). Prophylactic administration of tocainide in acute myocardial infarction. Workshop on Tocainide, pp 201–204

Corr PB, Sobel BE (1979) The importance of metabolites in the genesis of ventricular dysrhythmia induced by ischemia. Mod Concepts Cardiovasc Dis 48: 49–52

Coumel P, Fidelle J, Lucet V, Attuel P, Bouvrain Y (1978) Catecholamine-induced severe ventricular arrhythmias with Adams-Stokes syndrome in children: report of four cases. Br Heart J [Suppl] 40: 28–37

Editorial (1980) Torsades de Pointes. Eur Heart J 1: 70–71

Editorial Comment (1982) Long-term and short-term Beta-blockade after myocardial infarction. Lancet I: 1159–1161

El-Sherif N, Scherlag BJ, Lazzara R, Hope RR (1977) Re-entrant ventricular arrhythmias in the late myocardial infarction period. Circulation 56: 395–402

Heger JJ, Prystowsky EN, Jackman WM, Naccarelli GV, Warfel KA, Rinkenberger RL, Zipes DP (1981) Amiodarone: Clinical efficacy and electrophysiology during long-term therapy for recurrent ventricular tachycardia or ventricular fibrillation. N Engl J Med 305: 539–544

Josephson ME, Horowitz LN, Farshidi A, Kastor JA (1978) Recurrent sustained ventricular tachycardia. 1. Mechanisms. Circulation 57: 431–447

Kaski JC, Girotti LA, Messuti H, Rutitzky B, Rosenbaum MB (1981) Long-term management of sustained, recurrent, symptomatic ventricular tachycardia with amiodarone. Circulation 64: 273–279

Kastor JA, Horowitz LN, Harken AH, Josephson ME (1981) Clinical electrophysiology of ventricular tachycardia. N Engl J Med 304: 1004–1020

Kumana C, Hamer J (1979) Anti-arrhythmic drugs. In: Hamer J (ed) Drugs for heart disease. Chapman & Hall, London, pp 44–147

Lichtman J, O'Rourke A, Klein A, Karliner JS (1973) Electrocardiogram of the athlete. Alterations simulating those of organic heart disease. Arch Intern Med 132: 763–770

Lie KI, Wellens HJJ, von Capelle FJ, Durrer D (1974) Lidocaine in the prevention of primary ventricular fibrillation. N Engl J Med 29: 1324–1326

Moe GK, Jalife J, Mueller WJ (1977) Reciprocation between pacemaker sites: Re-entrant parasystole? In: Kulbertus HE (ed) Re-entrant arrhythmias. MPT Press, Lancaster, pp 271–280

Nademanee K, Hendrickson JA, Cannom DS, Goldreyer BN, Singh BN (1981) Control of refractory life-threatening ventricular tachyarrhythmias by amiodarone. Am Heart J 101: 759–768

Onions CT (ed) (1973) The shorter oxford english dictionary: on historical principles. A-Markworthy. Clarendon Oxford

Rosenbaum MB, Chiale PA, Halpern MS, Nau GJ, Przybylski J, Levi RJ, Lazzari JO, Elizari MV (1976) Clinical efficacy of Amiodarone as an antiarrhythmic agent. Am J Cardiol 38: 934–944

Rudolph W, Petri H, Kafka W, Hall D (1979) Effects of propafenon on the accessory pathway (AP) in patients with WPW syndrome (Abstr). Am J Cardiol 43: 430

Scheinman MM, Thorburn D, Abbott JA (1975) Use of atropine in patients with acute myocardial infarction and sinus bradycardia. Circulation 52: 627–633

Schwartz PJ, Periri M, Malliani A (1975) The long Q-T syndrome. Am Heart J 89: 378–390

Seipel L, Breithardt G (1980) Propafenone – a new antiarrhythmic drug. Eur Heart J 1: 309–313

Singh BN, Ellrodt G, Peter CT (1978) Verapamil: A review of its pharmacological properties and therapeutic use. Drugs 15: 169–197

Tonkin AM, Aylward PE, Joel SE, Heddle WF (1980) Verapamil in prophylaxis of paroxysmal atrioventricular nodal reentrant tachycardia. J Cardiovasc Pharmacol 2: 473–486

Vaughan Williams EM (1978) Some factors that influence the activity of antiarrhythmic drugs. Br Heart J [suppl] 40: 52–61

Waleffe A, Mary-Rabine L, De Rijbel R, Soyeur D, Legrand V, Kulbertus HE (1980) Electrophysiological effects of propafenone studied with programmed electrical stimulation of the heart in patients with recurrent paroxysmal supraventricular tachycardia. Eur Heart J 2: 345–352

Wellens HJ (1977) Modes of initiation of circus movement tachycardia in 139 Wolff-Parkinson-White syndrome studied by programmed electrical stimulation. In: Kulbertus HE ed) Re-Entrant arrhythmias. MPT Press, Lancaster; pp 135–169

Wit L Rosen MR (1981 a) Cellular electrophysiology of cardiac arrhythmias. (part 1). Mod Concepts Cardiovasc Dis 50: 1–6

Wit AL, Rosen MR (1981 b) Cellular electrophysiology of cardiac arrhythmias. (part 2). Mod Concepts Cardiovasc Dis 2: 7–11

Zilcher H, Glogar D, Kaindl F (1980) Torsades de Pointes: Occurrence in myocardial ischaemia as a separate entity. Multiform ventricular tachycardia or not. Eur Heart J 1: 63–71

Sudden Cardiac Death: Prognosis of Long-term Antiarrhythmic Therapy

M. Manz, G. Steinbeck and B. Lüderitz

Introduction

According to cause-of-death statistics in the Federal Republic of Germany for the year 1979, the percentage of deaths due to cardiovascular disease has risen from 39% to 49% over the past 20 years. This rise in cardiovascular mortality is attributed to an increase in ischemic heart disease from 22% to 35% during the same period (Cause-of-Death Statistics, 1981). Studies by Lovegrove and Thompson (1978) have shown that approximately 71% of these persons die within 30 minutes after the onset of symptoms, i.e., have what is termed a "sudden death." In 87% of persons who died within 1 h, evidence pointed to a cardiac arrhythmia as the immediate cause of death (Aspirin Myocardial Infarction Study Research Group, 1980). Death in such cases is due to a potentially treatable electrical instability of the heart, rather than to a terminal stage of organic failure. Much research, therefore, has been directed toward the recognition of patient groups that are at risk of sudden cardiac death, as well as toward the development of treatment regimes aimed at preventing such deaths.

Definition

Despite extensive research during the past 15 years, there is no generally accepted definition for the sudden death syndrome. In 1969 the International Society of Cardiology and the American Heart Association defined "sudden death" as unexpected death occurring suddenly or within 24 h after the onset of acute symptoms (Paul and Schatz 1971). Later the term was revised, and the exclusion of other causes such as acute myocardial infarction and pulmonary embolism was added to the temporal definition (International Society and Federation of Cardiology, WHO Task Force on Standardization of Clinical Nomenclature, 1979). However, such a definition has serious disadvantages if it is to be used as a working definition for studies on prevention. First, the time frame of 0–24 h is too imprecise. For questions relating to cardiac arrhythmias, studies with the shortest possible time frame (say, 30–60 min after symptom onset) would probably yield the most meaningful results. Second, the requirement of a diagnosis by exclusion to characterize sudden cardiac death creates diagnostic and organizational problems in prevention studies and contributes little to the interpretation of results, as pointed out in the ART study, among others (Tempel and Pledger 1980).

Groups at Risk of Sudden Death and Indications for Long-term Antiarrhythmic Therapy

The occurrence of sudden cardiac death has been correlated in epidemiologic studies with the presence of ventricular premature beats (VPB) in the resting ECG (Chiang et al. 1969; Kannel et al. 1979), and with coronary artery disease and left ventricular hypertrophy (Kannel et al. 1979). Studies of coronary cases have shown (Table 1) that patients with frequent, "complex" VPB (pairs or salvos) in their long-term ECGs are at significantly greater risk of sudden cardiac death than patients without VPB or with isolated VPB. Several studies have pointed to ventricular ectopic beats as a risk factor that is almost independent of hemodynamic parameters (Schulze et al. 1977; Hammermeister et al. 1979; Moss et al. 1979). These studies indicate that while the presence of "complex" VPB in the long-term ECG is a highly sensitive index, the specificity of this feature is limited, inasmuch as pairs and salvos can be demonstrated in a large percentage of the coronary population (Anderson et al. 1978; Cats et al. 1979).

Persons who have been successfully resuscitated out-of-hospital constitute yet another group that is at risk of sudden cardiac death. In the study done by Schaffer and Cobb (1975), for example, 26% of such patients suffered a recurrence or died suddenly during the year following the first resuscitation. Comparable results are reported by Liberthson (1974): Of the patients who survived prehospital resuscitation, 28% died suddenly during the 12.7 months following discharge.

Another condition that predisposes to sudden death is recurrent ventricular tachycardia. (Some patients with this condition were included in the aforementioned studies of prehospital resuscitation survivors.) According to studies by Armbrust (1950), 45% of patients with ventricular tachycardia died within 6 months after their condition was diagnosed. Despite the introduction of new therapeutic measures, the mortality from ventricular tachycardia occurring in the first 8 weeks after an infarction was approximately 83% after an average of 8 months, and 47% in the chronic phase of myocardial infarction after an average of 2.8 years (Wellens et al. 1982).

The foregoing studies were able to identify patient groups that were at high risk of sudden cardiac death. This risk, in turn, provides an indication for prophylactic antiarrhythmic therapy in these patient groups. Thus, prophylactic antiarrhythmic therapy is indicated in patients with coronary artery disease and complex VPB in their long-term

Table 1. Frequency of sudden death in patients with coronary heart disease

study		(pat.)	duration (years)	ECG (hour)	frequency of sudden deaths (%) without VPB	simple VPB	complex VPB	sig
Ruberman	(1977)	1739	3	1	4,3%	4,2%	15,5%	+
Vismara	(1975)	64	2	10		6%	12,0%	+
Kotler	(1973)	160	3	12		3%	13,0%	+
van Durme	(1976)	150	1	8	0%		8%	+
Davis	(1979)	940	3	6	4%	6,0%	15,0%	+
Schulze	(1977)	81	7 mO	24		0%	10,0%	+
Cats	(1979)	200	1	24		0,5%	1,5%	–

ECG, in patients who have been resuscitated out-of-hospital, and in patients with recurrent ventricular tachycardia.

In this paper we examine studies in which antiarrhythmic therapy was employed for the prevention of sudden cardiac death.

Antiarrhythmic Drug Therapy Following Myocardial Infarction

The first clinical study on the prevention of cardiac death in survivors of acute myocardial infarction was conducted with diphenylhydantoin (300–400 mg daily) (Collaborative Group 1971). A total of 568 patients were enrolled in the study and were followed over a 12-month period. The total mortality was 9%; no difference was noted between the placebo- and drug-treated groups.

Due to the large variability of diphenylhydantoin plasma levels in the study, a further study was carried out with 150 patients who had had a previous myocardial infarction. In this study plasma level monitoring was used as a means of establishing drug dosages. After 2 years the mortality was 24% in the diphenylhydantoin group and 18% in the placebo group. Hence, the drug was rated as ineffective in the prevention of cardiac death (Peter et al. 1978).

Another study was conducted with procainamide, administered in a dose of 1.5–2 g/day; 78 patients were enrolled. However, treatment had to be discontinued due to serious side effects, most notably the occurrence of a lupus erythematodus syndrome in 58% of the persons treated. Although a reduction in sudden cardiac death was noted after 6 months in the treated group, this drug is clearly unsuited for long-term prophylactic use (Kosowsky et al. 1973).

Additional studies were done in subgroups with a very high risk of sudden cardiac death. In a controlled study, the efficacy of 2.5 g procainamide per day was tested on 70 patients who had suffered a myocardial infarction and had frequent VPB or a history of ventricular tachycardia or ventricular fibrillation. The prognosis could not be improved with procainamide, and six patients experienced severe side effects that required a discontinuance of therapy (Nielsen et al. 1978). Thus, even in patients with a very high risk of sudden cardiac death, procainamide appears to be unsuited for prophylactic antiarrhythmic therapy.

Another study using aprindine was conducted in 305 patients with prior myocardial infarction and complex VPB. The dose of aprindine was 100–200 mg daily. While a statistically insignififant reduction in mortality was recorded (from 12.5% to 7.8%/year), serious dide effects caused 21% of the patients to be dropped from the study (van Durme and Bogaert 1980).

In a comparative study, 344 patients were treated with mexiletine, 600–750 mg/day, for 3 months following an acute myocardial infarction. While mexiletine was found to reduce the occurrence of complex VPB, it exhibited no effect on mortality over a 3-month period (mexiletine group 13%, control group 12%). Thirty patients in the drug-treated group had to be dropped from the study because of side effects (Chamberlain et al. 1980).

In surveying the results of the foregoing studies, we find that they have been unable to demonstrate a long-term antiarrhythmic regimen that is effective in preventing sudden death or improving total mortality in myocardial infarction patients. Even in the subgroups with complex VPB, no efficacy could be shown with the prophylactic antiarrhythmic regimens tested.

Survivors of Prehospital Resuscitation

Sixteen patients who were resuscitated after prehospital cardiac arrest were treated with procainamide (2–5 g/day) and quinidine (1.6–3 g/day). Of the 16, eight suffered no recurrent arrests over a 12-month period, while of eight who had recurrences, six died. This corresponds to a mortality of 37%. Patients who had no recurrences exhibited therapeutic plasma levels of the antiarrhythmic drugs, while the levels measured in patients with recurrences were mostly subtherapeutic. The effect of the drugs on VPB in the 24-h ECG was the same in both groups. Despite the fact that the authors, themselves, could not demonstrate a definite prognostic improvement, they concluded that a plasma level-monitored antiarrhythmic regimen is of potential benefit in the prevention of sudden cardiac death (Myerburg et al. 1979).

In another study, 31 patients who had been successfully resuscitated after out-of-hospital cardiac arrest were treated with various antiarrhythmic drugs with the aid of programmed ventricular stimulation. Ventricular arrhythmia was electrically inducible in 25 of the 31. Complete suppression of inducible ventricular arrhythmia was achieved with antiarrhythmic therapy in 19 of these 25 patients; ventricular arrhythmia could still be induced in the remaining six. None of the 19 patients in whom the inducible arrhythmia was suppressed had a recurrence after a mean follow-up of 12 months. Of the six patients in whom inducible arrhythmia could not be completely suppressed, three died suddenly. Accordingly, the incidence of sudden death was 9.6% after 12 months. As no additional patients died, this figure represents the total mortality (Ruskin et al. 1980).

Sustained Ventricular Tachycardia

The efficacy of a long-term antiarrhythmic regimen in patients with recurrent sustained ventricular tachycardia is difficult to assess for several reasons. First, the guarded prognosis and associated clinical symptoms make long-term therapy essential for this patient group; thus, the follow-up of an untreated control group is precluded on ethical grounds. Second, the patients enrolled in these studies display a marked heterogeneity, given the relatively small size of the study population. Third, the patients tend to represent a special subgroup; they are selected in terms of their response to a certain treatment modality (e.g., drugs) or method of regimen selection (e.g., programmed ventricular stimulation). These circumstances hamper both the assessment of the efficacy of antiarrhythmic therapy and the comparison of results.

Horowitz et al. (1978) conducted a study on 20 patients with sustained ventricular tachycardia that was inducible by programmed ventricular stimulation. In 14 patients an effective antiarrhythmic regimen involving various agents could be found, based on the response to programmed ventricular stimulation. In the remaining patients no complete suppression of inducible tachycardia could be achieved with any drug or drug combination tested. After a mean follow-up of 12 months, five patients died (25%), three of these from sudden cardiac death (15%).

In another study (Mason and Winkle 1980), ventricular stimulation was used to select antiarrhythmic drug regimens for 51 patients with recurrent ventricular tachycardia, who were then followed up for an average of 12 months. In 39 cases an effective regimen could be devised with various antiarrhythmic agents, while in 19 cases no effective therapy could be found. The total mortality was 25%, with sudden death occurring in 19% of cases (the outcome is unknown for five patients who were referred for cardiac surgery). After a mean follow-up of 12 months, four of 26 patients treated with effective drugs died suddenly, as opposed to six of 16 in the "ineffective drug" group.

Heger et al. (1981) treated 30 patients with amiodarone (mostly combined with additional drugs). The mean follow-up for these patients was 12 months. A total of five patients had died by the end of this period (16%), two of sudden cardiac death (7%).

In a study by Kaski et al. (1981), 23 patients were treated with amiodarone (200–1200 mg) in a long-term management program. After a mean follow-up of 24 months, the total mortality for this group was 43%, with sudden cardiac death occurring in a total of five cases (21%).

The results of the foregoing studies indicate that there is a strong correlation between favorable prognosis in patients who have been resuscitated out-of-hospital or patients with recurrent ventricular tachycardia, and the ability of antiarrhythmic drugs to prevent electrical induction of arrhythmia by programmed ventricular stimulation. Conversely, the persistence of an electrically inducible ventricular tachyarrhythmia is associated with a poor long-term prognosis, so other therapeutic options should be considered for such patients. Despite the stated limitations inherent in assessing the impact of drug therapy on total mortality, controlled antiarrhythmic therapy appears to improve the long-term prognosis of patients with recurrent ventricular tachycardia or ventricular fibrillation.

Beta-receptor Blocking Agents for Secondary Prophylaxis After Myocardial Infarction

The major prospective studies with beta-receptor blocking agents are listed in Table 2. The most meaningful of these are the timolol study and the metoprolol study, owing to the large study populations and the study designs. The results of the propranolol study (1981) will be considered preliminary until a scientific analysis can be made.

In the timolol study, a reduction was achieved both in overall mortality and in the number of sudden deaths. Sudden death, however, was defined as death occurring within 24 h after the onset of symptoms. This very long interval, together with a failure to analyze rhythms at the start of the study and during its course, prohibits meaningful interpretation of the mechanism of action and the influence of the drug on possible arrhyth-

Table 2. Prospective studies on betareceptor blockers

	Patients	duration (months)	overall mortality			sudden deaths		
			placebo	verum	P	placebo	verum	P
Alprenolol 1974	230	24	14	7	ns	11	2	< 0.05
Practolol 1975	3038	3–12	117	94	ns	52	30	< 0.02
Alprenolol	480	12	64	61	ns	–	–	
1979	(< 65y 282	12	29	13				< 0.01)
Propranolol 1980	720	9	27	28	ns	–	–	
Timolol 1981	1884	12–17	152	98	< 0.001	95	47	< 0.001
Metoprolol 1981	1395	3	62	40	0.03	–	–	
Propranolol 1981	3837	30	183	135		–	–	

mias. In the metoprolol study, the data pertain only to total mortality and not to sudden death.

Thus, it has been shown with statistical certainty that timolol is effective in the prevention of sudden death, although the mode of action of timolol, especially as it relates to presumed ventricular arrhythmias, remains unclear. Available evidence, then, does not prove that beta-receptor blocking drugs are effective in the long-term treatment of patients with ventricular arrhythmias.

Summary

Research to date indicates that patients who have been successfully resuscitated out-of-hospital, patients with recurrent ventricular tachycardia, and coronary patients with complex ventricular premature beats in their long-term ECG have an increased risk of sudden cardiac death. For this reason, prophylactic antiarrhythmic therapy is indicated for these patient groups. The efficacy of prophylactic antiarrhythmic treatment with diphenylhydantoin, procainamide, aprindine and mexiletine could not be established in the chronic postinfarction phase. The selection of an antiarrhythmic regimen by means of programmed ventricular stimulation in survivors of prehospital resuscitation and in patients with recurrent ventricular trachycardia appears to improve the long-term prognosis in these patient groups.

References

A multicentre international study (1975) Improvement in prognogis of myocardial infarction by long-term beta-adrenoreceptor blockade using practolol. Br Med J 3: 735–40

Anderson KP, DeCamilla J, Moss AJ (1978) Clinical significance of ventricular tachycardia (3 beats or longer) detected during ambulatory monitoring after myocardial infarction. Circulation 57: 890–896

Andersen MP, Bechsgaard P, Frederiksen J, Hansen DA, Jürgensen HJ, Nielsen B, Pedersen F, Pedersen-Bjergaard O, Rasmussen SL (1979) Effect of alprenolol on mortality among patients with definite or suspected acute myocardial infarction. Lancet 27: 865–867

Armbrust CA, Levine SA (1950) Paroxysmal ventricular tachycardia: A study of one hundred and seven cases. Circulation 1: 28–40

Aspirin Myocardial Infarction Study Research Group (1980) A randomized, controlled trial of aspirin in persons recovered from myocardial infarction. JAMA 243: 661–669

Baber NS, Wainwright Evans D, Howitt G, Thomas M, Wilson C, Lewis JA, Dawes PM, Handler K, Tuson R (1980) Multicentre post-infarction trial of propranolol in 49 hospitals in the United Kingdom, Italy, and Yogoslavia. Br Heart J 44: 96–100

Betablocker heart attack study group (1981) The betablocker heart attack trial. JAMA 246: 2073–2074

Cats VM, Lie KI, Van Capelle FJL, Durrer D (1979) Limitations of 24-hour ambulatory electrocardiographic recording in predicting coronary events after acute myocardial infarction. Am J Cardiol 44: 1257–1262

Chamberlain DA, Julian DG, Boyle DMcC, Jewitt DE, Campbell RWF, Shanks RG, and others (1980) Oral mexiletine in high-risk patients after myocardial infarction. Lancet 20/27: 1324–1327

Chiang BN, Perlam LV, Ostrander LD, Epstein FH (1969) Relationship of premature systoles to coronary heart disease and sudden death in the Tecumseh epidemiologic study. Ann Intern Med 70: 1159–1166

Collaborative Group (1971) Phenytoin after recovery from myocardial infarction. Lancet 2: 1055–1057

Davis HT, DeCamilla J, Bayer LW, Moss AJ (1979) Survivorship patterns in the posthospital phase of myocardial infarction. Circulation 60: 1252–1258

Hammermeister KE, DeRouen TA, Dodge HT (1979) Variables predictive of survival in patients with coronary disease. Circulation 59: 421–430

Heger JJ, Prystowsky EN, Jackman WM, Naccarelli GV, Warfel KA, Rinkenberger RL, Zipes DP (1981) Amiodarone: Clinical efficacy and electrophysiology during long-term therapy for recurrent ventricular tachycardia or ventricular fibrillation. N Engl J Med 305: 539–545

Hjalmarson Å, Elmfeldt D, Herlitz J, Holmberg S, Málek I, Nyberg G, Rydén L, Swedberg K, Vedin A, Waagstein F, Waldenström A, Waldenström J, Wedel H, Wilhelmsen L, Wilhelmsson C (1981) Effect on mortality of metoprolol in acute myocardial infarction: A double-blind randomised trial. Lancet 17: 823–827

Horowitz LN, Josephson ME, Farshidi A, Spielman SR, Michelson EL, Greenspan AM (1978) Recurrent sustained ventricular tachycardia 3. Role of the electrophysiologic study in selection of antiarrhythmic regimes. Circulation 58: 987–997

Kannel WB, Sorlie P, McNamara PM (1979) Prognosis after initial myocardial infarction: The Framingham Study. Am J Cardiol 44: 53–59

Kaski JC, Girotti L, Messuti H, Rutitzky B, Rosenbaum MB (1981) Long-term management of sustained, recurrent, symptomatic ventricular tachycardia with amiodarone. Circulation 64: 273–279

Kosowsky BD, Taylor J, Lown B, Ritchie RF (1971) Long-term use of procainamide following acute myocardial infarction. Circulation 47: 1204–1210

Kotler MN, Tabatznik B, Mower MM, Tominaga S (1973) Prognostic significance of ventricular ectopic beats with respect to sudden death in the late postinfarction period. Circulation 47: 959–966

Liberthson RR, Nagel EL, Hirschman JC, Nussenfeld SR (1974) Prehospital ventricular defibrillation. N Engl J Med 291: 317–321

Lovegrove T, Thompson P (1978) The role of acute myocardial infarction in sudden cardiac death – a statisticians's nightmare. Am Heart J 96: 711–713

Mason JW, Winkle RA (1980) Accuracy of the ventricular tachycardia-induction study for predicting long-term efficacy and inefficacy of antiarrhythmic drugs. N Engl J Med 303: 1073–1077

Moss AJ, Davis HT, DeCamilla J, Bayer LW (1979) Ventricular ectopic beats and their relation to sudden and nonsudden cardiac death after myocardial infarction. Circulation 60: 998–1003

Myerburg RJ, Conde C, Sheps DS, Appel RA, Kiem I, Sung RJ, Castellanos A (1979) Antiarrhythmic drug therapy in survivors of prehospital cardiac arrest: Comparison of effects on chronic ventricular arrhythmias and recurrent cardiac arrest. Circulation 59: 855–863

Nielsen BL, Nielsen JC, Nielsen JS (1978) Can procainamide improve the prognosis of patients with ventricular arrhythmias after myocardial infarction? Dan Med Bull 25: 121–125

Paul O, Schatz M (1971) On sudden death. Circulation 43: 7–10

Peter T, Ross D, Duffield A, Luxton M, Harper R, Hunt D, Sloman G (1978) Effect on survival after myocardial infarction of long-term treatment with phenytoin. Br Heart J 40: 1356–1360

Report of the Joint International Society and Federation of Cardiology World Health Organization Task Force on Standardization of Clinical Nomenclature (1979) Nomenclature and criteria for diagnosis of ischemic heart disease. Circulation 59: 607–609

Ruberman W, Weinblatt E, Goldberg GD, Frank CW, Shapiro S (1977) Ventricular premature beats and mortality after myocardial infarction. N Engl J Med 297: 750–759

Ruskin JN, DiMarco JP, Garan H (1980) Out-of-hospital cardiac arrest: Electrophysiologic observations and selection of longterm antiarrhythmic therapy. N Engl J Med 303: 607–613

Schaffer WA, Cobb LA (1975) Recurrent ventricular fibrillation and modes of death in survivors of out-of-hospital ventricular fibrillation. N Engl J Med 293: 259–262

Schulze RA, Strauss HW, Pitt B (1977) Sudden death in the year following myocardial infarction. Am J Med 62: 192–199

Temple R, Pledger GW (1980) The FDA's critique of the anturane reinfarction trial. N Engl J Med 303: 1488–1492

The Norwegian multicenter study group (1981) Timolol-induced reduction in mortality and reinfarction in patients surviving acute myocardial infarction. N Engl J Med 304: 801–807

Todesursachenstatistik (Cause-of-death statistics) (1981) Dtsch Med Wochenschr 106: 157–158

Van Durme JP, Pannier RH (1976) Prognostic significance of ventricular dysrhythmias 1 year after myocardial infarction. Am J Cardiol 37: 178

Van Durme JP, Bogaert MG (1980) Prevention of sudden death. The role of antiarrhythmic therapy. In: Kulbertus HE, Wellens HJJ (eds) Sudden death. Nyhoff, The Hague p 331

Vismara LA, Amsterdam EA, Mason DT (1975) Relation of ventricular arrhythmias in the late hospital phase of acute myocardial infarction to sudden death after hospital discharge. Am J Med 59: 6–12

Wellens HJ, Bär FWHM, Vanagt EJDM, Brugada P (1982) Medical treatment of ventricular tachycardia: Considerations in the selection of patients for surgical treatment. Am J Cardiol 49: 186–193

Wilhelmsson C, Vedin JA, Wilhelmsen L, Tibblin G, Werkö L (1974) Reduction of sudden deaths after myocardial infarction by treatment with alprenolol: preliminary results. Lancet 2: 1157–60

Basic Electrophysiological Actions of Propafenone in Heart Muscle

M. Kohlhardt

The excitability of atrial and ventricular myocardium under physiological conditions depends on the ability of the cardiac membrane to respond to suprathreshold stimuli with an increase in Na^+ permeability. This allows the occurrence of a fast Na^+ inward current. However, action potential generation is not exclusively related to the availability of the fast Na^+ system since Na^+ inactivation as it develops after decreasing the resting potential to about -50 mV (Weidmann 1955 a) does not abolish excitability (Engstfeld et al. 1961). In this particular situation, slow response action potentials can be generated (Mascher 1970) mediated by another inward conductance system, the slow channel. This maintains excitability but may also be involved in the development of certain cardiac arrythmias (for review see Kohlhardt 1980). The antiarrhythmic effect of a drug, therefore, does not arise only from its affinity for fast Na^+ channels – a fact which caused Vaughan Williams (1975) to introduce the classification of antiarrhythmics into four groups depending on the electrophysiological action. Class 1 compounds depress the fast Na^+ current (I_{Na}) and comprise different drugs such as local anesthetics, quinidine, or certain β-receptor blockers with side effects on excitable membranes. Propafenone represents another member of class 1 though it loses the virtual specifity for the Na^+ system when higher drug concentrations are applied. The latter phenomenon represents a widespread property of class 1 antiarrhythmics and is not peculiar to propafenone.

Based on the Hodgkin-Huxley framework (Hodgkin and Huxley 1952), a drug-induced I_{Na} blockade can result from either a plugging of the Na^+ pore or an interference with channel gating, i.e., activation and/or inactivation process. Local anesthetics and related compounds seem to affect predominantly Na^+ inactivation, at least in the nerve membrane, which finally prevents the Na^+ channel from attaining the open configuration needed for the Na^+ passage. Methodological limitations inherent in I_{Na} measurements in most of the commonly used multicellular cardiac preparations are the reason why the precise mechanism of drug action remains to be clarified in cardiac I_{Na} channels. More relevant experimental results originate from action potential studies (for review see Hauswirth and Singh 1979) where the maximal rate of rise ($\dot{V}_{max}$) has been taken as an estimate for I_{Na}.

I_{Na} Inhibition by Propafenone

Figure 1 demonstrates the characteristic effect of propafenone on the fast Na^+-dependent action potential of a guinea pig's ventricular myocardium. After exposure to a drug-containing (3×10^{-5} mol/liter) Tyrode's solution, $\dot{V}_{max}$ declined gradually. This inhibitory effect proved concentration dependent and in the presence of higher propafe-

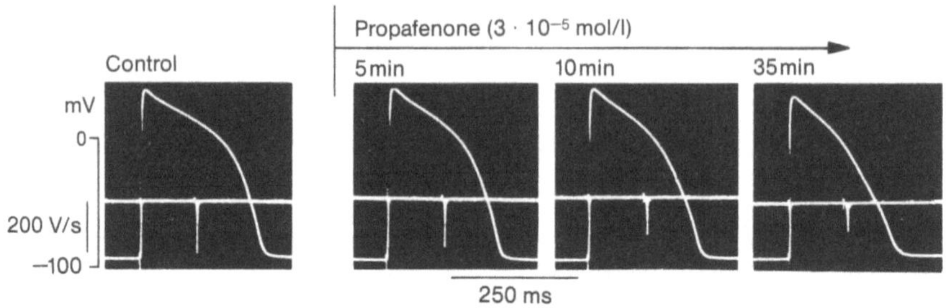

Fig. 1. Registrations of the fast Na^+-dependent action potential and the maximal rate of rise in a papillary muscle of a guinea pig prior to and after the addition of 3×10^{-5} mol/liter propafenone to Tyrode's solution. The preparation was continuously stimulated at a rate of 12/min. External K^+ concentration, 2.7 mmol/liter, pH 7.4. (Kohlhardt and Seifert 1980)

none concentrations ($6–8 \times 10^{-5}$ mol/liter) it evokes a complete loss of excitability. Changes in resting potential occur only if the drug concentration exceeds 8×10^{-5} mol/liter. Alterations of the action potential configuration also appeared, consisting of a plateau shift to less positive potentials and, less pronounced, an abbreviation on the level 90% repolarization.

In contrast to classical local anesthetics, the inhibitory propafenone effect on I_{Na} develops comparatively slowly, taking about 30 min for completion. The recovery from blockade on return to a drug-free solution also has a special characteristic; because washout periods of as long as 60 min do not restore $\dot{V}_{max}$ completely, a certain residual fraction of block persists.

Recovery from inactivation of the I_{Na} system can also be affected by antiarrhythmics. This process develops due to membrane repolarization and in restoring the channel conductance causes the Na^+ pore to regain its availability. The rate of recovery strongly declines in response to the application of the neuroleptic droperidol (Hauswirth 1968; Kern et al. 1971) after propranolol (Tarr et al. 1973) or quinidine (Luckstead and Tarr 1972) treatment. Double-pulse experiments with propafenone revealed that such an alteration of the recovery kinetics does not represent a feature common to all antiarrhythmics of class 1 (Kohlhardt and Seifert 1980). According to results of Gettes and Reuter (1974), time constants at a membrane potential close to -90 mV between 15 ms and 40 ms were obtained under normal conditions in a drug-free environment. Propafenone proved unable to affect the recovery kinetics even in concentrations which drastically suppressed $\dot{V}_{max}$ by 50% or more.

Is the Selectivity Filter of the I_{Na} Channel a Target for Propafenone?

Voltage clamp studies including the analysis of gating currents and TTX-binding experiments during the last decade have supplied insights into the structure and possible organization of I_{Na} channels in the nerve membrane. I_{Na} channels consist of proteins embedded in the double lipid matrix which span the membrane, and thus provide a hydrophilic pathway if changes in the electrical field across the membrane occur. Certain changes of the molecular arrangement will ultimately allow the formation of an open pore within the protein. According to the model of Hille (1975), a narrow part separates the outer broad channel mouth from the inner part of the pore; this is the selectivity filter, which acts as an energy barrier for the Na^+ passage because its diameter of 3–5 Å equals the diameter of a hydrated Na^+ ion. Negatively charged groups of the selectivity filter, being limited in number, are thought to be intimately involved in overcoming this energy barrier by interacting with the cation. The main experimental support for this model lies in the fact that I_{Na} does not obey the independence principle supposed by Hodgkin and Huxley (1952) for transmembrane ionic movements. Rather, I_{Na} depends nonlinearly on the extracellular Na^+ concentration and exhibits saturation characteristics (Hille 1975). If $\dot{V}_{max}$ of the cardiac fast-action potential is accepted as the estimate for I_{Na}, the same nonlinear Na^+ dependence exists in ventricular myocardium (Kohlhardt 1982). This strongly suggests a uniform organization of I_{Na} channels, regardless of their origin.

In blocking I_{Na}, propafenone could interact with those negatively charged groups of the selectivity filter gaining access to them via either the outer or the inner channel mouth. If this is true, a competitive interaction between propafenone and Na^+ ions should exist. In an attempt to test this hypothesis, I_{Na} saturation characteristics have been studied prior to and after drug application (Kohlhardt 1982). The Lineweaver-Burk analysis of the $\dot{V}_{max}$-$[Na^+]_o$ relation revealed an increase of the apparent K_m for Na^+ in the presence of propafenone. The y-intercept of the straight, however, was shifted to greater $\dot{V}_{max}$ values which is inconsistent with competitive interaction. The results of voltage clamp experiments should provide a definite answer.

Modification of I_{Na} Inactivation

As first demonstrated by Weidmann (1955b) in cardiac Purkinje fibers, local anesthetics and other related antiarrhythmic compounds can interfere with Na^+ inactivation. The same alteration of the voltage dependence of h_∞ appears after treatment with propafenone (Fig. 2). In these experiments with 1×10^{-5} mol/liter, half inactivation was shifted by 12 mV on the average, from -65 mV to -77 mV (Kohlhardt and Seifert 1980). The shape of the $h_\infty - E_m$ relation remained unaffected. Presupposing a drug-induced I_{Na}alteration to result from a drug – receptor interaction obeying the law of mass action, this voltage shift of h_∞ can only emerge from the drug-affected channels and, moreover, will be the stronger the more channels interact with the drug. This interpretation, however, is inconsistent with the assumption that two channel fractions exist after drug application, one of them being blocked and the other exhibiting the normal state, which consequently implies that the latter fraction has a normal voltage dependence of inactivation.

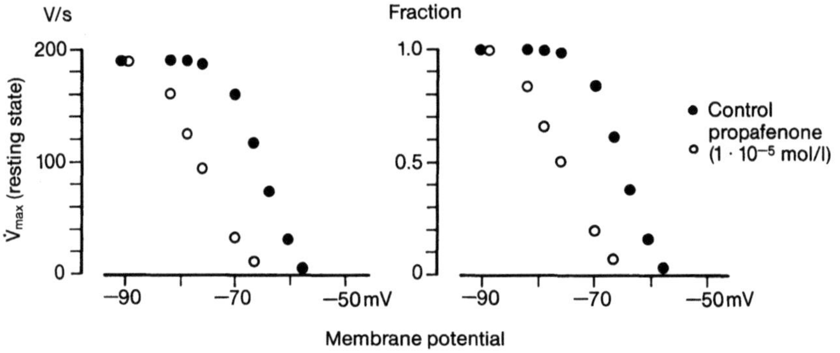

Fig. 2. The dependence of $\dot{V}_{max}$ as obtained after a resting period of 5 min, on membrane potential under control conditions *(filled circles)* and after treatment with 1×50^{-5} mol/liter propafenone *(open circles)*. In the *right diagram,* normalized $\dot{V}_{max}$ values are plotted against membrane potential in order to obtain virtual h_∞-curves. The changes in resting potential were evoked by a stepwise increase in external K^+concentration. (Kohlhardt and Seifert 1980)

Access Routes to the Receptor

The I_{Na}channels are supposed to possess a binding site or receptor structure for local anesthetics located within the pore somewhere between the inner channel mouth and the selectivity filter (Hille 1977). Depending on the ionization of the molecule, the drug can reach this receptor structure from the surrounding lipid matrix by using a lateral lipophilic route or via the inner channel mouth using a hydrophilic pathway. In order to determine the preferential pathway of propafenone, we increased the fraction of neutral drug molecules from 0% to 50% by an extracellular pH variation between 6.4 and 9.0 (Kohlhardt and Seifert 1980). Nevertheless, the inhibitory drug action remained unaffected suggesting that propafenone might reach its channel receptor via either of the two possible pathways.

Rate Dependence of the Inhibitory Propafenone Action on I_{Na}

The inhibitory potency of some class 1 antiarrhythmics can be strongly modulated by changes in the stimulation frequency (Tritthart et al. 1968; Heistracher 1971). Figure 3 demonstrates that propafenone represents another drug with a pronounced use-dependent efficacy. In this type of experiment, the preparations were kept under strictly resting conditions during drug application. After the usual equilibration period of 30 min, a chain of action potentials was triggered with a frequency of 12/min. The $\dot{V}_{max}$ of the first action potential was 200 V/s instead of 260 V/s under control conditions in a drug-free environment. During continuous stimulation, $\dot{V}_{max}$ declined gradually from beat to beat and at 165 V/s finally attained a new steady state. Cessation of repetitive activity caused $\dot{V}_{max}$ to recover from inhibition within 50–60 s. However, a complete restoration did not

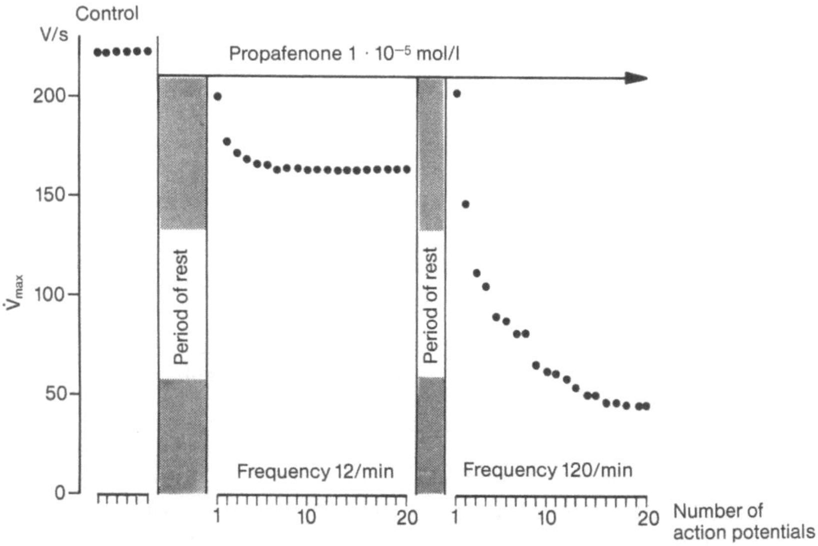

Fig. 3. Drug-induced tonic and phasic $\dot{V}_{max}$ block in mammalian ventricular myocardium. During drug application, several stimulation periods with different rates were performed, separated from each other by periods of rest as symbolized by the *shadowed columns*. Taking the control values of $\dot{V}_{max}$ as a reference level, the tonic $\dot{V}_{max}$ block results from the percentage of $\dot{V}_{max}$ decrease in the first beat. The phasic block emerges from the steady state decrease at a given stimulation frequency when $\dot{V}_{max}$ of the first of a chain of action potentials serves as another reference level. External K^+concentration, 5.4 mmol/liter. (Kohlhardt and Seifert 1980)

occur because $\dot{V}_{max}$ attained only 200 V/s, i. e., the value of the first in a chain of action potentials. This experiment proved the existence of two different forms of $\dot{V}_{max}$ inhibition, tonic and phasic blockade. The tonic block develops during the resting state and is independent of the history. The phasic block results from repetitive activity and is a function of the length of the interstimulus interval (Fig. 4). In the presence of a given drug concentration this allows for the occurrence of any strenght of I_{Na} inhibition.

The development kinetics of the propafenone-induced phasic $\dot{V}_{max}$ block exhibit the expected characteristics of a first-order reaction and are determined like the quinidine-induced phasic $\dot{V}_{max}$ block (Grant et al. 1982) by the interstimulus interval. The shorter the interstimulus interval is the faster the $\dot{V}_{max}$ block develops, and vice versa. When the kinetics are regarded as an event-dependent process, the rate constant declines with a decrease in interstimulus interval indicating that the fraction of total phasic block which can be installed per beat is smaller at higher stimulation freqences than at lower ones.

A comparative study by Courtney (1979) of some local anesthetics revealed a correlation between the molecular weight and the onset rate of phasic I_{Na} block in that smaller molecules produce faster block development than larger molecules do. This is noteworthy because the on-kinetics of the propafenone- and ajmaline-induced (Heistracher 1971) phasic $\dot{V}_{max}$ blocks are quite similar although the molecular weights of the drugs differ by 52 daltons.

The length of the interstimulus interval seems to be the most important determinant factor for the development kinetics of the propafenone-induced phasic $\dot{V}_{max}$ blockade.

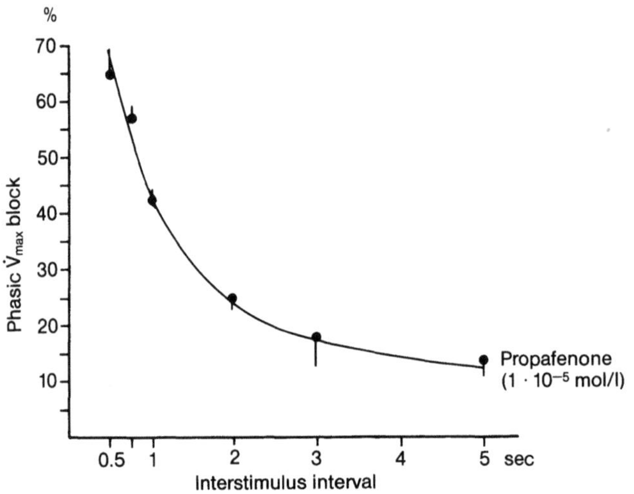

Fig. 4. The dependence of the propafenone-induced phasic $\dot{V}_{max}$ block in mammalian ventricular myocardium on the length of the interstimulus interval. Each *point* is the mean of five experiments, *vertical bars* indicate SEM. The curve fits the function $y = ax^b$ with $r = 0.981$. External K^+ concentration, 5.4 mmol/liter

Changes of resting potential as tested in a range between −90 mV and −79 mV, and variations in temperature or in the pH of the bulk solution proved ineffective and did not modify the onset rate (Kohlhardt and Seifert 1980).

Voltage Dependence of the Inhibitory Propafenone Action on I_{Na}

It is well known that anodal polarization strongly attenuates or even abolishes the inhibitory action of local anesthetics on I_{Na} channels while a decrease in resting potential accentuates the drug effect. Figure 5 indicates that the interaction of propafenone with cardiac I_{Na} channels can also be modified by variations of the membrane potential. In this type of experiment, the resting potential was lowered stepwise from −90 mV to −70 mV by elevating the K^+ concentration in the drug-containing solution. This caused an intensification of the $\dot{V}_{max}$ inhibition. After discrimination between tonic and phasic $\dot{V}_{max}$ block, a different voltage sensitivity of each block form becomes evident. The tonic $\dot{V}_{max}$ block increases in response to this 20 mV depolarization from about 10% to more than 60%. The phasic $\dot{V}_{max}$ block reacted less sensitively and rose only from 20% to 40%. Moreover, the shapes of the curves relating tonic and phasic $\dot{V}_{max}$ block to membrane potential differ tremendously from each other: the tonic block has a sigmoid voltage dependence but that of the phasic block is almost exponential.

The voltage dependence of drug action explains why hypoxia (Hondeghem et al. 1974) or ischemia (Chen et al. 1975) intensifies inhibitory drug effects on I_{Na}. Because of their enhanced sensitivity, I_{Na} of hypoxic cells can even be selectively blocked (Hondeghem et al. 1974) while I_{Na} channels in metabolically normal tissue remain unaffected.

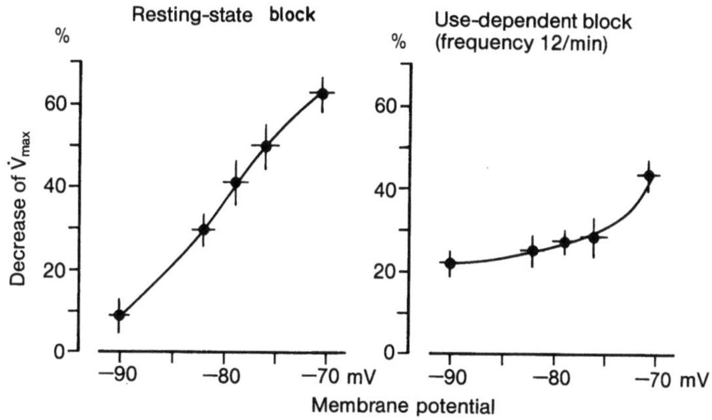

Fig. 5. The voltage dependence of propafenone-induced tonic *(left)* and phasic *(right)* $\dot{V}_{max}$ block in mammalian ventricular myocardium. Drug concentration: 1×10^{-5} mol/liter. Each *point* is the mean of five experiments, *vertical* and *horizontal bars* indicate SEM. (Kohlhardt and Seifert 1980)

Consequently, an antiarrhythmic effect of identical strength will not develop in the whole myocardium when regional disturbances of myocardial perfusion exist provided that the reduction in coronary flow rate still guarantees a sufficient drug concentration in the extracullular space of this myocardial area but cannot maintain a normal resting potential. One conclusion from these regional differences in the I_{Na} drug sensitivity is that the effect no longer correlates with the plasma concentration of antiarrhythmics when factors modulating the drug efficacy do not uniformly affect all myocardial cells.

Na^+ Dependence of the Inhibitory Propafenone Effect on I_{Na}

Extracellular Na^+ withdrawal modifies the efficacy of propafenone and intensifies the $\dot{V}_{max}$ inhibition (Kohlhardt 1982). As can be seen in Fig. 6, both tonic and phasic $\dot{V}_{max}$-block increase in response to a decrease in the Na^+ concentration in the Tyrode's solution from 150 mmol/liter to 50 mmol/liter. However, tonic and phasic $\dot{V}_{max}$ block exhibit quite different individual Na^+ sensitivities as the former reacts more strongly than the latter. Withdrawal of Na^+ seems to facilitate the drug-receptor interaction underlying the $\dot{V}_{max}$ inhibition. Thus, the apparent K_m value for the tonic $\dot{V}_{max}$ blockade decreases from 5×10^{-5} mol/liter at 150 mmol/liter Na^+ to 1.4×10^{-5} mol/liter at 50 mmol/liter Na^+. The decline of the apparent K_m for the phasic block (stimulation frequency 12/min) from 3.8×10^{-5} mol/liter to 2.3×10^{-5} mol/liter was less pronounced. Experiments with lidocaine and procaine revealed that this Na^+ dependence of drug action is not specific for propafenone (Kohlhardt 1982).

After treatment with compounds such as propafenone capable of altering the voltage dependence of h_∞, the (h_∞ − E_m) relation becomes sensitive towards external Na^+ variations. Na^+ withdrawal causes the h_∞ curve to shift further in the hyperpolarizing direction (Fig. 7) which consequently changes the voltage dependence of the I_{Na} blockade.

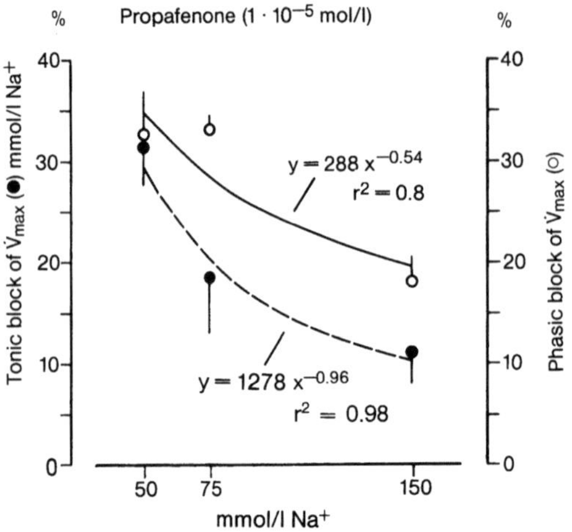

Fig. 6. The dependence of propafenone-induced tonic *(filled circles)* and phasic *(open circles)* $\dot{V}_{max}$ block in mammalian ventricular myocardium on external Na^+ concentration. Each point is the mean of three experiments, *vertical bars* indicate SEM. The slopes of both calculated curves as expressed by the exponents −0.96 and −0.54 differ significantly from each other. Osmotic replacement of Na^+ by sucrose; external K^+ concentration, 5.4 mmol/liter. (Kohlhardt 1982)

Figure 7 demonstrates such an experiment. Under normal environmental conditions, half blockade appeared at −66 mV, but at −74 mV when the preparation was exposed to an Na^+-poor solution. The shape of the curve relating h_∞ and $\dot{V}_{max}$ inhibition to membrane potential remained virtually unaffected.

The decline of the apparent K_m in Na^+-poor solutions strongly suggests an enhanced affinity of the drug receptor for propafenone provided that the pharmacon concentration in the space closely surrounding the receptor area does not change. Considering the proposed localization within the I_{Na} channel, the receptor cannot sense the extracellular Na^+ concentration except during the open configuration of the channel when I_{Na} flows. A sensitization would be a transient, very short state of the receptor of 1 ms or less. Cahalan and Almers (1979) had the idea that the Na^+ ions passing the pore could alternatively control the access of the drug to the receptor. Thus, the probability of a drug-receptor interaction rises with a decrease in the number of I_{Na} charge carriers, and vice versa.

Do I_{Na} Channels Possess a Single Drug Receptor?

On the premise that the drug – receptor interaction underlying the I_{Na} inhibition follows the law of mass action, the inhibitory propafenone effect can be defined by

$$[\text{Drug}]+[\text{Receptor}] \underset{k_2}{\overset{k_1}{\rightleftharpoons}} [\text{P R}] \overset{k_3}{\rightharpoonup} \text{biological effect}$$

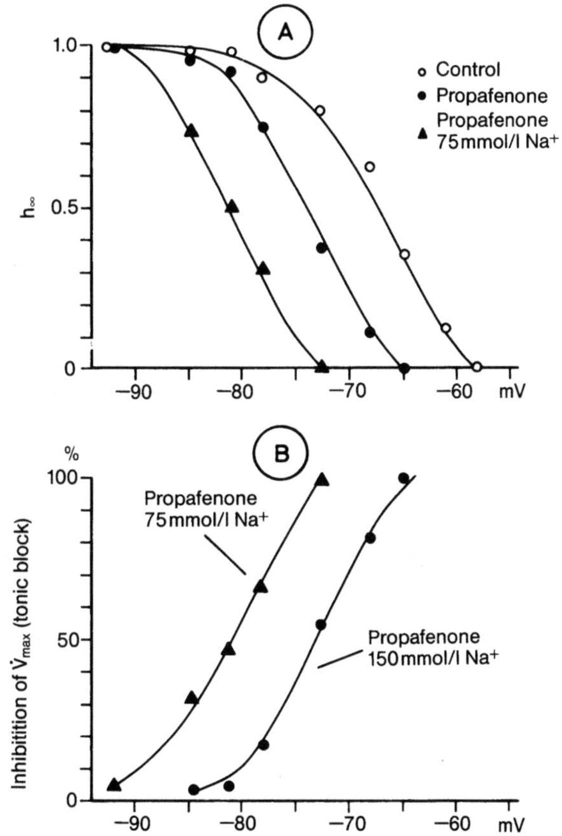

Fig. 7. A Virtual h_∞ curves under control conditions *(open circles)*, after propafenone treatment (1×10^{-5} mol/liter; *filled circles*), and in the continued drug presence after Na^+ withdrawal from 150 mmol/liter to 75 mmol/liter *(filled triangles)* in mammalian ventricular myocardium. **B** Voltage-dependence of the tonic $\dot{V}_{max}$ block at normal *(filled circles)* and reduced *(filled triangles)* external Na^+ concentrations. (Kohlhardt 1982)

if the step labeled with k_3 is not rate limiting. This implies the existence of a single drug receptor which seems, however, inconsistent with the experimental results mentioned above, namely the individual voltage dependence and the individual Na^+ sensitivity of tonic and phasic $\dot{V}_{max}$blockade. Similar discrepancies have been observed by Khodorov et al. (1976) in voltage clamp experiments with the local anesthetic trimecaine. The apparent K_m for the drug-induced decline of P_{Na} differed greatly from the dissociation constant for the delay in slow I_{Na} inactivation. These authors, therefore, postulated the existence of two binding sites within the I_{Na} channel for local anesthetics. The assumption of more than one receptor – one involved in the development of tonic blockade and the other in the installation of phasic blockade – could explain why the two block forms respond to changes in membrane potential or external Na^+ concentration quantitatively in quite a different manner. Nevertheless, the individual response of both types of I_{Na} block does not invalidate the concept of a single drug receptor. According to the modulated receptor model of Hille (1977), configuration and, thus, affinity of the binding site for drugs depends on the state of the channel, resting, activated or inactivated. Such a conformational rearrangement could also modify the receptor sensitivity to changes in membrane potential or external Na^+ concentration.

Nonselective I_{Na} Inhibition by Propafenone

The changes in the shape of the action potential, particularly as they occur at drug concentrations higher than 1×10^{-5} mol/liter, clearly indicate that propafenone affects not only I_{Na}. The depression of the plateau suggests an inhibition of I_{si} which has been demonstrated in voltage clamp experiments on the ventricular myocardium of cats (Kohlhardt 1977). This I_{si} sensitivity explains why higher propafenone concentrations (8×10^{-5} mol/liter) exert an inhibitory effect on the sinoatrial node. The I_{si}-mediated sinoatrial action potential responds with a decrease of overshoot and upstroke velocity regardless of the cell type, primary or secondary pacemaker. In a few cases, the depression was so strong that only miniature action potentials of some 20 mV in amplitude persisted (Kohlhardt, unpublished). Since I_{si} also plays the key role in the excitation process in N- and NH-cells of the atrioventricular node, AV-node action potentials should exhibit a similar low sensitivity.

This susceptibility of I_{si} to propafenone proves that in higher concentrations the drug gains properties of class 4 antiarrhythmics. Propafenone thus resembles drugs like prenylamine or quinidine.

References

Cahalan MD, Almers W (1979) Interactions between quaternary lidocaine, the sodium channel gates, and tetrodotoxin. Biophys J 27: 39–56

Chen CM, Gettes LS, Katzung BG (1975) Effect of lidocaine and quinidine on steady-state characteristics and recovery kinetics of dV/dt_{max} in guinea-pig ventricular myocardium. Circ Res 37: 20–29

Courtney KR (1979) Fast frequency-dependent block of action potential upstroke in rabbit atrium by small local anesthetics. Life Sci 24: 1581–1588

Engstfeld G, Antoni H, Fleckenstein A (1961) Die Restitution der Erregungsfortleitung und Kontraktionskraft des K^+-gelähmten Frosch- und Säugetiermyokards durch Adrenalin. Pflügers Arch 145–163

Gettes LS, Reuter H (1974) Slow recovery from inactivation of inward currents in mammalian myocardial fibres. J Physiol 240: 703–724

Grant AO, Trantham JL, Brown KK, Strauss HC (1982) pH-dependent effects of quinidine on the kinetics of dV/dt_{max} in guinea pig ventricular myocardium. Circ Res 50: 210–217

Hauswirth O (1968) Effects of droperidol on sheep Purkinje fibers. Naunyn-Schmiedebergs Arch Pharmacol 261: 133–142

Hauswirth O, Singh BN (1979) Ionic mechanisms in heart muscle in relation to the genesis and the pharmacological control of cardiac arrhythmias. Pharmacol Rev 30: 5–63

Heistracher P (1971) Mechanisms of action of antifibrillatory drugs. Naunyn-Schmiedebergs Arch Pharmacol 269: 199–212

Hille B (1975) Ionic selectivity, saturation, and block in sodium channels. A four-barrier model. J Gen Physiol 66: 535–560
Hille B (1977) Local anesthetics: hydrophilic and hydrophophobic pathways for the drug-receptor reaction. J Gen Physiol 69: 497–515
Hodgkin AL, Huxley AF (1952) Currents carried by sodium and potassium through the membrane of giant axon of Loligo. J Physiol 116: 449–472
Hondeghem LW, Grant AO, Jensen RA (1974) Antiarrhythmic drug action: selective depression of hypoxic cardiac cells. Am Heart J 87: 602–605
Kern R, Einwächter HM, Haas HG, Lack EG (1971) Cardiac membrane currents as affected by a neuroleptic agent: Droperidol. Pfluegers Arch 325: 262–278
Khodorov BI, Shishkova L, Peganov E, Revenko S (1976) Inhibition of sodium currents in frog Ranvier node treated with local anesthetics. Role of slow sodium inactivation. Biochim Biophys Acta 433: 409–435
Kohlhardt M (1977) Der Einfluß von Propafenon auf den transmembranären Na^+- und Ca^{++} -Strom der Warmblüter-Myokardfasermembran. In: Fortschritte in der Pharmakotherapie von Herzrhythmusstörungen. Fischer, Stuttgart New York
Kohlhardt M (1980) Genese, Eigenschaften und funktionelle Bedeutung des Slow-response-Aktionspotentials am Herzen. Z Kardiol 69: 307–315
Kohlhardt M (1982) A quantitative analysis of the Na^+-dependence of $\dot{V}_{max}$ of the fast action potential in mammalian ventricular myocardium. Saturation characteristics and the modulation of a druginduced I_{Na} blockade by $[Na^+]$ o. Pflügers Arch 392: 379–387
Kohlhardt M, Seifert C (1980) Inhibition of $\dot{V}_{max}$ of the action potential by propafenone and its voltage-, time- and pH-dependence in mammalian ventricular myocardium. Naunyn-Schmiedebergs Arch Pharmacol 315: 55–62
Luckstead EF, Tarr M (1972) Comparison of quinidine and bretylium tosylate effects on cardiac ionic currents. Fed Proc 31: 818
Mascher D (1970) Electrical and mechanical responses from ventricular muscle fibres after inactivation of the sodium carrying system. Pfluegers Arch 317: 359–372
Tarr M, Luckstead EF, Jurewics PA, Haas HG (1973) Effect of propranolol on the fast inward sodium current in frog atrial muscle. J Pharmacol Exp Ther 184: 599–610
Tritthart H, Fleckenstein B, Fleckenstein A, Krause H (1968) Frequenzabhängige Einflüsse von antiarrhythmisch-wirksamen Substanzen auf die Aufstrichsgeschwindigkeit des Aktionspotentials (Versuche an isolierten Meerschweinchenpapillarmuskeln). Pfluegers Arch 300: 52
Vaughan Williams EM (1975) Classification of antidysrhythmic drugs. Pharmacol Ther [B] 1: 115–138
Weidmann S (1955 a) The effect of cardiac membrane potential on the rapid availability of the sodium-carrying system. J Physiol 127: 213–224
Weidmann S (1955 b) Effects of calcium and local anesthetics on electrical properties of Purkinje fibres. J Physiol 129: 568–582

The Pharmacology of Propafenone

H. Scholz

Propafenone is an antiarrhythmic drug that has been shown to be clinically effective in the treatment of supraventricular and ventricular premature beats (see Hochrein et al. 1977, Lüderitz 1978, 1981, Neuss and Buss 1978, Theisen 1978, Petri and Rudolph 1979, Schmitz 1980, Seipel and Breithardt 1980, Scholz 1981). In this paper I shall briefly summarize the pharmacologic properties of propafenone as determined in animal experiments in vitro and in vivo. The pharmacokinetic properties of the drug and the results of toxicologic studies are also presented.

Pharmacologic Effects of Propafenone

Details on the pharmacologic actions of propafenone as determined in both in vivo and in vitro animal experiments are presented by Hapke and Prigge (1976), Hapke (1977), Ledda et al. (1981), and von Philipsborn (1981).

Antiarrhythmic Action of Propafenone

The antiarrhythmic action of propafenone in intact animals has been demonstrated in dogs, cats, guinea pigs, rats, and rabbits using numerous model arrhythmias (electrical stimulation, chloroform inhalation plus epinephrine infusion; infusion of $CaCl_2$, cardiac glycosides or aconitine; coronary ligation). The minimum doses necessary for this action were 1 mg/kg body wt. i. v. and 5–10 mg/kg body wt. by intraduodenal or peroral administration. In isolated cardiac preparations (guinea pig atria), propafenone in concentrations beginning at 0.5 μg/ml led to a concentration-dependent decrease in the maximum following frequency (i. e., the maximum frequency at which the preparation can follow electrical stimulation) and to a lengthening of the functional refractory period as determined by the paired stimulus method of Govier (1965). These effects were fully developed 20–40 min after application of the drug. It is noteworthy in this connection that the antiarrhythmically effective plasma levels observed in man (0.2–5.3 μg/ml; mean value approx. 0.8 μg/ml) are of the same order of magnitude, although interindividual variations are great (Wiebringhaus et al. 1977, Keller et al. 1978, Meyer-Estorf et al. 1978, 1980, Blanke et al. 1979).

The decrease in the maximum following frequency in isolated guinea pig atria was also taken as an index for comparing the potency of propafenone and other antiarrhythmic agents. In the study of von Philipsborn (1981), an average of 2.35 μg/ml propafenone was necessary to decrease the maximum following frequency by 50%. Under the same conditions quinidine, procainamide, mexiletine, lidocaine, and disopyramide were less potent than propafenone, while ajmaline and aprindine had about the same potency, and prajmalium was more potent.

Mechanism of the Antiarrhythmic Action of Propafenone

According to electrophysiologic studies by Kohlhardt (1977), Bergmann and Bolte (1977), Kohlhardt and Seifert (1980), and Ledda et al. (1981), propafenone inhibits the fast sodium current and so can be classified as a membrane-stabilizing antiarrhythmic drug, i. e., as a class I agent (Vaughan Williams 1975), of which quinidine and lidocaine are prototypes. Propafenone defies clear-cut classification, however. On the one hand it reduces the depolarization rate of the fast action potential at low (less negative) resting potentials more than at normal ones. Moreover it shortens the duration of the action potential; in this respect it is similar to lidocaine. On the other hand propafenone, like quinidine, apparently has no significant effect on the recovery of the fast Na^+ current from inactivation. For this reason, and because the drug does not prolong the action potential, at least the *effective* refractory period is not significantly influenced by propafenone.

In rabbit Purkinje fibers and ventricular myocardium, the effective refractory period was increased by about 10% in only 50% of the preparations and only by high propafenone concentrations (Bergmann and Bolte 1977). Ledda et al. (1981) observed a shortening of the effective refractory period in sheep Purkinje fibers treated with propafenone. Thus one might expect that the *total* refractory period is not appreciably altered by propafenone neither, although I know of no direct studies that have been done on this question. Finally, it is worth noting that the aforementioned electrophysiologic effects are more pronounced in Purkinje fibers than in the working myocardium (Bergmann and Bolte 1977, Ledda et al. 1981).

Higher concentrations of propafenone were also found to have an inhibitory effect on the slow Ca^{++} inward current (Kohlhardt 1977). Moreover, propafenone exerts a beta-receptor blocking action. The latter has been reported to be more pronounced in tracheal and vascular muscle than in the heart (Kukovetz et al. 1977, Paietta et al. 1977). Nevertheless, it appears to contribute to the antiarrhythmic action of propafenone, in contrast to the "Ca^{++} antagonist" effect of the drug. These points will be discussed in greater detail below.

Beta-sympatholytic Action of Propafenone

Figure 1, taken from a study by Ledda et al. (1981), shows that propafenone inhibits the positive inotropic and positive chronotropic effect of isoprenaline in isolated guinea pig atria. The propafenone concentrations of 0.5 and 1 μg/ml correspond to those that are antiarrhythmically effective in the same preparations, as mentioned above. Thus is appears not unlikely that the beta-sympatholytic effect of propafenone plays a part in its antiarrhythmic action. Quantitatively, 1 μg/ml propafenone shifts the concentration-response curve by more than one order of magnitude to the right. For the inhibition of the positive inotropic effect of isoprenaline by propafenone, Ledda et al. (1981) calculat-

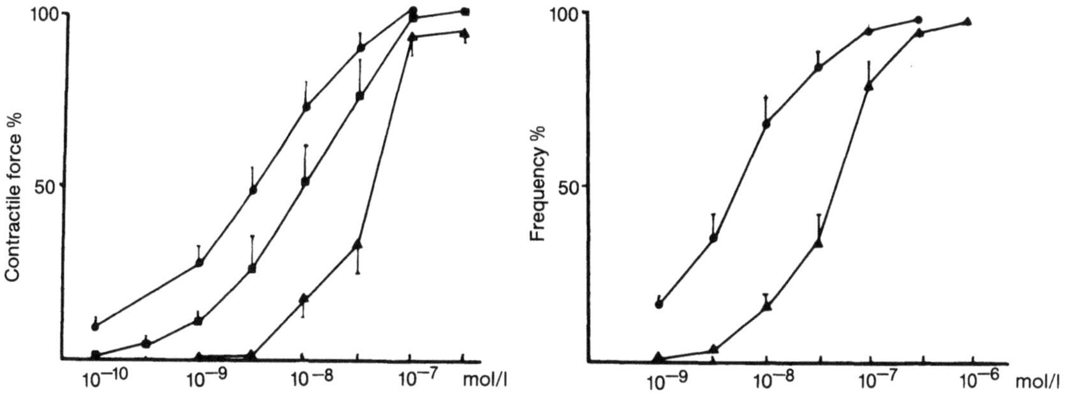

Fig. 1. Influence of propafenone on the positive inotropic effect (*left*) and on the positive chronotropic effect (*right*) of isoprenaline in isolated cardiac preparations from guinea pigs (*left:* ventricular strips electrically stimulated at 2.5 Hz; *right:* spontaneously beating atria). *Circles:* control; *squares:* propafenone 0.5 μg/ml; *triangles:* propafenone 1 μg/ml; ordinates: percentage of maximum response; abscissae: concentration of isoprenaline. The incubation time for propafenone was 30 min in all cases; isoprenaline application was cumulative. (From Ledda et al. 1981)

ed a mean pA_2 value of 6.49, i.e., approximately 0.12 μg/ml propafenone reduces the response to isoprenaline by 50%. In earlier investigations by Kukovetz et al. (1977) on spontaneously beating guineapig hearts perfused by the method of Langendorff, propafenone was approximately three times less potent, and there was no clear-cut shift to the right of the concentration-response curve for the positive inotropic effect of isoprenaline.

As mentioned above, a beta-sympatholytic effect of propafenone has been observed not only in the heart, but also in isolated bovine coronary artery and tracheal muscle strips (Kukovetz et al. 1977, Paietta et al. 1977). Propafenone inhibited the relaxant effect of isoprenaline in these preparations (stimulation of $beta_2$-adrenoceptors), and proved to be about five times more potent in the coronary arteries than in the myocardium, and some 50 times more potent in tracheal muscle. Thus, at least in these studies, propafenone affected mainly the $beta_2$-receptors. In vivo in the rat, however, the $beta_1$- and $beta_2$-sympatholytic effects of propafenone were not different (ED_{50} was in each case 3.2 mg/kg i.v.; von Philipsborn 1981). The relevance of this beta-sympatholytic action of propafenone in vivo, e.g. in patients with bronchial asthma, remains unclear. It is conceivable that the $beta_2$-sympatholytic action of propafenone is compensated by a direct spasmolytic effect (cf. Kukovetz et al. 1977).

Calcium Antagonist Effect of Propafenone

As mentioned above, high concentrations of propafenone (25 μg/ml) inhibited the slow Ca^{++} inward current in cat ventricular myocardial preparations (Kohlhardt 1977). In the same study the propafenone concentrations necessary to inhibit the fast Na^+ influx were about 20 times lower, indicating that the effect of the drug on the slow Ca^{++} channel is relatively weak, while that on the fast Na^+ channel clearly predominates. Similar

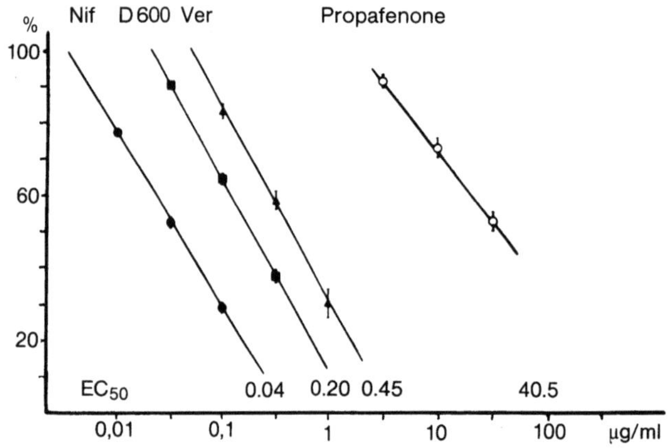

Fig. 2. Influence of (*from left to right*) nifedipine, D 600, verapamil, and propafenone on the force of contraction of K^+-depolarized (22 m*M*) ventricular strips from guinea pigs. Contractions were evoked by electrical stimulation (0.2 Hz) in the presence of 10 µ*M* histamine, i. e., by slow Ca^{++}-dependent action potentials. Ordinate: force of contraction as percentage of initial value before addition of drug; abscissa: drug concentrations. (From Ledda et al. 1981)

conclusions were reached by Ledda et al. (1981), who studied the inhibitory effect of propafenone on contractions initiated by slow Ca^{++}-dependent action potentials. Nifedipine, verapamil, and D600 were investigated for comparison. The results are summarized in Fig. 2. All drugs exerted a negative inotropic effect under these conditions. The corresponding EC_{50} values (µg/ml) were 0.04 for nifedipine, 0.2 for D600, 0.45 for verapamil and 40.5 for propafenone. This means that a "calcium antagonist" effect – in contrast to the beta-sympatholytic effect – probably plays no significant role in the antiarrhythmic action of propafenone. In this respect propafenone is about 100 times less potent than verapamil for example. In addition, the "calcium antagonist" effect of propafenone is observed only at concentrations considerably greater than those that are antiarrhythmically effective in the same preparation.

Other Cardiovascular Effects of Propafenone

The antiarrhythmic action of propafenone is accompanied by negative inotropic and negative chronotropic effects. The propafenone concentrations which in isolated guinea pig atria led to a 50% decrease in the maximum following frequency on the one hand and to a 25% reduction each in the spontaneous rate and the force of contraction (in this case in electrically stimulated preparations) on the other were similar, amounting respectively to 2.35, 1.36, and 4.85 µg/ml (von Philipsborn 1981). Similar results were obtained by Hapke and Prigge (1976) and Ledda et al. (1981). In the study of Ledda et al. (1981), for example, 3 µg/ml propafenone in isolated guinea pig atria and ventricular strips led to reductions in the spontaneous rate and force of contraction of 36.7% and 31.6% respectively.

In isolated perfused guinea pig hearts, 1–10 µg propafenone led to a 67%–240% increase in coronary flow. The stroke amplitude of the spontaneously beating preparations was not altered at these doses (Hapke and Prigge 1976, Hapke 1977).

In the in vivo studies of Hapke and Prigge (1976) and Hapke (1977) in anesthetized dogs, the intravenous administration of propafenone had the following hemodynamic effects: There was only a transient and relatively slight fall in blood pressure. A dose of 1 mg/kg produced no appreciable blood pressure change. When the dose was increased to 3 mg/kg, the systolic pressure fell by an average of 15 mmHg and the diastolic pressure by 25 mmHg for a period of 3–5 minutes. The enteral administration of propafenone in doses of 10 mg/kg did not alter the blood pressure. The maximum rate of pressure rise in the left ventricle was not significantly affected by doses of 0.3 and 1 mg/kg propafenone. Doses of 3 and 6 mg/kg lowered this parameter by 27% and 47% respectively; similarly, the left ventricular systolic pressure fell by 20 and 40 mmHg respectively. At the same time, doses of 1–6 mg/kg propafenone led to an increase in the left ventricular end-diastolic pressure by 5–18 mmHg which persisted for up to 30 min or longer, depending on the dose. The stroke volume decreased by 12%–14% after 2–4 mg/kg propafenone and remained low for 10 min to 1 h. The coronary flow increased by 20%–70% after 1–5 mg/kg propafenone. The heart rate was not appreciably influenced by 1 mg/kg propafenone. After 5 mg/kg the heart rate increased from an average of 85 to 120 beats/min, probably representing a reflex response to the blood pressure fall.

On the whole, these findings show that propafenone like other antiarrhythmic agents can exert a negative inotropic effect when administered in antiarrhythmically effective doses similar to the effects observed in man (cf. Seipel and Breithardt 1980).

Spasmolytic Effect of Propafenone

It has already been mentioned that propafenone leads to an increase in coronary flow. Kukovetz et al. (1977) have also described a relaxant effect of propafenone in isolated bovine coronary artery and tracheal muscle strips and in isolated guinea pig colon. In coronary arteries propafenone had an EC_{50} of $1.5 \cdot 10^{-4}$ mol/l (=56 μg/ml) and so was less potent than etafenone or papaverine, but more potent than theophylline. In tracheal muscle and guineapig colon the spasmolytic effect of propafenone corresponded roughly to that of papaverine, with an EC_{50} of $1.5 \cdot 10^{-5}$ mol/l. Hapke and Prigge (1976) and Hapke (1977) have demonstrated a spasmolytic effect of propafenone in vivo by means of pressure measurements in the duodenum of the dog. The basal tone of the bowel decreased after doses of 2 and 4 mg/kg propafenone. The level of peristalsis, i. e., the amplitude of the bowel movements, was in all cases markedly reduced after doses higher than 0.5 mg/kg. The duration of this effect was about 10–30 min following 1 mg/kg.

The mechanism of the spasmolytic action of propafenone is unknown. It may be assumed, however, that this action (as in the case of verapamil) does not result from an inhibition of phosphodiesterase (PDE) with the subsequent accumulation of cAMP in the cell, for propafenone inhibits PDE only in concentrations some 100 times higher than the spasmolytically active levels (Kukovetz et al. 1977).

Local Anesthetic Effect of Propafenone

Propafenone exerts a local anesthetic action. In the guinea pig cornea, a 0.5% solution of propafenone was roughly equivalent to a 0.7% procaine solution (Hapke and Prigge

1976; Hapke 1977). Thus, the local anesthetic effect of propafenone corresponds at least to that of procaine and is readily explained by the membrane-stabilizing action of the drug.

Pharmacokinetic Properties of Propafenone

The following data on the pharmacokinetics of propafenone relate to human beings. They are based on investigations by Keller et al. (1978), Meyer-Estorf et al. (1978, 1980), and Blanke et al. (1979), as well as on information furnished by the manufacturer (Brode and Bühler 1981).

The absorption of propafenone after oral administration is concentration-dependent. Its bioavailability is 49%. This suggests that propafenone is subject to a high first-pass metabolism. Plasma levels are maximal 2–3 h after oral administration. The therapeutic plasma levels are highly variable from one individual to the next; values ranging from 0.2 to 5.3 μg/ml with a mean of about 0.8 μg/ml are reported in the literature. The distribution volume is 2–4.5 liters/kg, and plasma protein binding is 87%–97%. The elimination half-life is 2.5–3.6 h and agrees well with the decrease of the antiarrhythmic effect of the drug (change in P-Q interval). Propafenone is intensely metabolized; only about 1% is excreted unchanged in the urine within 24 h.

Toxicology of Propafenone

The following information on the toxicology of propafenone is based essentially on studies and data supplied by the manufacturer (Dieckmann et al. 1981).

Acute Toxicity

The mean LD_{50} of propafenone in mice, rats, and dogs ranges from 10.0 to 31.1 mg/kg i.v. and from 315 to 3556 mg/kg orally. In cats a mean LD_{50} ranging from 60 to 80 mg/kg is reported with oral administration.

Subacute and Chronic Toxicity

The subacute (3–4 weeks) and chronic toxicity (6–12 months) of propafenone have been tested in rats, dogs, and rabbits. The doses which caused no systemic adverse signs and no appreciable chemical or histopathologic changes in the rat were 90–150 mg/kg orally and 1.75 mg/kg i.v. The corresponding values in the dog were 30–50 mg/kg orally and 1 mg/kg i.v. In rabbits, however, in the course of these toxicologic studies, the intravenous administration of 0.3–1.0 mg/kg propafenone over a 3-week period caused an inhibition of spermiogenesis, which also occurred in dogs and Rhesus monkeys which had been given 2–5 mg/kg i. v. for 4 weeks. The inhibition of spermiogenesis was reversible within 4–8 weeks following discontinuance of propafenone and has not been observed in dogs that were given the drug orally for 6–12 months. The cause and significance of this disturbance are not fully understood. It is known only that, according to information from the manufacturer (Brode and Bühler 1981), propafenone is eliminated in the rat more slowly from the testes (half-life about 9 h) than from the plasma and other tissues (half-life about 4 h). However, according to Kleinsorge and Pfennigsdorf (1980), no drug-related damage to the spermatogenetic germinal epithelium was found in light- and electron-microscopic examinations of testis and epididymis of rabbits and dogs after repeated administration of propafenone for up to 4 weeks.

At least one case of probably propafenone-induced impotence and impaired spermiogenesis has been described in man (Körst et al. 1980). This side effect of propafenone, which recurred after reexposure, was also reversible within 6–7 weeks. The authors, who recommend caution during long-term use of propafenone, attributed the oligospermia to direct tubular damage, endocrine causes having been ruled out by hormone assays. However, this particular conclusion was not substantiated by adequate data. For instance, quantitative data about ejaculation and glandular secretion are missing, as well as tests of the motility and morphology of the sperm cells, as has been pointed out by Kleinsorge and Pfennigsdorf (1980) in their above-mentioned commentary.

Other Toxicologic Investigations

Teratologic investigations in rabbits (up to 150 mg/kg orally and 4.5 mg/kg i. v.) and rats (up to 600 mg/kg orally and 6 mg/kg i. v.) have shown no evidence of teratogenic or embryotoxic effects of propafenone. Tests in rabbits and rats showed no influence on fertility or sexual behavior (up to 120 and 150 mg/kg respectively, orally for 10 weeks) and tests in mice, hamsters, and rats revealed no signs of propafenone-related mutagenicity or carcinogenicity.

Summary

The antiarrhythmic effect of propafenone was demonstrated experimentally, both in vivo and in vitro, in numerous animal models. It is probably based chiefly on a partly lidocaine-like and partly quinidine-like inhibition of the fast Na^+ inward current (membrane-stabilizing antiarrhythmic drug of class I after Vaughan Williams). In addition, propafenone exerts a beta-sympatholytic action that presumably contributes to its antiarrhythmic effectiveness. It is doubtful that a "calcium antagonist" effect, which is observed only at high concentrations, contributes materially to the antiarrhythmic activity of the drug. As with other antiarrhythmic drugs, the antiarrhythmic action of propafenone is associated with a negative inotropic effect. The bioavailability of propafenone in man is approximately 50%. The drug is probably subject to a high first-pass metabolism. It is almost completely metabolized and has a mean elimination half-life of 2.5–3.6 h.

Toxicologic studies revealed that propafenone can inhibit spermiogenesis. However, this disturbance occurred in animals only after several weeks of intravenous use and was reversible. At least one case of probably propafenone-induced impotence with oligospermia in man has been reported; the cause is not definitely established, and further clarification is necessary.

References

Bergmann M, Bolte HD (1977) Elektrophysiologische Untersuchungen mit Propafenon an myokardialen Einzelfasern. In: Hochrein H, Hapke H-J, Beck OA (eds) Fortschritte in der Pharmakotherapie von Herzrhythmusstörungen. Fischer, Stuttgart New York, pp 29–34

Blanke H, Aschbrenner B, Karsch KR, Kreuzer H (1979) Plasmaspiegel-Wirkungs-Beziehung und Organverteilung von Propafenon. Dtsch Med Wochenschr 104: 587–591

Brode E, Bühler V (1981) Zur Pharmakokinetik von Propafenon. Internal report. Knoll AG, Ludwigshafen

Dieckmann W, Fischer A, Heimann W, Schnitzlein W, Träger H (1981) Exposé of propafenone HCl. Toxicological part. Internal report VP/FBA 8126. Knoll AG, Ludwigshafen

Govier WC (1965) The mechanism of the atrial refractory period change produced by ouabain. J Pharmacol Exp Ther 148: 100–105

Hapke H-J (1977) Pharmakologische Wirkungen von Propafenon. In: Hochrein H, Hapke H-J, Beck OA (eds) Fortschritte in der Pharmakotherapie von Herzrhythmusstörungen. Fischer, Stuttgart New York, pp 2–8

Hapke H-J, Prigge E (1976) Zur Pharmakologie von 2′-[2-Hydroxy-3-(propylamino)-propoxy]-3-phenylpropiophenon (Propafenon, SA 79)-hydrochlorid. Arzneimittelforsch 26: 1849–1857

Hochrein H, Hapke H-J, Beck OA (1977) Fortschritte in der Pharmakotherapie von Herzrhythmusstörungen. Fischer, Stuttgart New York

Keller K, Meyer-Estorf G, Beck OA, Hochrein H (1978) Correlation between serum concentration and pharmacological effect on atrioventricular conduction time of the antiarrhythmic drug propafenone. Eur J Clin Pharmacol 13: 17–20

Kleinsorge H, Pfennigsdorf G (1980) Potenz- und Spermiogenesestörungen durch Propafenon. Dtsch Med Wochenschr 105: 1395–1396

Körst HA, Brandes J-W, Littmann K-P (1980) Potenz- und Spermiogenesestörungen durch Propafenon. Dtsch Med Wochenschr 105: 1187–1189

Kohlhardt M (1977) Der Einfluß von Propafenon auf den transmembranären Na^{+}- und Ca^{++}-Strom der Warmblüter-Myokardfasermembran. In: Hochrein H, Hapke H-J, Beck OA (eds) Fortschritte in der Pharmakotherapie von Herzrhythmusstörungen. Fischer, Stuttgart New York, pp 35–38

Kohlhardt M, Seifert C (1980) Inhibition von $\dot{V}_{max}$ of the action potential by propafenon and its voltage-, time and pH-dependence in mammalian ventricular myocardium. Naunyn-Schmiedebergs Arch Pharmacol 315: 55–62

Kukovetz WR, Pöch G, Holzmann S, Wurm A, Paietta E (1977) Wirkung von Propafenon auf Phosphodiesterase, Koronararterien und Herz. In: Hochrein H, Hapke H-J, Beck OA (eds) Fortschritte in der Pharmakotherapie von Herzrhythmusstörungen. Fischer, Stuttgart New York, pp 9–19

Ledda F, Mantelli L, Manzini S, Amerini S, Mugelli A (1981) Electrophysiological and antiarrhythmic properties of propafenone in isolated cardiac preparations. J Cardiovasc Pharmacol 3: 1162–1173

Lüderitz B (1978) Fortschritte in der medikamentösen Arrhythmiebehandlung. Herz Kreisl 10: 99–106

Lüderitz B (1981) Therapie der Herzrhythmusstörungen. Springer, Berlin Heidelberg New York

Meyer-Estorf G, Keller K, Beck OA, Hochrein H (1978) Antiarrhythmische Wirksamkeit von Propafenon in Abhängigkeit von Serumkonzentration und Erregungsleitungshemmung. Z Kardiol 67: 352–356

Meyer-Estorf G, Keller K, Beck OA, Hochrein H (1980) Serumkonzentration und AV-Überleitungszeit unter mehrtägiger oraler Behandlung mit Propafenon. Z Kardiol 69: 417–420

Neuss H, Buss J (1978) Wirkungsspektrum neuer Antiarrhythmika. Internist 19: 234–240

Paietta E, Pöch G, Kukovetz WR (1977) Analyse der β-Blockerwirkung von Propafenon (SA 79). In: Hochrein H, Hapke H-J, Beck OA (eds) Fortschritte in der Pharmakotherapie von Herzrhythmusstörungen. Fischer, Stuttgart New York, pp 20–28

Petri H, Rudolph W (1979) Medikamentöse Therapie tachykarder Rhythmusstörungen. Herz 4: 344–358

Philipsborn G von (1981) Überblick über pharmakologische Arbeiten mit Propafenon. Internal report VP/FBP 8109. Knoll AG, Ludwigshafen

Schmitz W (1980) Klassifizierung neuerer Antiarrhythmika nach elektrophysiologischen Gesichtspunkten. Klin Wochenschr 58: 907–918

Scholz H (1981) Therapie der Arrhythmien. Neue Antiarrhythmika. Verh Dtsch Ges Herz Kreislaufforsch 47: 18–33

Seipel L, Breithardt G (1980) Propafenone – a new antiarrhythmic drug. Eur Heart J 1: 309–313

Theisen K (1978) Medikamentöse Therapie tachykarder Herzrhythmusstörungen. Klin Wochenschr 56: 153–168

Vaughan Williams EM (1975) Classification of antidysrhythmic drugs. Pharmacol Ther B 1: 115–138

Wiebringhaus E, Seipel L, Breithardt G, Loogen F (1977) Langzeitergebnisse mit dem neuen Antiarrhythmikum Propafenon unter Berücksichtigung der Plasmaspiegel. Z Kardiol 66: 625–632

Clinical Pharmacology of Propafenone

H. Neuss and M. Schlepper

Some aspects of the clinical pharmacology of propafenone are presented in other reports in this volume. This chapter will therefore be limited to a discussion of clinicoelectrophysiological findings and to questions of clinical effectiveness and the occurrence of side effects.

Clinicoelectrophysiological Findings

The clinical electrophysiology of propafenone will be presented in the light of our own findings, which were derived from His-bundle electrography in 41 patients (23 men and 18 women, aged 18–73 years: Table 1). Each patient received propafenone in a dose of 2 mg/kg body wt in the form of an i.v. bolus, and in most cases the investigation was concluded 20 min after administration.

Influence of Sinus Node Function

In contrast to reports from other authors (Beck et al. 1975; Seipel et al. 1975) we found no significant influence on sinus rate (Table 2), although in eight patients a lengthening of sinus interval of over 100 ms was determined. Sinus node recovery time and conduction time were not systematically investigated in our study group, but isolated observations were in agreement with the observations of the Düsseldorf team (Breithardt et al. 1975) on an increase in this parameter (Fig. 1).

Table 1. Material for the electrophysiological study

Diagnosis	No. of patients
Wolff-Parkinson-White syndrome	18
AV node reentry tachycardia	13
Intraventricular conduction disturbances (incl. three patients with documented complete AV block)	8
Ectopic atrial tachycardia	2

Table 2. AV conduction times and refraction parameter

Parameter (ms)	*n*	Control	Propafenone	Increase (%)	*P*
PA interval	41	34 ± 11	47 ± 17	38	0.001
ERP A	38	223 ± 27	247 ± 29	11	0.001
FRP A	38	263 ± 30	287 ± 31	9	0.001
PP interval	41	758 ± 119	760 ± 120	0	n.s.
AH interval	35	79 ± 23	96 ± 26	22	0.01
Wenckebach point	21	294 ± 72	387 ± 53	32	0.01
FRP	26	392 ± 47	432 ± 54	9	0.01
ERP AVN	14	283 ± 34	322 ± 29	14	0.05
HV interval	35	44 ± 10	57 ± 12	29	0.001
QRS	35	98 ± 22	144 ± 26	16	0.001
QT_c	35	395 ± 36	423 ± 16	7	0.05
ERP V	32	209 ± 17	233 ± 10	11	0.001

Abbreviations: PA interval, intra-atrial conduction time; ERPA, ERP AVN, ERP V, effective refractory period of atrial myocardium (A), AV node (AVN), ventricular myocardium (V); FRP, functional refractory period; PP interval, sinus interval; AH interval, nodal conduction time; Wenckebach point, atrial stimulation interval at which a supra-His grade II AV block occurs; HV interval, conduction time in His-Purkinje system; QRS, width of ventricular complex; QT_c rate-corrected QT interval

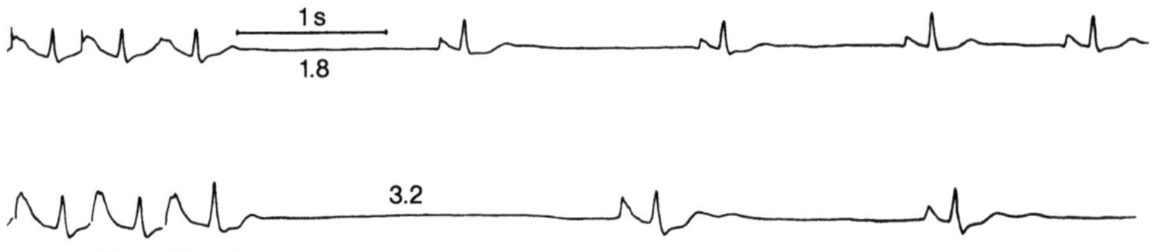

Fig. 1. ECG (lead I) after atrial overdrive before *(above)* and after *(below)* i.v. administration of 140 mg propafenone. Increase in sinus node recovery time from 1.8 to 3.2 s

Effect at Atrial Level

At atrial level significant increases in conduction time, i.e., PA interval (Fig. 2), and in functional and effective refractory period could be established. The changes were most marked approximately 5 min after the bolus injection, but the effect had still not worn off completely by the conclusion of the investigation.

Effect on the AV Node

A similar clear lengthening of conduction time, i.e., of AH interval, was evident at AV node level (Fig. 2). Grade II AV blocks occurred at a significantly reduced stimulation rate. The functional and effective refractory period of the AV node was also clearly extended (Table 2).

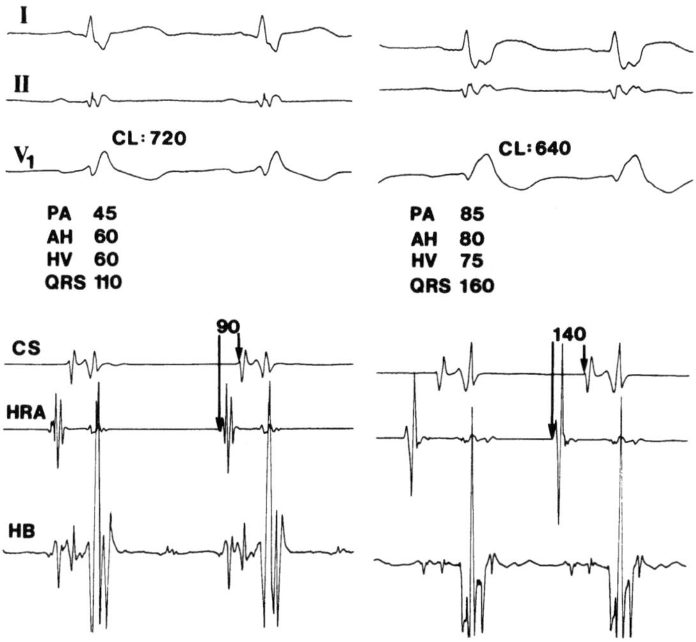

Fig. 2. ECG (leads I, II, and V_1) and electrogram of left atrium *(CS)*, high right atrium *(HRA)*, and His bundle *(HB)* in a 49-year-old male patient with ectopic atrial tachycardia. After propafenone *(right)* all intracardial conduction times increase. All intervals in milliseconds

Effect at Ventricular Level

At ventricular level clear increases in HV interval and QRS duration were found. The increase in QT_c may well have been due essentially to a QRS widening, as the JT interval showed no significant change. In the ventricular myocardium as at atrial level there was a lengthening of the effective refractory period (Table 2).

Propafenone in AV Node Reentry

In all 13 patients with AV node reentry propafenone led to a reduction in tachycardia rate; the RR interval increased from 339 ± 55 ms to 400 ± 50 ms. In 11 of the 13, tachycardia ceased immediately after the bolus injection (Fig. 3), in ten cases through a block in the retrograde limb of the reentry pathway. In addition to a depression of the retrograde-conducting pathway (VA block at a stimulation interval of 281 ± 27 ms before propafenone, 449 ± 94 ms after propafenone) a depression of the anterograde-conducting limb was determined (1 : 1 AV conduction to a stimulation interval of 268 ± 54 ms before propafenone, 392 ± 49 ms after propafenone). In eight of the 13 patients the echo zone disappeared. In four patients tachycardia could be initiated again within 20 min, in some cases with a clearly widened echo zone (Fig. 4).

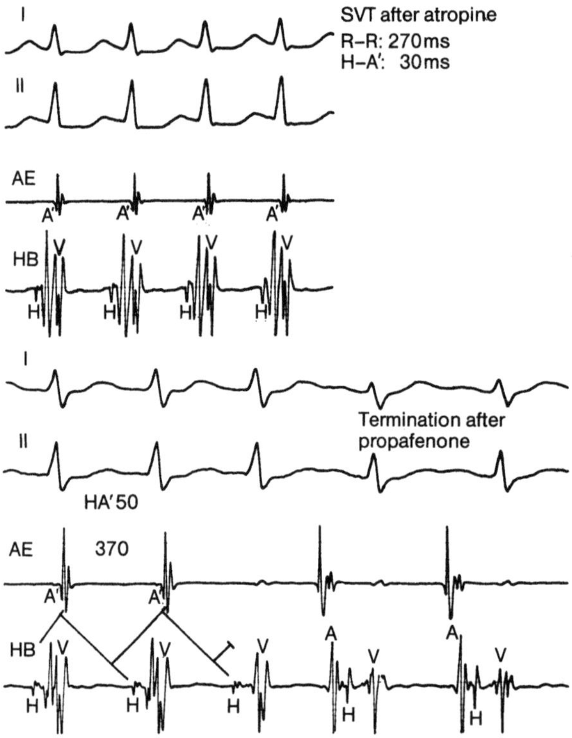

Fig. 3. ECG (leads I and II) and electrogram of high right atrium *(AE)* and His bundle *(HB)* of a 27-year-old female patient with AV node reentry tachycardia. *Above:* stable tachycardia (after atropine premedication) with an RR interval of 270 ms. *Below:* after propafenone, a clear decrease in tachycardia rate (RR interval 370 ms) through preferential increase of conduction time in the anterograde limb of the reentry pathway (increase of AH interval from 240 to 320 ms) and termination through block in the retrograde conducting pathway (ending of tachycardia with a ventricular complex which is followed by no retrograde atrial depolarisation)

Propafenone in WPW Syndrome

Propafenone also led to a reduction in tachycardia rate in the 12 patients with WPW syndrome and supraventricular reentry tachycardia (RR interval 318 ± 34 ms before propafenone, 397 ± 66 ms after propafenone), and in ten patients effected a termination through a block in the accessory pathway. A depression in the retrograde conducting capacity of the accessory pathway could be determined by rapid ventricular stimulation (1 : 1 AV conduction to a stimulation interval of 275 ± 29 ms before propafenone, 418 ± 104 ms after propafenone). Furthermore, the effective refractory period of the accessory VA conduction clearly increased (286 ± 24 ms before propafenone, 338 ± 43 ms after propafenone). The anterograde conduction capacity of the accessory pathway was also clearly depressed. In six cases an accessory pathway block occurred in sinus rhythm (under control conditions at 335 ± 100 ms) and in nine patients the stimulation rate which

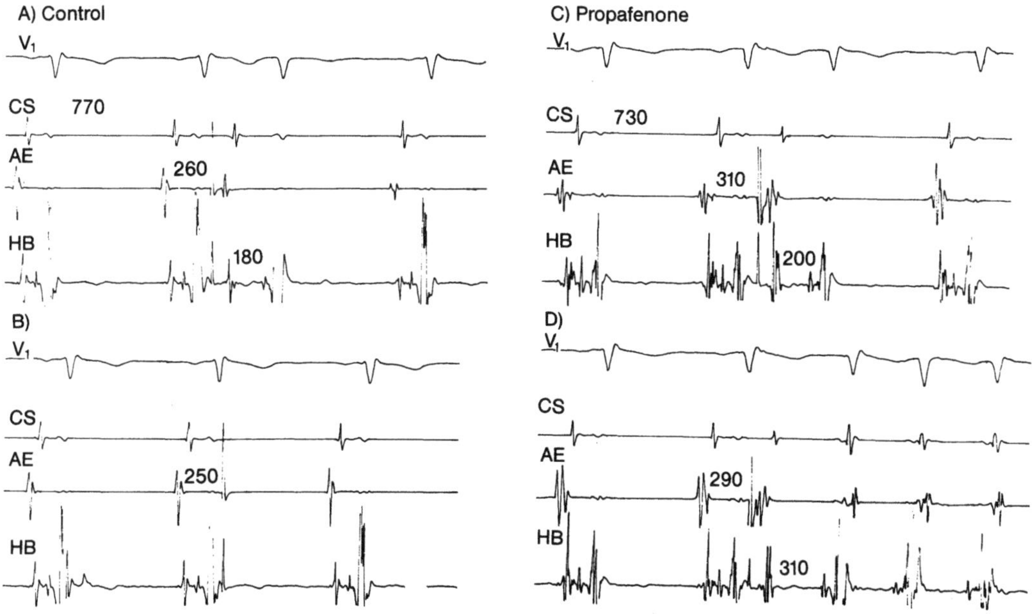

Fig. 4. **A** ECG (lead V_1) and electrogram of coronary sinus *(CS)*, high right atrium *(AE)* and His bundle *(HB)* in a 30-year-old male patient with AV node reentry tachycardia. Under control conditions, no paroxysm could be triggered in sinus rhythm; until attainment of the effective atrial refractory period (**B**) only an insufficient increase in the AH interval of induced atrial premature beats could be achieved. After propafenone (**C, D**), a coupling interval of 290 ms leads to a sharp increase in the AH interval of the atrial premature beats (the effective refractory period of the fast-conducting AV pathway is reached) and tachycardia starts

led to an accessory pathway block was clearly lower than under control conditions (control 227 ± 26 ms, propafenone 494 ± 125 ms; Fig. 5).

In induced atrial fibrillation (nine patients), propafenone clearly decreased the mean ventricular rate; the mean RR interval was 375 ± 66 ms before propafenone, 525 ± 118 ms after propafenone (Fig. 6).

Despite a clear depression in the conduction capacity of the accessory pathway, alleviation of tachycardia in 2 patients resulted from widening of the echo zone (Fig. 7).

Propafenone in Intraventricular Conduction Disturbances

Particularly marked increases of HV interval and QRS width were observed in the eight patients with intraventricular conduction disturbances. Only in one of three patients with documented paroxysmal AV block did a complete trifascicular block develop (Fig. 8, 9).

The electrophysiological findings described show propafenone to be an antiarrhythmic substance which leads to depression of conduction and lengthening of refractory periods in all sectors of the heart. This undoubtedly explains the wide range of clinical indications.

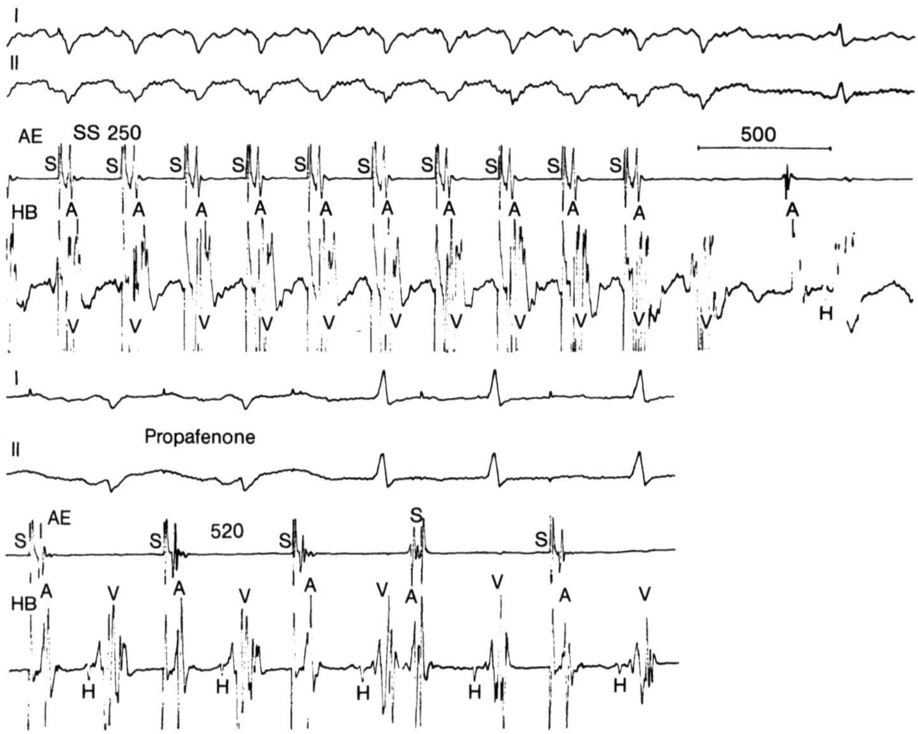

Fig. 5. ECG (leads I and II) and electrogram of high right atrium *(AE)* and His bundle *(HB)*. *Above:* under control conditions, 1:1 AV conduction over an accessory pathway until a stimulation interval of 250 ms was reached. *Below:* after propafenone treatment a block of accessory AV conduction under atrial stimulation first occurred at a stimulation interval of 520 ms

Nevertheless, in isolated cases these actions can have an arrhythmogenic effect, especially when in reentry the lengthening of refractory periods is neutralized by a considerable increase in conduction times in the reentry circuit.

The clinicoelectrophysiological findings indicate a risk for patients with manifest or latent lesions of sinus node function and AV conduction. The clinical significance of these side effects cannot yet be assessed.

Therapeutic Effectiveness of Propafenone

Noncontrolled clinical studies speak for therapeutic effectiveness in the conversion of atrial fibrillation (Beck et al. 1978; Ivancic and Goldner 1977), termination and prevention of supraventricular tachycardias present in WPW syndrome or produced by AV node reentry (Wiebringhaus et al. 1978; Neuss et al. 1979; Petri et al. 1978), termination and prevention of ventricular tachycardias (Baedeker et al. 1977; Theisen et al. 1977;

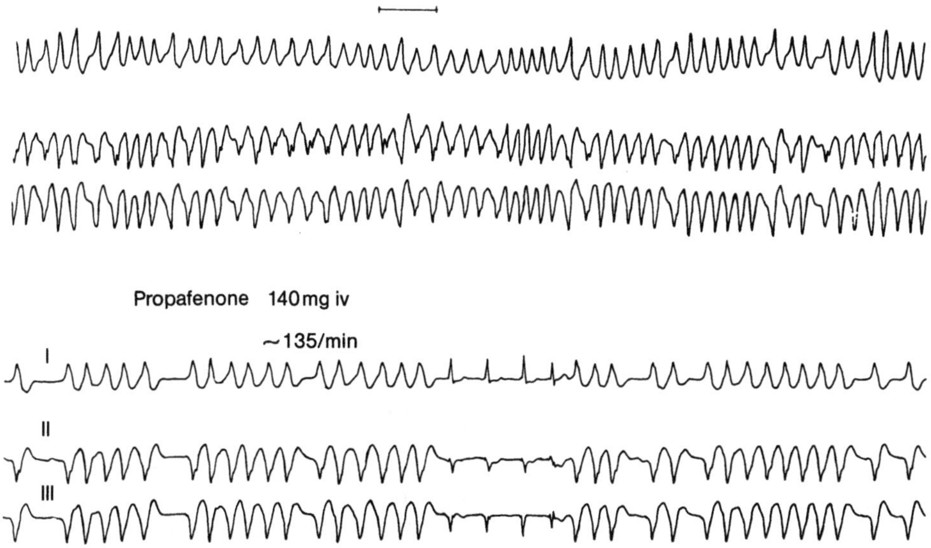

Fig. 6. ECG (leads I, II, and III) of a male patient with atrial fibrillation in WPW syndrome. *Above:* under control conditions the mean ventricular rate is about 220/min. *Below:* propafenone administration lowers the ventricular rate to an average 135/min by depression of the accessory pathway

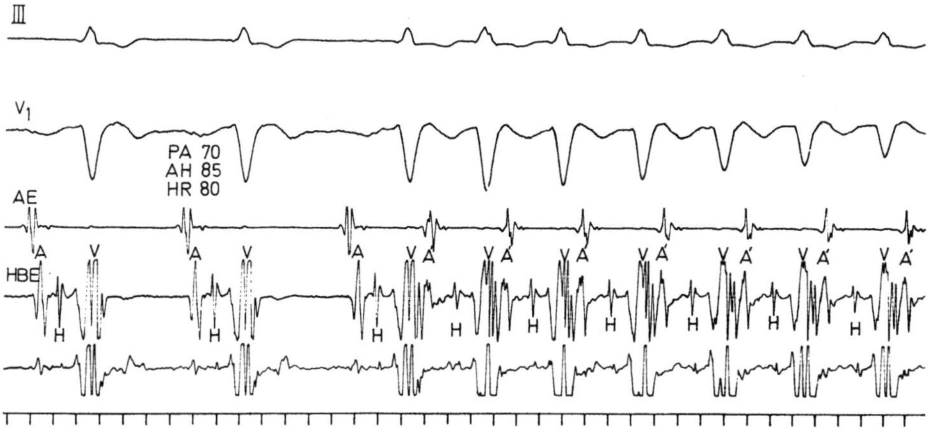

Fig. 7. Alleviation of onset of tachycardia in WPW syndrome. ECG (leads III and V_1) and electrogram of high right atrium *(AE)* and His bundle *(HBE)* in a 28-year-old male patient. After propafenone administration the accessory pathway ist blocked anterogradely during sinus rhythm (the signs of preexcitation have disappeared). Through the increase in AV conduction times (increase in PA, AH, and HV and occurrence of a left bundle-branch block) an excitation of sinus origin may reach the atrial myocardium (via the accessory pathway) outside its refractory period and initiate a reentry tachycardia

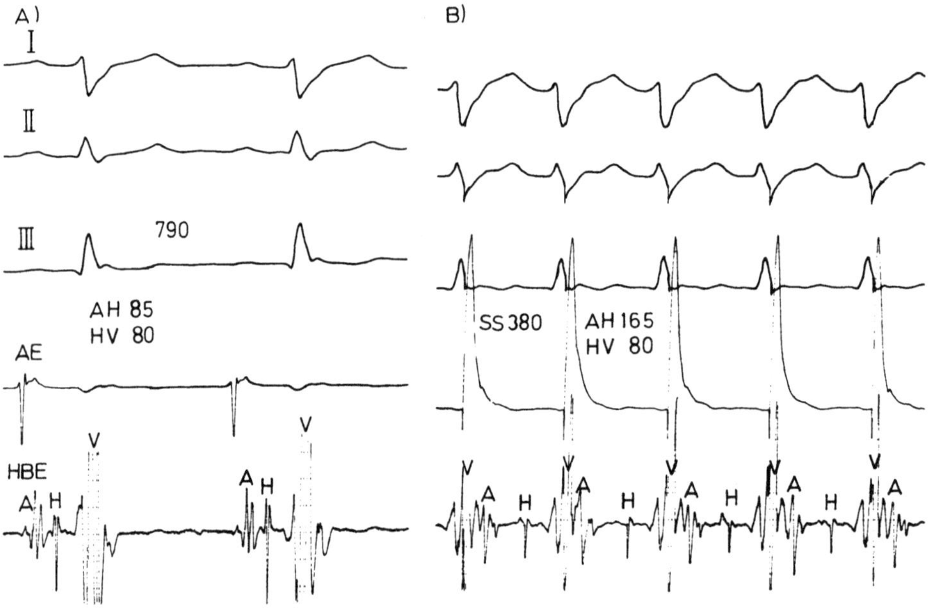

Fig. 8 A, B. ECG (leads I, II, and III) and electrogram of high right atrium *(AE)* and His bundle *(HBE)* in a male patient with documented complete AV block. Under control conditions, the ECG shows the signs of a bifascicular block; the HV interval is increased to 80 ms (**A**). During incremental pacing (**B**) no further disturbance of intraventricular conduction can be determined until attainment of the conduction capacity of the AV node (stimulation interval of 380 ms)

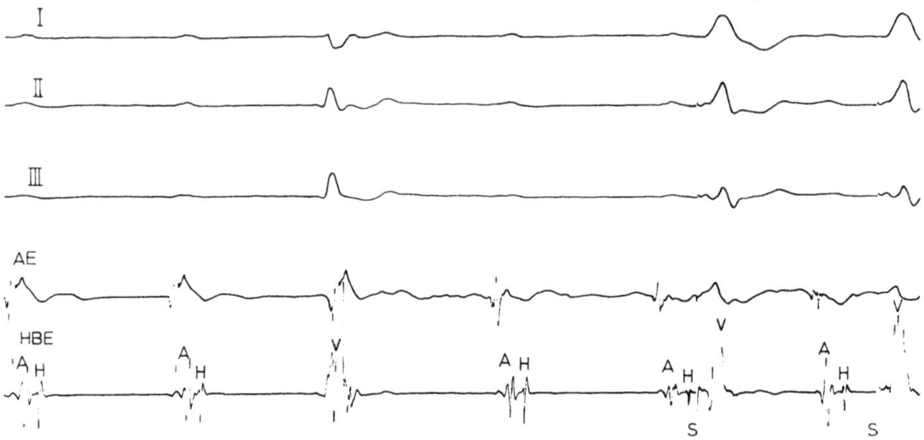

Fig. 9. Same patient as in Fig. 8. After injection of propafenone a complete trifascicular block appears; all atrial stimulation is blocked below the His bundle

Breithardt et al. 1980), and reduction or elimination of ventricular premature beats (Aldor and Heeger 1976; Beck et al. 1977; Fischer and Seipel 1977; Koch 1977).

The number of controlled clinical studies published is still small (Klein et al. 1980; Wieser et al. 1979; Rutsch 1978), and in some cases there are reservations about the methods, so the question of the value of the drug in the treatment of arrhythmias is difficult to answer.

Two problems arising from the discussion of the results of two of our own controlled studies should be addressed.

Comparison of Propafenone and Disopyramide

In a randomized, single-blind, crossover trial we investigated the antiarrhythmic effectiveness of propafenone (3 × 150 mg/day) and disopyramide (4 × 150 mg/day) in stable ventricular premature beats (> 300 VPB/h). Figure 10 gives the study protocol.

The two agents showed themselves to be of comparable effectiveness (Table 3). Individual results indicated that propafenone at the chosen dose level did not afford complete protection against arrhythmia over 24 h; in a few cases (four patients) it displayed a loss of effect 4–6 h after administration. This can best be explained by its relatively short elimination half-life of about 3–4 h. It is probable that at the low dosage chosen the plasma concentration falls to subtherapeutic levels toward the end of the 8-h dose interval.

Comparison of Propafenone and Tocainide

The second study had the same structure (Fig. 10): Propafenone (3 × 300 mg/day for 6 days) was compared with tocainide (3 × 400 mg/day for 6 days) for effect on chronic ventricular premature beats. As expected, the higher dose achieved an extensive decrease of ventricular premature beats (Table 4). The antiarrhythmic effect was also more constant through the day. There were no longer any important fluctuations in the hourly frequency of premature beats, and no relationship with dose interval could be shown.

However, the higher doses had clear side effects. One patient complained of orthopnea and displayed obvious signs of lung congestion. A second developed sinoatrial block with pauses of up to 3 s and a third suffered ventricular fibrillation after the second dose.

Table 3. Propafenone vs disopyramide: randomized single-blind trial in 12 patients with stable ventricular premature beats (> 300/h)

Group	VPB/h	Reduction (%)
Control	1096 ± 544	–
Propafenone	612 ± 503	44
Disopyramide	560 ± 471	49

Control against propafenone: $P < 0.01$
Control against disopyramide: $P < 0.005$
Disopyramide against propafenone: n.s.

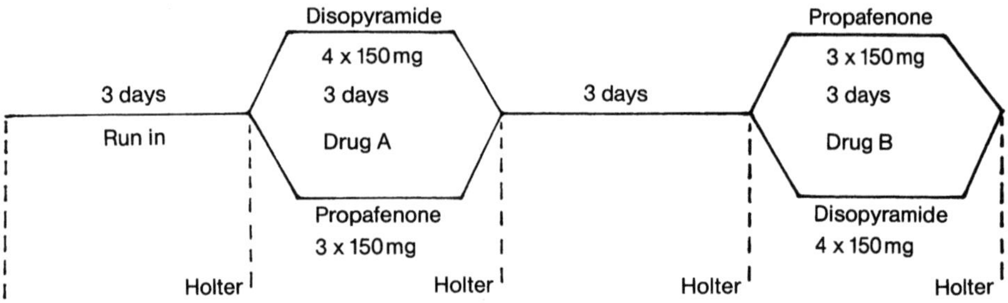

Fig. 10. Protocol of a controlled study to compare the antiarrhythmic effect of propafenone and disopyramide on patients with stable ventricular premature beats. The study comparing propafenone and tocainide was similarly organized, but the drugs were given for 6 days each and the daily doses were different (propafenone 3 × 300 mg and tocainide 3 × 400 mg)

Table 4. Propafenone vs tocainide: double-blind trial in 12 patients with coronary heart disease and stable ventricular premature beats (> 300/h)

Group	VPB/h	Reduction (%)
Control	689 ± 351	–
Propafenone	151 ± 198	78
Tocainide	191 ± 221	72

Control against propafenone: $P < 0.001$
Control against tocainide: $P < 0.001$
Tocainide against propafenone: n. s.

Table 5. Reported side effects (report on clinical investigation, Knoll AG, 1980)

Side effects	No. of cases
Cardiac	223 (of 1723 patients)
1. Depression of sinus node function	38
2. AV block	46
3. Triggering of arrhythmia	3
4. Cardiac failure	4
5. Hypotension	8
Extracardiac	88 (of 614 patients)
1. Anorexia, nausea, vomiting	23
2. Dizziness	20
3. Taste disturbances	18
4. Blurred vision	11
5. Constipation	13
6. Cholostatic hepatitis	2

Side Effects of Propafenone Therapy

In view of the conflicting opinions on the prognostic value of antiarrhythmic therapy, the risk of antiarrhythmic therapy may be an important means of selection between the various agents.

The side effects reported during propafenone therapy hardly differ in type or frequency from those of other group I antiarrhythmics (Table 5). Again there are no controlled studies, and therefore evaluation of propafenone is impossible. Of special significance here would be studies involving patients with prognostically relevant arrhythmias, which often yield hemodynamic and electrocardiographic evidence of more or less diffuse myocardial damage. It is in the treatment of these patients, and not in the therapy of, e.g., ventricular premature beats with no organopathological substrate, that the value and risk of antiarrhythmic agents will best be assessed.

References

Aldor E, Heeger H (1976) Propafenon – ein neues Antiarrhythmikum. Dtsch Med Wochenschr 101: 1318

Baedeker W, Wirtzfeld A, Sack D, Oversohl K (1977) Die antiarrhythmische Wirkung von Propafenon bei ventrikulären Tachykardien. Herz Kreislauf 9: 348

Beck OA, Witt E, Hochrein H (1975) Der Einfluß des Antiarrhythmikums Propafenon auf die intrakardiale Erregungsleitung. Z Kardiol 64: 179

Beck OA, Abdulla S, Hochrein H (1977) Wirkung und Dosis-Wirkungs-Beziehung von Propafenon nach peroraler Anwendung. In: Hochrein H, Hapke H-J, Beck OA (Hrsg) Fortschritte in der Pharmakotherapie von Herzrhythmusstörungen. Fischer, Stuttgart

Beck OA, Lehmann H-U, Hochrein H (1978) Propafenon und Lidoflazin bei chronischem Vorhofflimmern und -flattern. Dtsch Med Wochenschr 103: 1068

Breithardt G, Seipel L, Höhfeld E, Both A, Loogen F (1975) Pharmakologische Beeinflussung der "sinu-atrialen Leitungszeit" und der Sinusknotenautomatie beim Menschen. Z Kardiol 64: 895

Breithardt G, Seipel L, Abendroth RR, Loogen F (1980) Serial electrophysiological testing of antiarrhythmic drug efficacy in patients with recurrent ventricular tachycardia. Eur Heart J 1: 11

Fischer G, Seipel L (1977) Klinische Erfahrung mit der oralen Propafenon-Therapie. In: Hochrein H, Hapke H-H, Beck OA (Hrsg) Fortschritte in der Pharmakotherapie von Herzrhythmusstörungen. Fischer, Stuttgart

Ivancić R, Goldner V (1977) Propafenon in der Therapie der Extrasystolien – unsere Erfahrungen. In: Hochrein H, Hapke H-H, Beck OA (Hrsg) Fortschritte in der Pharmakotherapie von Herzrhythmusstörungen. Fischer, Stuttgart

Klein G, Wirtzfeld A, Schlegel J, Himmler C, Neiß A (1980) Antiarrhythmika bei chronischer ventrikulärer Extrasystolie. Dtsch Med Wochenschr 105: 189

Koch R (1977) Zur Propafenon-Wirkung bei ventrikulärer Arrhythmie. In: Hochrein H, Hapke H-H, Beck OA (Hrsg) Fortschritte in der Pharmakotherapie von Herzrhythmusstörungen. Fischer, Stuttgart

Neuss H, Mitrovíc V, Schlepper M, Thormann J (1979) Propafenon bei supraventrikulären Tachykardien durch Re-entry in der AV-Region. Z Kardiol 68: 256

Petri H, Kafka W, Rudolph W (1978) Der Einfluß von Propafenon auf das akzessorische Bündel (AB) bei Patienten mit WPW-Syndrom. Z Kardiol [Suppl] 5: 50

Rutsch W (1978) Beeinflussung der ventrikulären Extrasystolie durch Propafenon. Herz Kreislauf 10: 183

Seipel L, Breithardt G, Both A (1975) Elektrophysiologische Effekte der Antiarrhythmika Disopyramid und Propafenon auf das menschliche Reizleitungssystem. Z Kardiol 64: 731

Theisen F, Theisen K, Jahrmärker H, Rackwitz R (1977) Elektrophysiologische und therapeutische Beobachtungen bei lebensbedrohlichen Tachykardien. Z Kardiol [Suppl] 4: 39

Wiebringhaus E, Seipel L, Breithardt G (1978) Antiarrhythmische Therapie beim WPW-Syndrom mit Propafenon. Z Kardiol [Suppl] 5: 49

Wieser H, Philippi M, Schuler CF (1979) Die antiarrhythmische Wirkung von Propafenon bei stabiler ventrikulärer Extrasystolie. Herz Kreislauf 11: 71

Pharmacokinetic and Metabolic Studies on Propafenone in Volunteers*

M. Hollmann, H. G. Hege, E. Brode, V. Bühler, D. Hotz, S. Kaumeier, O. H. Kehrhahn, H. Lietz, J. A. Schwarz, B. Stieren and J. Weymann

Knowledge of the pharmacokinetic and metabolic behavior of propafenone in humans has been limited mainly by difficulties in analysis and in using radioactively labeled substances. In earlier studies by Wiebringhaus, Keller, and Blanke et al. in Düsseldorf, Berlin, and Göttingen and in our research center in Ludwigshafen, the method used allowed sufficiently precise determinations only above a concentration of 200 ng/ml, which left some uncertainty about the selectivity of the method and the process of elimination, especially regarding the terminal elimination phase.

The data presented here are the results of several pharmacokinetic and metabolic studies on propafenone undertaken during 1981 with volunteers; by that time a very sensitive assay for propafenone quantification and a new system for structural evaluation of metabolites had been developed and established. The paper focuses on kinetic data on the elimination of the drug after intravenous administration and on its metabolism.

Pharmacokinetics of Propafenone

The following results are based on a high-pressure liquid chromatographic assay with internal analogue standardization; with 2-ml plasma samples it allows determination of levels as low as 5 ng/ml with high precision and accuracy. Metabolites were studied using deuterated substance in a number of volunteers and in a patient with a biliary fistula in whom the use of radioactivity could be avoided.

Most of the volunteers – whose physical characteristics are shown in Fig. 1 – were members of our research center, where the study was undertaken after the participants had given their written consent.

The results of experiments are illustrated in Fig. 2. The curve representing plasma concentration versus time was obtained after injecting 16 people intravenously with 70 mg propafenone each, and is expressed as median values with confidence limits. Analysis of the curves from the various participants showed that an open two-compartment model could be used in all subjects. After a short initial distribution phase the 2-min peak values of ca. 1 000 ng/ml rapidly dropped to levels between 200 and 300 ng/ml and then decreased with a half-life of about 3 h. After 24 h only four subjects had plasma levels above 5 ng/ml.

Table 1 presents the mean and median values for the apparent volume of the central compartment (V_c) and for the volume after distribution (V_B). The values for the latter

---

* The chapter on pharmacokinetics was presented by M. Hollmann et al., the chapter on metabolic studies by H. G. Hege

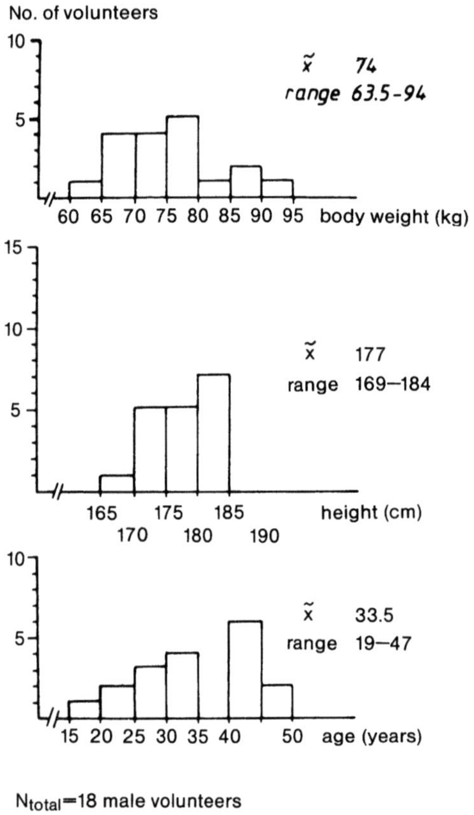

Fig. 1. Distribution, medians (x̃) and ranges for body weight, height, and age of volunteers in propafenone studies

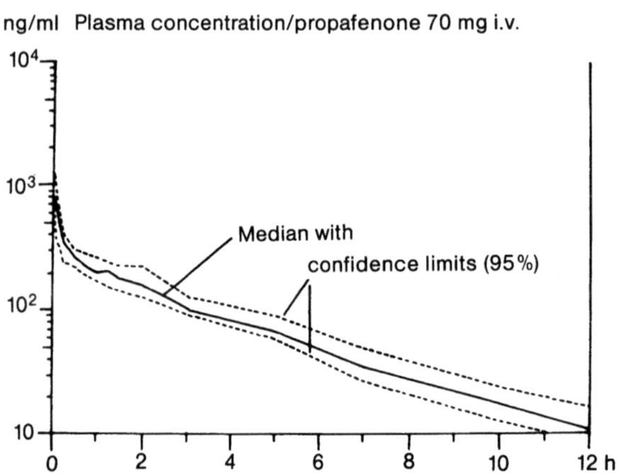

Fig. 2. Plasma concentration of propafenone after i. v. injection of 70 mg per volunteer

Table 1. Pharmacokinetics of propafenone (70 mg i. v.)

$n = 16$	$\bar{x}$ (mean)	$\tilde{x}$ (median)	range
$T_{½}$ (h)	2.83	2.48	2.09–5.21
V_C (liter/kg)	1.23	1.01	0.45–3.45
V_B (liter/kg)	3.44	3.10	2.40–5.61
Total $clearance_{iv}$ (ml/min)	1061	1129	441–1375

Table 2. Comparison of half-life and total clearance for propafenone injected (70 mg i. v.) before and after 12 days of oral administration (300 mg/day)

$n = 8$		$\bar{x}$ (mean)	$\tilde{x}$ (median)	range
$T_{½}$ (h)	Before	2.82	2.48	2.31– 5.21
	After	3.92	2.64	2.10– 9.42
Total $clearance_{iv}$ (ml/min)	Before	1012	1075	441 –1375
	After	895	1054	239 –1271

(3–4 liters/kg) exceed any real space; thus, one can assume that, in addition to plasma protein binding of more than 95%, considerable binding takes place within the tissues. The total clearance value representing all metabolic and excretory processes was calculated to be more than 1 liter/min.

Taking into account the plasma/blood distribution ratio of more than 1.2, the total clearance value approaches the average hepatic blood flow value of 1.5 liters/min. Since only very small amounts of propafenone are excreted unchanged via urine and feces total clearance is handled largely by metabolism, most probably in the liver and dependent upon its blood flow.

In order to check on possible changes in the pharmacokinetic behavior of propafenone under steady-state conditions, intravenous injections were repeated after oral doses had been given for several days (Table 2). The change in half-life did not reach statistical significance. Neither was the slight decrease in total clearance significant, although it decreased further to 239 and 308 ml/min respectively in the two volunteers who had had the lowest initial clearance values.

On the whole, the results confirm earlier data and define them more precisely. Based on the total clearance values and extraction rate, which numerically exceed the unbound fraction of the plasma concentration of the drug, the elimination of propafenone is characterized by intensive metabolism, unrestricted by plasma protein binding.

The Metabolism of Propafenone in Man

An has been pointed out, total clearance of propafenone is dominated by hepatic metabolism and only very small amounts of propafenone are excreted unchanged via urine and feces. After oral administration, propafenone accounts for only 10% of the total me-

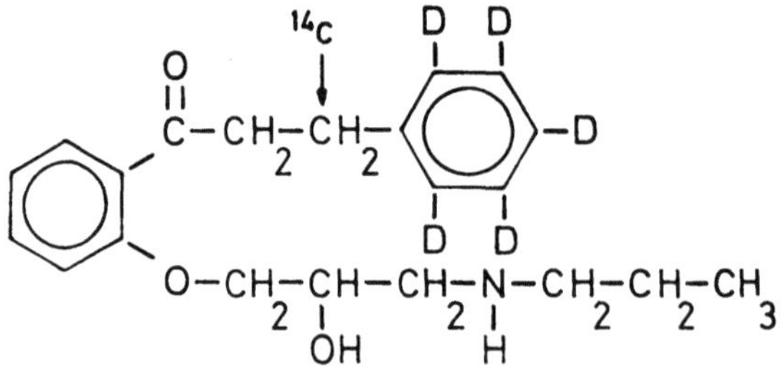

Propafenone [^{14}C, ^{2}H]

Fig. 3. Labeling sites for carbon-14 and deuterium in the propafenone molecule

tabolites in plasma at the peak plasma level; the other 90% are conjugated or in the form of polar metabolites at this time. This raises a question as to the structure and quantity of the metabolites.

In animals, investigations of absorption, distribution, metabolism and excretion are normally carried out after administration of the radioactively labeled substance. The fate of the drug and its metabolites can thus be monitored rather simply by measuring the radioactive tracer in the biological material. For this purpose propafenone labeled with carbon-14 was synthesized, and blood level time curves and the excretion of propafenone and its metabolites were measured in different animal species. The structure of the excretion products was elucidated by means of mass spectrometry.

There are obvious restrictions on the administration of radioactive isotopes to man, and a large amount of work must be done with animals before studies with humans can be started. In man, therefore, metabolic studies with stable isotopes have recently been given preference. The microwave plasma detector in combination with chromatographic methods, in our experience, is very well suited following the fate of deuterated substances in biological material. Using this detector after administration of the deuterated drug, we were able to perform all the metabolic studies in man which have previously been carried out in animals using the radioactive labeled substance.

Figure 3 shows the labeling sites in the propafenone molecule. In order to achieve clear-cut conclusions the labeling sites should be metabolically as stable as possible. For the synthesis of carbon-14-labeled and deuterium-labeled compounds we therefore chose sites in the propiophenone part of the molecule which were most likely to meet this requirement. Labeling with deuterium is effected in the phenyl ring on the right side of the molecule, where all five hydrogen atoms are exchanged for deuterium.

Table 3. Studies performed on the metabolism of propafenone in man

Study	Method(s)	Aim
Excretion	Measurement of total deuterium (MPD)	Amount and route of excretion
Metabolic pattern	Chromatography (TLC, LC, GC)	Comparison with other species
Isolation of metabolites	Mass spectroscopy (MS)	Elucidation of structure

MPD, microwave plasma detector; TLC, thin-layer chromatography; LC, liquid chromatography; GC, gas chromatography

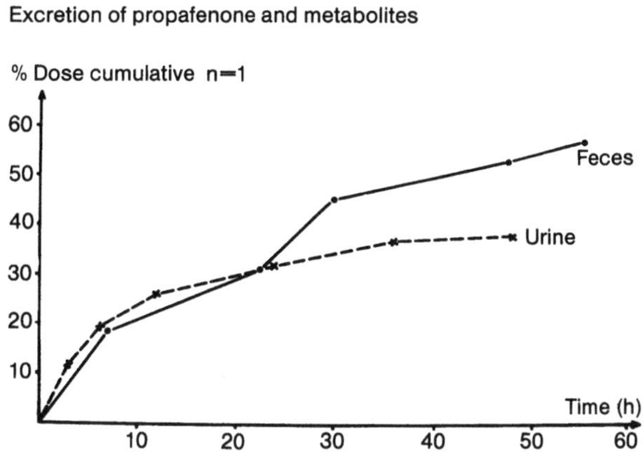

Fig. 4. Excretion of propafenone and its metabolites via urine and feces

Table 3 lists studies done in man on the metabolism of propafenone. The preferred route and duration of excretion were determined by measuring the total deuterium content of the excretion products with the microwave plasma detector. Next a metabolic pattern of the excretion products was established in order to determine the number of separate metabolites formed and their quantities, compared with other species. This required chromatographic separation of the metabolites. Finally the metabolites were isolated and their structures were determined by means of mass spectrometry and by comparison of chromatographic and spectroscopic data with available reference substances.

Excretion

The main route of excretion is via the feces (see Fig. 4); 57% of the dose is excreted within 55 h by this route, 38% via the urine. Excretion is rapid; 77% is eliminated as early as 30 h after administration and 91% after 48 h.

Metabolic pattern

Figure 5 shows on the left the metabolic pattern before enzymatic cleavage and on the right after. Metabolic profiles similar to this one are obtained in the urine and bile as well. It should be emphasized that plasma and both excreta contain predominantly conjugated metabolites. Only about 10% of the metabolites in plasma, urine, and bile are unconjugated.

Structure elucidation

Figure 6 shows the structure of the propafenone molecule. In analogy to other compounds with similar structure, the following enzymatic reactions can be expected:

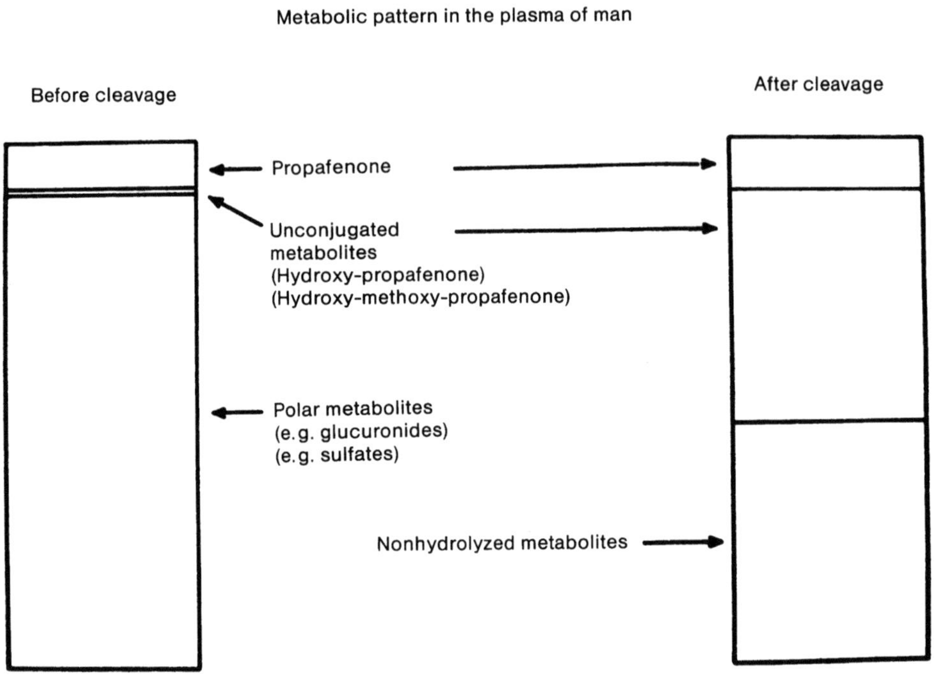

Fig. 5. Metabolic pattern in human plasma before (*left*) and after (*right*) cleavage

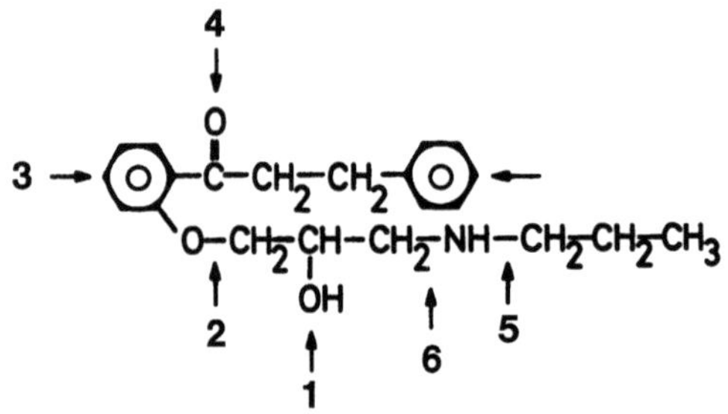

Fig. 6. Possible enzymatic attack on the propafenone molecule

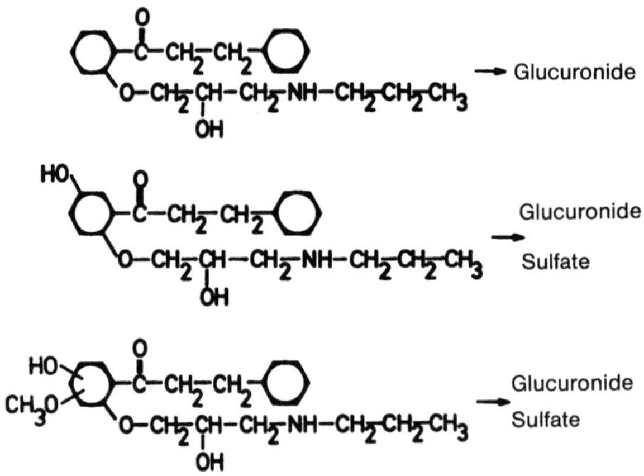

Fig. 7. The main metabolites which have been found in man

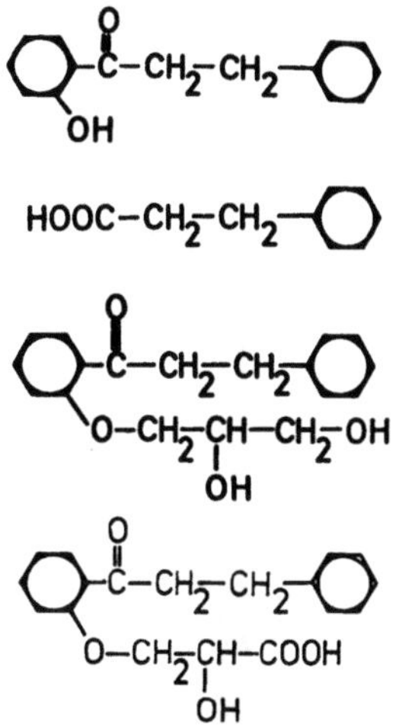

Fig. 8. Metabolites which are primarily excreted unconjugated, and are present only in small quantities

1. The alcohol group can be conjugated directly, e.g., with glucuronic acid or sulphuric acid.
2. Ether cleavage.
3. Oxydation reactions at the aromatic rings.
4. The keto group can be affected by enzymes.
5. Dealkylation.
6. Oxydative deamination.

Figure 7 and Figure 8 show the molecular structures of metabolites which have in fact been found in man. Figure 7 represents the major metabolites that account for more than 80% of the dose in plasma, urine, bile and feces. As already mentioned, these compounds occur in plasma and excreta mainly in the form of conjugates, only about 10% of the dose being excreted in the form of free, unconjugated metabolites. Propafenone, for example, is bound to glucuronic acid in the alcohol group. The two metabolites hydroxylated in the phenylene ring have been shown to be bound to both glucuronic acid and sulphuric acid. Most important in the quantitative sense is the metabolite hydroxylated in paraposition to ether oxygen.

A corresponding compound with a single hydroxy substitution in metaposition has not yet been found. On the other hand, two isomers of hydroxy-methoxy metabolites have been identified. We still do not know the exact positions of the hydroxy and methoxy groups. The two isomers are probably formed via a dihydroxy compound as a common precursor which is then O-methylated – probably similar to O-methylation of catecholamines. The quantitative ratio of hydroxy-propafenone to hydroxy-methoxy-propafenone to propafenone is about 3:2:1.

Surprisingly, the aromatic ring on the right side of the molecule is not affected in man. Species-related differences to the rat and the dog are evident here. The rat oxydizes the final ring almost exclusively, while the dog is capable of oxydizing both aromatic rings.

Ether cleavage leading to the first structure in Fig. 8 plays a subordinate role in the metabolism of propafenone in man. Cleavage adjacent to the keto group results in 3-phenylpropionic acid. The mechanism of this reaction is still unclear. The fact that this metabolite is found primarily in the feces, and only in negligible quantities in urine and

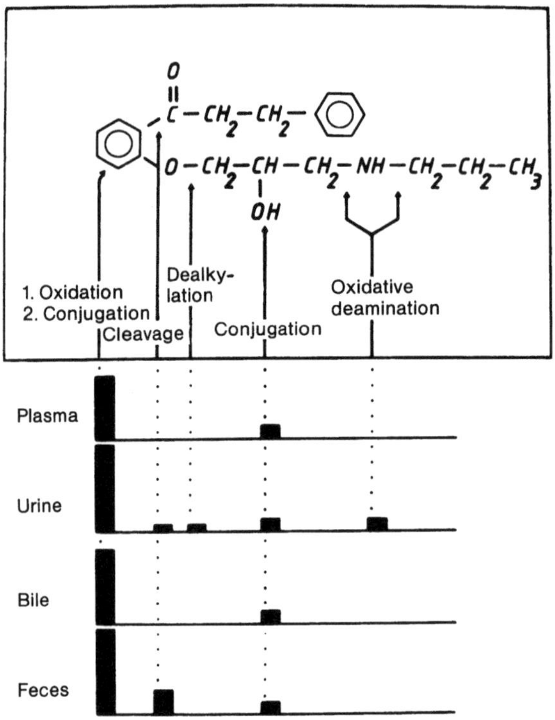

Fig. 9. Summary of the metabolic reactions of propafenone in man

bile, indicates that it might not be formed in the liver but rather by attack of intestinal bacteria on enterally excreted metabolites.

None of the two metabolic products formed by oxydative deamination shown as structures 3 and 4 of Fig. 8 is of any great quantitative importance. This reaction probably leads to an aldehyde which is reduced to an alcohol and/or oxidized to the corresponding acid. A glycol derivative and a substituted lactic acid were shown to be the end products of this type of reaction.

The metabolic reactions of propafenone in man are summarized in Fig. 9.

The quantitative importance of the different metabolites can be estimated from the lower part of Fig. 9.

Metabolically, propafenone fits very well into the group of lipophilic drugs with a similar ether side chain. Hydroxylation and conjugation reactions are the main metabolic pathways in the metabolism of propafenone in man.

Acknowledgements: We wish to thank E. Brode, V. Bühler, D. Hotz, S. Kaumeier, O. H. Kehrhahn, H. Lietz, J. A. Schwarz, B. Stieren, and J. Weymann – all members of the biochemical, human pharmacology, and biometric departments of BASF/KNOLL – for their contributions to the results of this study.

Effects of Propafenone on Hemodynamics and Cardiac Inotropy

M. Schlepper and H. Neuss

The aim of antiarrhythmic treatment is to prevent dangerous arrhythmias which might cause sudden death, to abolish or to minimize disturbing subjective symptoms, but also to improve haemodynamics by abolishing existing cardiac arrhythmias. The suppression of such haemodynamically significant arrhythmias may have a net effect on cardiac pump function that masks possible negative inotropic actions. When trying to unmask these unwanted effects one faces several difficulties, since antiarrhythmic drugs can alter certain haemodynamic parameters, which in turn can either diminish or enhance the direct action such a drug may have on the contractile performance. Ideally, the components influencing the heart's overall pump function, such as pre- and afterload, contractility, and heart rate, should be analysed separately. However, in comparison to the animal model these factors are difficult to assess in the clinical setting, and their influence and complex interaction often can only be speculated upon.

The investigation of healthy individuals is important, but results obtained from these groups are generally unacceptable, if not misleading, since arrhythmias do not occur in such a group. Arrhythmias with hazardous haemodynamic consequences are, however, only found in diseased hearts with very few exceptions, i. e. tachycardias confined to the atria and the AV node with and without the existence of accessory pathways. Hence, studies should be carried out with priority on patients with impaired ventricular function. Particular attention has to be paid to haemodynamic and negative inotropic side effects, when tachycardia persists in spite of lege artis administration of antiarrhythmic drugs.

According to theoretical standpoint haemodynamic and inotropic effects of antiarrhythmic drugs should be investigated in various groups:

1) In volunteers or patients without arrhythmias
   a) with apparently healthy and
   b) with diseased hearts.
2) In patients in whom the arrhythmia can be abolished, thus improving their circulatory condition.
3) In patients whose arrhythmias cannot be abolished in spite of proper administration of antiarrhythmic drugs.

In groups 2 and 3 the tachycardia may occur in patients with apparently healthy hearts. Some of the arrhythmias in these groups can be simulated by special stimulation techniques. Assessment of contractility and overall pump function as well as the components influencing this function requires different methodological approaches.

Similar to the beta-blockers and calcium antagonists with antiarrhythmic properties membrane active antiarrhythmic drugs of class 1 have to be considered as potentially negative inotropic agents. The negative inotropic effect differs, however, in degree. Mexilitine, tocainide and encainide are reported to elicit far less negative inotropic action than disopyramide (Jewitt 1980). The negative inotropic effects of this drug seem well established in patients under acute and chronic treatment with disopyramide. In a placebo – controlled study on 18 patients with recent myocardial infarction, 100 mg of disopyramide i.v. over 5 min significantly prolonged pre-ejection period (PEP), thus increasing the ratio of PEP to LV ejection time (Hillis et al. 1976). In 4 patients with impaired ventricular function and 6 with normally functioning hearts disopyramide in a dose of 1.5 mg/kg i.v. over 2 min significantly reduced cardiac index and stroke work index and to a greater degree in patients with an abnormal left ventricular function both during sinus rhythm and at a stable heart rate achieved by atrial pacing (Sutton 1976). Of 100 patients consecutively treated with oral disopyramide, 16 developed cardiac failure. The majority of these 16 patients had a history of previous congestive failure (Podrid et al. 1980). Following administration of disopyramide electromechanical dissociation was observed in patients with severe congestive failure and renal insufficiency (Desai et al. 1978).

Compared with investigations of other antiarrhythmic drugs, studies on propafenone have only been carried out in a few instances. Breithardt et al. (1978) examined the systolic time intervals in healthy volunteers before and after oral administration of various antiarrhythmic drugs. A dose dependent alteration of these parameters by propafenone indicating a negative inotropic action was demonstrated. Possinger et al. (1980) reported on one patient in whom signs of pulmonary congestion occurred concomitantly with an increase of the PEP/LVET ratio after oral administration of both N-prajmalinebitartrate (60 mg/die) and propafenone (450 mg/die). These reactions were not elicited by mexilitine (600 mg/die).

In 5 patients with unimpaired ventricular function Probst and Pachinger (1976) demonstrated a slight decrease in the left ventricular systolic pressure and a moderate increase in LVEDP, neither of them significant. Contractility, however, as measured by dp/dt max significantly decreased by 22.3%. The maximum effect was noted 10 min after the injection of 2 mg/kg propafenone administered over a period of 2 min. In a more extensive study, patients with coronary heart disease, 60% of whom had a history of previous myocardial infarction, were investigated by Bachour et al. (1974). Following i.v. injection of 70 mg propafenone there was a decrease in systolic blood pressure, while PC-wedge pressure and mean pulmonary artery pressure increased by 17% and 8% respectively. Cardiac output was reduced by 15%. The maximum effect was observed between 5 and 15 min post injection, with an average duration of 16 min. Apparently the negative haemodynamic effect prevailed over the antiarrhythmic effect, and thus a second cardio-circulatory depressive effect could be observed when dysrhythmias reccurred.

From the reviewed literature it becomes obvious that relatively few studies have been undertaken to clarify the haemodynamic and inotropic effects of propafenone. These results, however, definitely indicate potential negative inotropic side effects of the drug, which is not surprising.

Investigations comparing various antiarrhythmic drugs with regard to their ratio of antiarrhythmic efficacy/negative inotropic action are practically nonexistent. Jewitt (1980) draws his conclusion from data collected from the literature. Breithardt et al. (1978) compared the negative inotropic effects of several antiarrhythmic drugs administered in the usual therapeutic oral dosage by measuring systolic time intervals in healthy individuals who naturally did not exhibit any arrhythmias. 4 class 1 antiarrhythmic substances (chinidinsulfate 3 × 250 mg; N-prajmaline-bitratrate 4 × 20 mg; disopyramide

4 × 100 mg, and propafenone 4 × 150 mg) were administered in comparable time intervals and 4 h after the last application measurements were taken. There were no differences in the degree of the negative inotropic effects of these 4 drugs, which increased PEP to the same extent and left LVET unaffected. Prolongation of PEP was not related to increased intraventricular conduction as measured by the width of QRS. Therefore the alterations of PEP really reflect changes in inotropy, and this all the more so since this parameter is independent of alterations of pre- and afterload. LVET was not affected by the dosage applied. A dosage-dependent increase of the negative inotropic effect could only be observed when propafenone was administered in the unusually high dose of 4 × 300 mg/die, while comparably high dosages of other antiarrhythmic agents were not used.

If the data from the literature are judged against the theoretical "prerequisites" given at the beginning, the lack of knowledge regarding negative inotropic side effects of antiarrhythmic drugs becomes apparent. The extent to which the results obtained depend on the methodological approach of the studies will be demonstrated by results from our own, as yet incomplete investigations.

8 patients suffering from aortic regurgitation (grade II NYHA) underwent exercise testing as part of the routine diagnostic procedure. These patients were exercised with an individually chosen submaximal work load (75–125 W) on a bicycle ergometer until steady state was reached. At rest and during steady state cardiac output (CO) was determined according to the Fick principle, and mean pulmonary artery pressure (PAP_m), blood pressure and heart rate were measured at the same time. The patients were then allowed to rest until all parameters were back to the initial rest values. Thereafter, with the consent of the patients a bolus of 2 mg/kg propafenone was injected over 5 min and a second identical course of exercise tests was started during which ⅙ of the initial bolus dosage was administered by constant infusion. When the random data of all participants before (abscissa) and after (ordinate) propafenone administration are arranged on a 45° identity line, it shows that the drug does not appear to have any effect on the four parameters (Fig. 1). No statistically significant differences were obtained by using the t-test on the data.

When CO and PAP_m were correlated (Fig. 2) the mean values of both did not significantly differ from those before and after propafenone application, either at rest or during exercise in steady state. However, the standard deviation is considerable and for that reason not included in Fig. 2.

In spite of the diseased hearts and a relatively high dosage of Propafenone these investigations (Gigler et al.) do not point to an evident or even marked negative inotropic effect of the drug. Since effects on pre- and afterload are apparently missing, counterbalance by alterations of these parameters cannot be considered. Even though this method serves as a routine diagnostic procedure, it might be insensitive so that cardiac depressive effects can only be excluded tentatively. The wide deviation of values and the different starting points of the patients have to be considered as well. In 4 out of the 8 patients propafenone increased PAP_m with an additional rise during exercise in comparison to the values before propafenone application and a smaller increase of CO.

In order to obtain results on a potentially negative inotropic action when propafenone is "unsuccessful" in abolishing arrhythmias with haemodynamic consequences, these situations were simulated in patients routinely undergoing electrophysiological treatment for paroxysmal supraventricular tachycardias by sequential AV-pacing tech-

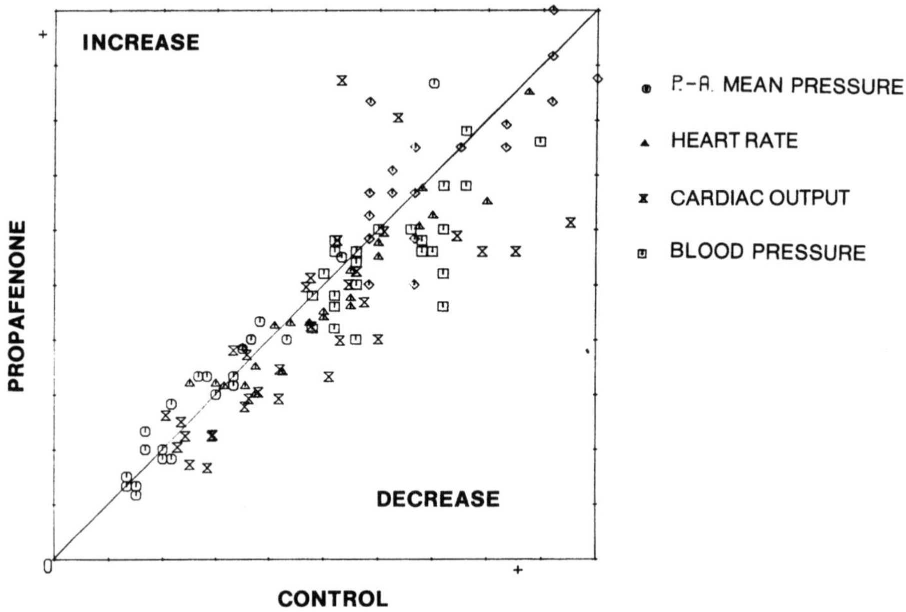

Fig. 1. Values of mean pulmonary arterial pressure, heart rate, blood pressure and cardiac output before and after propafenone arranged on a 45° identity line. No statistically significant difference could be ascertained for the 4 parameters

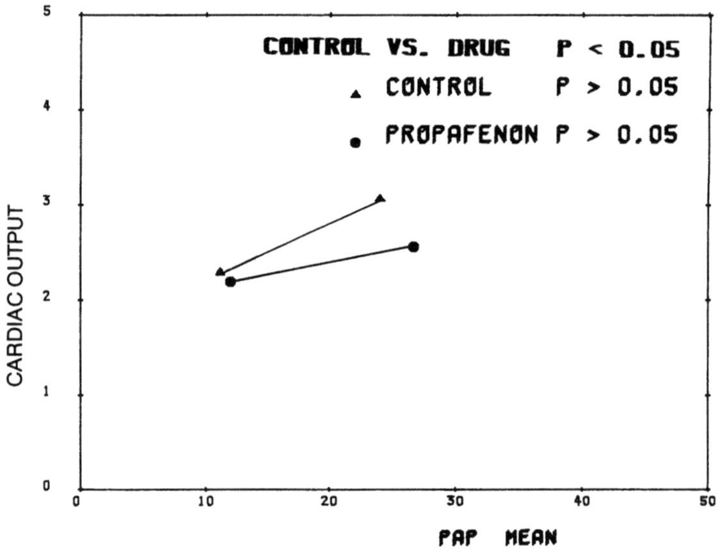

Fig. 2. Mean values of cardiac output and mean pulmonary artery pressure of 8 patients with aortic regurgitation grade II. At rest and during exercise before and after propafenone there is no statistically significant difference. No SD is given (see text)

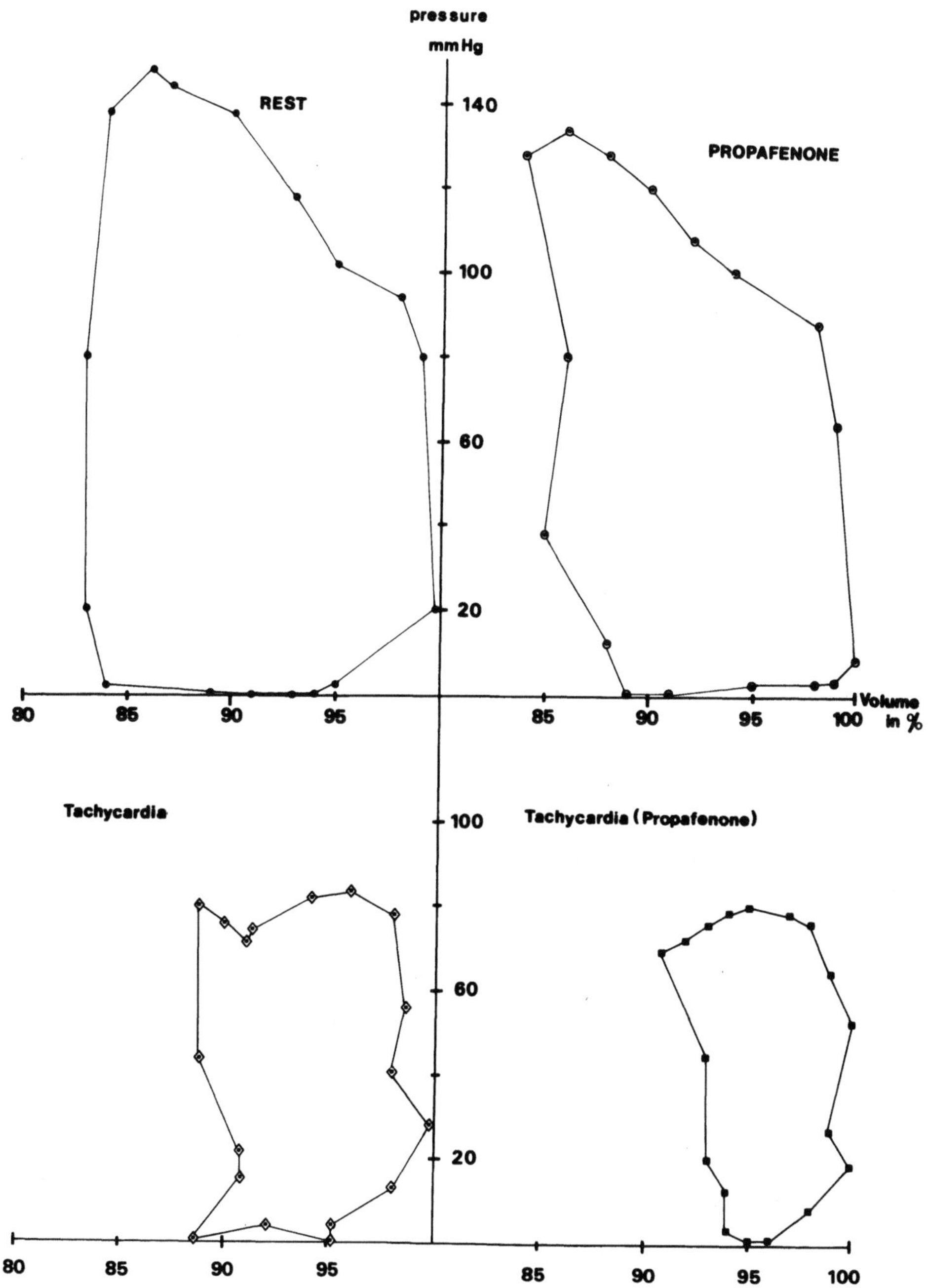

Fig. 3. Computer assisted pressure volume diagrams of the left ventricle of a 32 year old patient without heart disease. In the upper pannel the influence of propafenone at an AV sequentially paced heart rate of 75/min is demonstrated, the lower panel exhibits the effects of a heart rate of 180/min and the effects of propafenone (see text)

nique. At various heart rates the AV interval was altered from 10 ms to a "normal" value of 130 ms. Left ventricular pressure and its derivatives were recorded by "tip" catheters, and changes in left ventricular volume were measured by technetium radionucleid ventriculography. From these values computer-assisted pressure volume diagrams of the left ventricle were constructed.

As an example part of the results obtained in a 32 year old female patient with no apparent heart disease are shown.

At a stimulated heart rate of 75/min with an AV interval of 130 ms, left ventricular pressure was found to be 145/0–6 mmHg and dp/dt max 1400 mmHg/s. The value for t – dp/dt max was 150 ms, EF 54%. Following a bolus injection of 2 mg/kg propafenone over 3 min and under an additional dosage of 0.7 mg/kg constantly infused, left ventricular systolic pressure (LVSP) decreased to 135 mmHg, while LVEDP was elevated to 12 mmHg. dp/dt max decreased to 950 mmHg/s and t – dp/dt max increased to 205 ms. EF was reduced by 17% to 45%.

Without propafenone augmentation of paced heart rate to 180/min with an unchanged AV interval caused an alteration of left ventricular pressure to 85/0–10 mmHg. Propafenone elicited a further decrease of LVSP to 75 mmHg and elevation of LVEDP to 15 mmHg. During induced tachycardia dp/dt max measured 1300 mmHg/s, EF was decreased to 43%. Propafenone further decreased dp/dt max to 850 mmHg/s and EF by 50% to 21%. While at a paced heart rate of 75/min propafenone increased t – dp/dt max by 36%, the increase of this parameter under "induced" tachycardia was found to be 50%.

When pressure volume diagrams are constructed, the unfavourable conditions produced by propafenone become apparent. The area under the curve represents cardiac work or cardiac power when the volume change per unit of time and the pressure created are considered. The reduction of the area under the curve following propafenone administration indicates a reduced contractile state (Fig. 3).

All these effects were more pronounced when the atrial booster pump function became ineffective because the AV interval was shortened, making it thus resemble ventricular tachycardia with 1 : 1 VA conduction even more.

These results point to the fact that findings regarding negative inotropic side effects of propafenone or other antiarrhythmic drugs are highly dependent on the method applied. Moreover, the functional state of the heart and the presence or absence of arrhythmias may play a key role. Without question propafenone must be regarded as a negative inotropic agent. Due to incomplete investigations its mechanism is poorly understood and no prognostic statements can be made. This lack of knowledge is by no means specific to propafenone, but also exists regarding other antiarrhythmic agents. Furthermore comparative studies confined to a certain condition in which the individual serves as his own control have not been undertaken.

From the haemodynamic point of view a warning against uncritical use of antiarrhythmic drugs seems therefore justified. It is necessary for the physician to balance electrophysiological benefits and possible haemodynamic improvements against haemodynamic hazards which these drugs may present.

References

1. Breithardt G, Jochum E, Kuhn H, Seipel L (1978) Die Wirkung verschiedener Antiarrhythmika auf die systolischen Zeitintervalle bei Normalpersonen. Z Kardiol 67: 680
2. Bachour G, Bender F, Beck OA, Wolf R, Hochrein H (1974) Untersuchungen zur Hämodynamik des Antiarrhythmikums Propafenon bei koronarer Herzkrankheit. Therapiewoche 24: 4979
3. Desai J, Hirschfeld D, Peters R, Scheinmann M, Gonzales R (1978) Electromedical dissociation associated with disopyramide. Circulation 58 (Suppl. II) 178
4. Gigler G, Bilgin Y, Schlepper M: Unpublished research.
5. Hillis WS, Tweddel A, Lorimer AR, Lawrie TDV (1976) Some aspects of the clinical pharmacology of intravenous disopyramide after myocardial infarction. J Int Med Res 4 (Suppl.) 74
6. Jewitt DE (1980) Hemodynamic effects of newer antiarrhythmic drugs. Am Heart J 100: 984
7. Neuss H, Schlepper M: Unpublished research.
8. Possinger K, Hegemann F, Engelhardt D (1980) Systolische Herzzeitintervalle bei Patienten mit Linksherzinsuffizienz. Intensivmed 17: 175
9. Probst P, Pachinger O (1976) Einflüsse von Propafenon auf die Hämodynamik des linken Ventrikels und die atrioventrikuläre Überleitung unter besonderer Berücksichtigung des WPW-Syndroms.
10. Podrid PJ, Schoenberger A, Lown B (1980) Congestive cardiac failure caused by oral disopyramide. N Engl J Med 302: 614
11. Sutton R (1976) Hemodynamics of intravenous disopyramide. J Int Med Res 4 (Suppl.) 46

Interaction Between Propafenone and Other Drugs

K. Steinbach, K. Frohner, F. Meisl and G. Unger

No studies have yet been done on the percentage of patients who are treated concurrently with two, three, or more drugs for a single disease or for several coexisting diseases. Thus, the danger of drug interaction – a potentiation or diminution of effect – exists for a large patient population whose number is beyond estimation. Obviously, the innumerable possibilities of drug combination make a systemic investigation of interaction impossible. It is hardly surprising, then, that of the 12 large pharmaceutical firms that were contacted and questioned during the preparation of this paper, none was in the practice of systematically testing newly-developed drugs for possible interactions. As a result, drug interactions are for the most part disclosed through clinical observation.

Taking the antiarrhythmic drug propafenone as an example, we shall endeavor to examine the mechanism of drug interaction, the methodologic problems inherent in investing interactions, and the clinical significance of the interactions, especially with respect to drug combination used in daily practice.

Mechanism

The attempt to describe the process of drug interaction represents a simplification of a highly complex phenomenon. The following general classification is suitable for our purposes, however.

Pharmacologic Interaction

This interaction can result from synergism or antagonism between two drugs. In both cases this effect may, but need not, come about owing to a common receptor site on the target organ. Experimental studies have been done by Doering on the sarcolemma of sheep hearts and by Straub on a sodium-potassium ATPase preparation of bovine hearts. Using different experimental setups, each author obtained different results concerning the displacement of digitalis from the receptor by quinidine [2, 9]. The change in the distribution volume of digoxin under the influence of quinidine demonstrated in vivo by Schenck-Gustaffson points, as do the results of Straub, to a direct competitive action of digitalis and quinidine on the heart muscle [8]. No studies have yet been done on the pharmacologic interaction of propafenone with other drugs in the heart.

Pharmacokinetic Interaction

Absorption, distribution, protein binding, metabolism, and elimination are, singly or combined, processes during which drug interactions can occur [1]. Investigations with the whole-body counter provide the best means of analayzing pharmacokinetics, while equilibrium dialysis following the administration of radioactive substances is best for the assessment of protein binding. These costly methods, which necessitate a degree of patient exposure to radiation, are generally unavailable for clinical studies of possible drug interactions. With a binding rate of 98%, however, it can be assumed that propafenone enters into no clinically relevant interactions with other drugs in terms of protein binding [7]. No data have yet been published on the binding of propafenone to tissue proteins, due to difficulties of methodology. However, its relatively large distribution volume of approximately 250 liters is a strong indication that propafenone also binds to tissue proteins. The extent to which propafenone can interact with another antiarrhythmic drug, disopyramide, for which the proportion of free drug ranges from 0.19 to 0.46 depending on the total plasma level (2–8 mg/liter), is difficult to judge [6]. So far the only available clinical data are based on determinations of serum concentration, which give only a global picture, and provide no information on individual pharmacokinetic stages.

Clinical Methods

Pharmacologic Interaction

Interaction in the heart can be recognized by changes in the sinus node rhythm, AV conduction, and duration of the main ventricular deflection in the body-surface ECG, as well as by effects on the AV node and bundle of His in the intracardiac ECG. This interaction could have clinical significance in patients who are taking several antiarrhythmic drugs concurrently. The combination of a class-I antiarrhythmic agent with a class-III agent would be possible. Among our own patients, a decline in the sinus node rhythm to 45/min was observed in three who were taking a combination of propafenone and amiodorone.

Determination of Serum Concentration

The serum concentration indicates the amount of antiarrhythmic drug that is available in the serum at the time the determination is made. It is affected by absorption, distribution, metabolism, or elimination. If we are to use the serum concentration as an index for assessing a possible interaction, there must be a rise or fall of the serum concentration after a second drug is administered that goes beyond any fluctuation attributable to other causes. For this we must know the therapeutic range of a drug, which naturally is subject to much variation, as well as the fluctuations of the serum levels in a given patient [10]. In 15 patients that were taking propafenone for Lown type-IV ventricular arrhythmias (900 mg/day for ten patients, 600 mg/day for five), and in whom between 3 and 15 serum level determinations were made on different days with no change in dosage, we found deviations of 75% from the mean value and deviations of −302% to +332% from the previous value (Table 1, Fig. 1). This illustrates the difficulties inherent in using this parameter for the assessment of possible interactions.

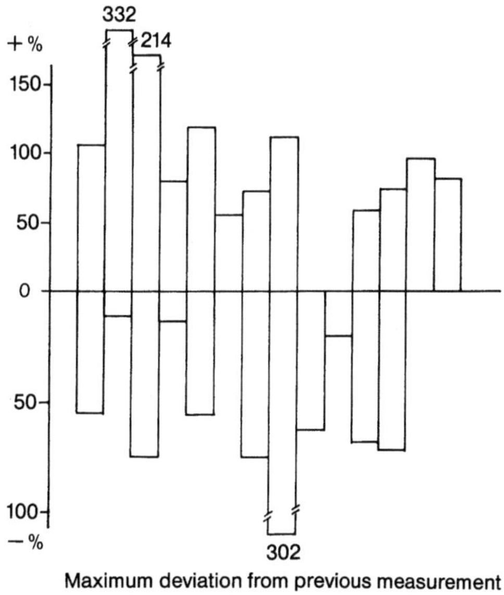

Fig. 1. Maximum deviation of propafenone concentration relative to previous value (propafenone dose 450–1 200 mg/day)

Table 1. Mean, maximum, and minimum serum concentrations measured in 15 patients during treatment with propafenone

Patient no.	Mean	Maximum	Minimum	No. of samples	H	Dose
1	1328	2688	655	6	3	3 × 300
2	941	1338	309	4	3	3 × 300
3	1443	1861	1025	5	3	3 × 300
4	682	1144	578	9	3	3 × 300
5	307	599	144	5	3	3 × 300
6	1969	3692	433	3	3–5	3 × 300
7	829	1702	465	4	3–5	3 × 300
8	998	1139	824	3	3–5	3 × 300
9	1592	2229	748	4	3	3 × 300
10	2385	2976	1377	4	3–5	3 × 300
11	192	318	64	4	10	3 × 300
12	1458	3056	624	8	3	4 × 300
13	1388	2244	809	14	3	4 × 150
14	229	372	156	9	3	4 × 150
15	336	571	150	4	3–5	3 × 150
	1072			86		

Abbreviation: H, interval between drug intake and blood sampling in hours

Determination of Urine Concentration

This test will reveal any effects at the elimination stage. For propafenone, which is almost entirely metabolized in the liver, this analysis has no relevance.

Indirect Detection of Drug Interactions

The parameters of blood coagulation can provide indirect evidence of a change in the kinetics of oral anticoagulants brought about by interaction with other drugs.

Propafenone Interactions

Studies on propafenone interaction are useful only if they relate to drug combinations that are used in daily medical practice. The following drugs are among those used most frequently in combination with propafenone.

Digitalis

Neither of the two drugs, digoxin and propafenone, had any effect on the serum concentration of the other in five patients. This is consistent with the results of Doering, who found that propafenone exerted no effect on the serum digoxin level [2].

Beta-Blocking Agents

The effect of propranolol on the serum propafenone concentration was tested in four patients; no interaction was observed. In one patient whose propafenone level was tested during i. v. infusion (70 mg/h) before and during propranolol (3×40 mg orally), the propafenone concentration was found to be markedly higher than the control level 60 and 90 min after the start of the i. v. infusion (Fig. 2). Of course a single observation provides no valid grounds for concluding an effect on pharmacokinetics, especially since propranolol should enter into the determination of the serum propafenone concentration. In the remaining three patients the serum levels 1248 mg/ml $\pm$ 248) did not exceed those of the control period before propranolol (1123 mg/ml $\pm$ 201).

Anticoagulants

An interaction of propafenone with warfarin is assumed; an interaction between disopyramide and warfarin has also been reported [3]. In three of five patients treated with warfarin, the prothrombin time decreased under a constant anticoagulant dosage and in two patients it was necessary to discontinue therapy. An interaction between propafenone and anticoagulants was also reported by Körst [4].

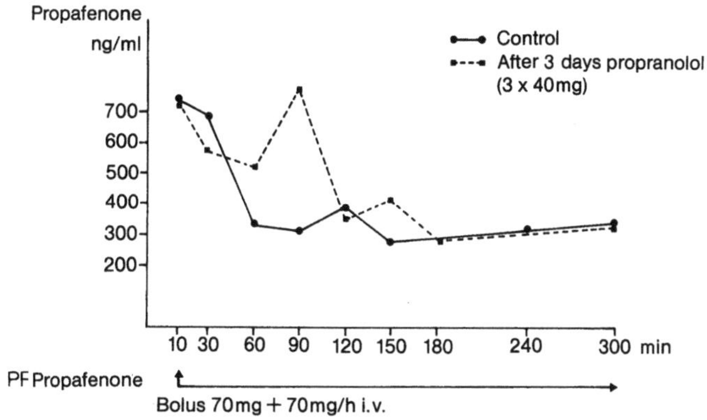

Fig. 2. Propafenone concentration after i.v. administration before and during treatment with 3 × 40 mg propranolol

Diuretics

An assessment of possible diuretic effects on the pharmacokinetics of propafenone requires that radiolabeled drugs be used to ascertain the distribution volume and its possible change by the diuretic. For technical reasons, no such investigations have yet been carried out [11].

Antiarrhythmic Agents with a Different Pharmacologic Action

Three patients in whom propafenone (900 mg/day) alone was insufficient to suppress ventricular tachycardia and who therefore received it in combination with amiodarone (600 mg/day) experienced a critical decline in heart rate (Fig. 3) and had to be stimulated with a temporary pacemaker. The heart rate normalized after propafenone was withdrawn. Because the malignant ventricular arrhythmia could be suppressed only with a combination of antiarrhythmic agents, a sequential AV pacemaker was implanted in two of the patients; one of them has been free of ventricular tachycardia for a period of 8 months, and the other for 10 months.

Problems in the Detection of Drug Interaction

It is understandably difficult to evaluate clinically a phenomenon that cannot be adequately studied by any method currently available. What is more, the occurrence of interactions is dependent on patient-specific factors and so cannot be considered strictly a pharmacologic and pharmacokinetic phenomenon. Foremost among these factors are diseases of the gastrointestinal tract, liver, and kidney, as well as an abnormal composition of the serum proteins.

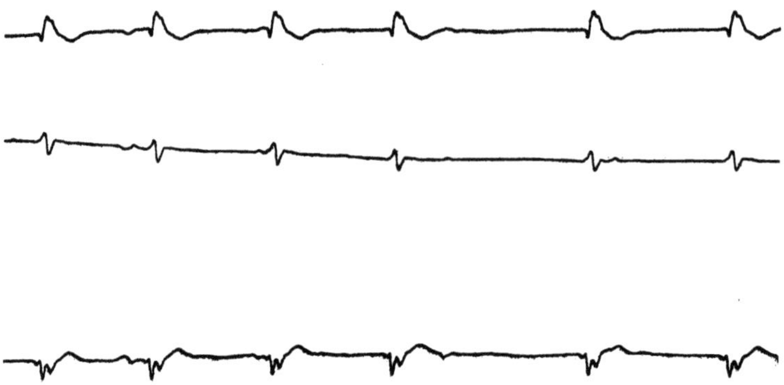

Fig. 3. Patient R. L., male, aged 60 years. Diagnosis: dilative cardiomyopathy. Under oral therapy with 3 × 300 mg propafenone and 2 × 200 mg amiodarone sinus rhythm falls to 40/min; dissociation with interference

In addition, interactions vary with the mode of administration (oral or i. v.), and demonstration in a given case is likely to prove difficult under clinical conditions.

This multiplicity of possible influences demonstrates the methodologic problems that are inherent in any systematic study of drug interactions in a clinical setting.

Conclusions

It is assumed that propafenone interacts both with amiodarone and warfarin. The process of interaction is a complex one and is influenced by many factors that are extremely difficult to pinpoint in any given case; the role of patient-specific factors with respect to the occurrence of interactions makes it likely that these interactions cannot be viewed strictly as pharmacologic or pharmacokinetic events.

Prospective clinical studies on the detection of interactions are not possible due to methodologic problems and ethical considerations. At present, therefore, interactions are detected "incidentally" through clinical observation, and reported case numbers are small. Determining the serum concentration of a drug is of little value for the detection of interactions.

References

1. Chien YW, Akers MJ, Yonan PK (1975) Effect of pKb on lipophilic binding of disopyramide derivates to human plasma. J Pharm Sci 64: 1632–1635
2. Doering (1979) Chinidine-digoxin interaction. N Engl J Med 301: 400–404
3. Haworth E, Burroughs (1977) Disopyramide and warfarin interaction. Br Med J 84: 866–867
4. Körst HA, Brandes JW, Littmann KP (1981) Propafenon potenziert Wirkung von oralen Antikoagulanzien. Med Klin 51: 349–350

5. Matos JA, Fischer JD, Kim SG (1981) Disopyramide – phenytoin interaction. Circulation [Suppl] 64: 4–264
6. Meffin JM, Robert EW, Winkler RA, Harapat SFA, Harrison DC (1979) Role of concentration-dependent plasma protein binding in disopyramide disposition. J Pharmacokinet Biopharm 7: 29–46
7. Neumann B (1978) Bindung von Propafenon an Plasmaproteine. Project report (unpublished) BASF, Sparte Plasma
8. Schenck-Gustafsson K, Jogestrand T, Nordlaner R, Dahlquist R (1981) Effect of guinidine in digoxin concentration in skeletal muscle and serum in patients with atrial fibrillation. N Engl J Med 305: 209–211
9. Straub KD, Kane JJ, Bissett JK (1978) Alterations of digitalis binding by chinidine: A mechanism of digitalis-guinidine interaction. Circulation 58 [Suppl] 2: 11–58
10. Wiebinghaus E, Seipel L, Breithardt G, Loogen F (1977) Langzeitergebnisse mit dem neuen Antiarrhythmicum Propafenon unter Berücksichtigung der Plasmaspiegel. Z Kardiol 66: 625–632
11. Wilkenson RD (1981) Acute effects of intravenous furosemide administration on serum digoxin concentration. Am Heart J 102: 63–65

Comparison of the Efficacy of Propafenone and Lidocaine in Patients with Acute Myocardial Infarction and Ventricular Extrasystoles: Result of a 24-h Holter Monitoring

N. Rehnqvist

Therapeutic traditions concerning ventricular arrhythmias in acute myocardial infarction have changed over the years. There are fewer indications for therapy now than previously. Lidocaine is the drug normally used in patients with acute myocardial infarction and ventricular arrhythmias; however, it can be given only by intravenous infusion. Therefore, drugs with specific antiarrhythmic action which can also be administered orally add to the therapeutic arsenal. If a drug can be shown to be as effective and safe as lidocaine in patients with acute myocardial infarction, it will probably also be of benefit to some of the patients suffering from ventricular arrhythmias of other origins. These patients present particular problems today, and development and improvement of antiarrhythmic drugs will help them. The purpose of this study was to compare the efficacy of lidocaine, given by a standard method, to the new class I antiarrhythmic drug, propafenone.

Methods

Patients below 70 years of age admitted because of chest pain suggestive of acute myocardial infarction, who showed higher grades of ventricular arrhythmias during routine monitoring (i.e., Lown grades 2–5) were considered for the study. Exclusion criteria were the usual for antiarrhythmic testing, that is, significant cardiac insufficiency, cardiogenic shock, severe bradycardia, sick sinus syndrome, sinoatrial ventricular and intraventricular disorders of impulse conduction, hypersensitivity to local anesthetics, treatment with antiarrhythmic agents other than digitalis or beta-blockers, hypotension, severe obstructive pulmonary disease, or severe renal or hepatic failure.

After 1 h of observation the patients were randomized for propafenone or lidocaine therapy. The randomization was based on whether there was concomitant medication with beta-blockers. Lidocaine was given as a bolus of 1 mg/kg bodyfollowed by an infusion of 3000 mg/24 h. Propafenone was given as a bolus injection of 1 mg/kg bodyup to 70 mg. This was followed by 150 mg propafenone 1 h later, and 150 mg every 6 h thereafter. During the study the one-lead ECG was printed out at a paper speed of 10 mm/s. The arrhythmias were thereafter interpreted manually. Therapy covered 24 h, and every hour blood pressure and heart rate were registered, as well as the QT interval in patients on propafenone.

Results

The study included 20 patients; at the time of writing, eight had completed the study four in each group. The mean ages were 62 years in the lidocaine group and 61 in the propafenone group. All patients had AMI. The mean reduction in VPCs was 79% in the lidocaine group and 81% in the propafenone group; therefore, both drugs significantly reduced the occurrence of serious arrhythmia during the 24 h. The number of 5-min periods containing high grades of arrhythmia was equally reduced in the two therapy groups.

Side Effects

Two patients complained of sweating during the bolus injection of propafenone. One patient had to be withdrawn from the study because of periods of sinus arrest during the oral period of propafenone therapy. One patient in the lidocaine group complained of ringing in the ears and in another the dose had to be reduced because of central nervous system symptoms. One patient in the lidocaine group developed ventricular fibrillation about 55 min after the start of therapy. One additional patient, not presented in this study, developed torsade-de-pointe ventricular tachycardia during Propafenone therapy which was further aggravated as the Propafenone dose was increased. In this patient the arrhythmias disappeared completely after treatment with Lidocaine.

Discussion

These data indicate that propafenone seems to be an effective antiarrhythmic drug. It also seems that it can be given safely during acute myocardial infarction. In addition, patients on beta-blockers can be given propafenone in these dosages. However, these data are preliminary and 20 patients need to complete the study before definite conclusions can be drawn.

Observations on the Antiarrhythmic Effects of Rytmonorm

Ku Fu-sheng, Lin Jui-Chin, Liu Pei-Tsun, Li Qing-lang, Chang Jang-thi, Shen Lu-hua and Yang Shi Hau

Propafenone hydrochloride, known commercially as Rytmonorm, is a synthetic antiarrhythmic drug produced by Helopharm, Federal Republic of Germany. Its chemical formula is 2'-(2-hydroxy-3-propylaminopropoxy)-3-phenylpropiophenone hydrochloride. It is available in the form of 150- and 300 mg oral tablets and as a parenteral preparation (70 mg per vial). The antiarrhythmic properties of this drug were reported by the Berlin Pharmaceutical Institute in 1979, after experiments with animals and human beings. It was demonstrated to be quite effective in the treatment of both ventricular and supraventricular arrhythmias.

Beginning in May 1980, we used Rytmonorm on 97 patients in 106 trials at Peking Friedship Hospital. We found that it was noticeably effective in treatment of frequent premature beats and tachyarrhythmias originating in the junctional area, the AV accessory pathway, and the intraventricular conductive system. The clinical indications for the drug, as well as its antiarrhythmic effects and its side effects, was investigated.

Method

We chose 97 cases from our cardiac clinic and cardiac wards. They were 40 patients with functional or idiopathic arrhythmias and 57 cases of arrhythmia in organic heart disease. While eight patients were suffering from congestive heart failure, most had normal cardiac function. All were examined thoroughly by experienced cardiologists. Most patients with refractory PVCs resistant to all other antiarrhythmic drugs were carefully followed up after administration of Rytmonorm, in order to evaluate the drug's long-term therapeutic effects. In addition, special attention was paid to those in patients whose arrhythmias were complicated by hypokalemia, and to those in the acute stage of myocardial infarction.

Clinical Observations

Of the 97 patients, 35 were inpatients, while the others were treated in a special cardiac clinic with facilities for telemetric ECG monitoring. All antiarrhythmic medications were withheld prior to observation. Continuous ECG monitoring was done for half an hour before and immediately after administration of Rytmonorm. The ECG data from each trial were analyzed by electrocardiograph specialists. Both the immediate effect after a single dose, and the long-term therapeutic effect were observed. In 51 cases there was immediate positive response, and treatment was continued for 2 weeks. Follow-ups of these patients were done on days 2, 3, 7, and 14 of treatment, and they were monitored by telemetric ECG. They were then examined on day 2 after withdrawal of the drug.

Rytmonorm was given either intravenously or orally. All patients suffering from various kinds of paroxysmal tachycardia were treated via i.v. injections, while those with chronic arrhythmias received oral therapy. In the i.v. injection group, antiarrhythmic medications were withdrawn 2 h prior to the administration of Rytmonorm. An initial dose of 70 mg dissolved in 20 ml dextrose was injected slowly (for 3–5 min) into each patient. Most of the patients in this group responded immediately. Injections were withheld as soon as tachyarrhythmias were converted to sinus rhythm. The dosage required varied greatly with the individual. Some patients' doses were smaller than 70 mg, i.e., 10–35 mg for infants and children, and 35–50 mg among adults. In cases where 70 mg was insufficient to control the tachyarrhythmia, a second dose of 70 mg was given after an interval of 10–20 min. In three cases, doses up to 350 mg were required; however, sinus rhythm was resumed without any side effect.

All antiarrhythmic drugs were withheld for at least 1 week from patients with chronic arrhythmia who were treated with oral tablets. They then received Rytmonorm according to their body weight, i.e. initial doses of 600 mg and maintenance doses ranging from 150 mg to 300 mg b.i.d. or t.i.d.

The following criteria were used to assess degrees of therapeutic effectiveness:

1. Markedly effective
   a) For the i.v. group if tachyrhythmias were abolished immediately or within 30 min after intravenous injection of Rytmonorm.
   b) For the oral group if arrhythmias disappeared completely within 7 h after the initial dose
2. Effective – the arrhythmias were not abolished by a single dose of rytmonorm but improvements in symptoms were observed, e.g.:
   a) In chronic atrial fibrillation the ventricular rate slowed by more than 20 beats per min.
   b) In Wolff-Parkinson-White (WPW) syndrome with atrial fibrillation the phenomenon of preexcitation was abolished.
   c) The frequency of extrasystoles in cases of persistent PVCs was reduced by 50%.
3. Ineffective – no response to the administration of Rytmonorm.

Results

Paroxysmal Tachycardia

As Table 1 shows intravenous injection of Rytmonorm was highly effective, converting all 23 cases of supraventricular tachycardia (SVT) and five cases of ventricular tachycardia (VT) to sinus rhythm. These results were the more impressive in that 14 of the 27 patients were suffering from organic diseases. The youngest patient was only 40 days old and had an attack of SVT with a heart rate of 230 beats per min. The tachycardia stopped as soon as 10 mg Rytmonorm was injected. In four cases SVT was abolished with a bolus dose of less than 70 mg; however, most patients required 70 – 140 mg, while two of the five cases of VT were converted.

Table 1. Immediate therapeutic effect of Rytmonorm (i.v. in 50 cases)

Diagnosed arrhythmia	No. of cases	Therapeutic effects		Dose required for conversion (mg i.v.)					
		Assess-ment	No. of cases	< 70	70	140	210	280	> 280
Supraventricular tachycardia	23	A	23	4	9	7	/	2	
Ventricular tachycardia	5	A	5	0	1	1	1	0	(350 mg) 2
W-P-W c̄ atrial fibrillation	3	A	2	0	0	0	0	0	
		B	1	0	1Δ				
Atrila fibrillation	10	A	3	0	1	1	0	1	
		B	2	0	2	0	0	0	
		C	5	0	1	0	0	3	(420 mg) 1
Atrial flutter	3	C	3	0	0	1	1	1	
Atrial tachycardia	3	A	1	0	1	0	0	0	
		C	2	0	2	0	0	0	
W-P-W	3	A	3	0	3	0	0	0	

W-P-W, Wolff-Parkinson-White syndrome; A, markedly effective; B, effective; C, ineffective

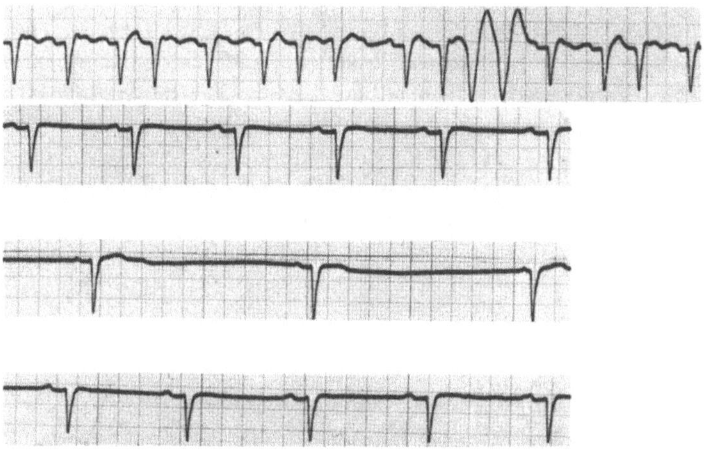

Fig. 1. Atrial fibrillation is converted to sinus rhythm by i.v. application of 4 × 70 mg Rytmonorm. Widening F-waves and QRS are shown in the 1st stripe

Atrial Fibrillation

Of 13 cases of paroxysmal atrial fibrillation, five resumed sinus rhythm following i.v. injection of Rytmonorm (Fig. 1). Among these five, two cases were associated with W-P-W syndrome. Six other cases failed to respond. Two cases were listed as "effective" since their W-P-W syndrome was abolished, but sinus rhythm was not resumed (Fig. 2). Only one of six cases of paroxysmal atrial flutter responded well to this drug. During treatment of this rapid atrial arrhythmia, a reduction in the frequency of the F wave was ob-

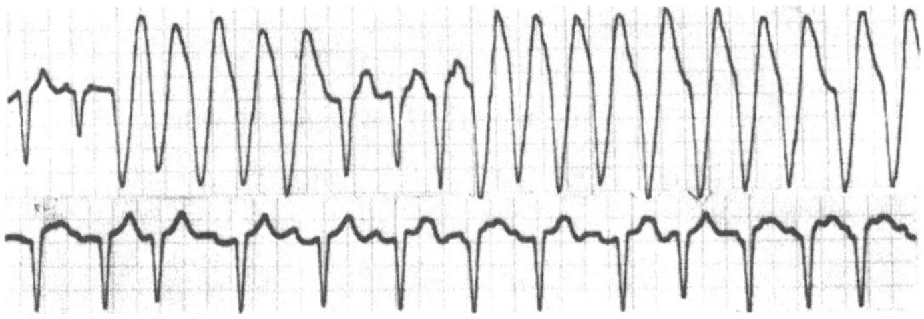

Fig. 2. Preexcitation is abolished by i.v. application of 70 mg Rytmonorm in a case of W-P-W and atrial fibrillation. The heart rate slowed down from 171 beats/min to 88 beats/min

served even though sinus rhythm was not resumed. The atrial flutter was converted to atrial tachycardia with a slower ventricular rate, which indicated that Rytmonorm had inhibited the atrial conductive system.

Response of Chronic Arrhythmias to Single Oral Doses of Rytmonorm

Each of 53 patients with various arrhythmias was given a single oral dose of Rytmonorm under telemetric monitoring of his or her ECG (Table 2). The most remarkable responses were in patients with junctional and ventricular premature beats. The ectopic beats disappeared in 39 of 40 such cases. The therapeutic effect ussually appeared 1½–2 h following administration of the drug. On the whole, the therapeutic responses to doses of both 300 and 600 mg of Rytmonorm were quite similar. In six cases the therapeutic effects manifested as early as 1 h after a dose of 600 mg, yet in other cases with the same dose the therapeutic responses appeared rather late. As side effects were seen more often with the 600-mg single dose, it was our impression that a 300-mg single dose of Rytmonorm usually yielded satisfactory therapeutic results for Chinese people.

The Long-term Therapeutic Effect of Rytmonorm

Oral therapy was continued 51 patients following the observation of immediate antiarrhythmic effects of Rytmonorm. They were kept on such therapy for 1–4 weeks, averaging 2 weeks (Table 3).

The therapeutic effect was again most prominent among those with PVCs which disappeared completely while Rytmonorm treatment was maintained. In four cases of SVT converted to sinus rhythm by i.v. injections of Rytmonorm, the arrhythmias did not reappear as long as the patients kept on taking the drug orally. In one case of preexcitation syndrome, the complication of atrial fibrillation did not recur during a half – year period of Rytmonorm maintenance therapy. In this particular case, the patient's atrial fibrillation had been refractory to various known therapies prior to the administration of Rytmonorm. However, during relatively long-term therapy it was again shown that Rytmonorm was ineffective in controlling most of the other atrial arrhythmias.

It is evident from Tables 2 and 3 that orally administered Rytmonorm was less effective in controlling atrial premature beat and fibrillation. For patients with preexcitation syndrome, oral Rytmonorm was effective in eliminating the preexcitation phenomenon in three cases and failed in one.

Table 2. Immediate therapeutic effect of oral Rytmonorm in 53 cases

Diagnosed arrhythmia	No. of cases	Dosage (mg)	Therapeutic effect									
			Appearance of marked effect								Effective	Ineffective
			1 h	1½ h	2 h	2½ h	3 h	4 h	6 h	7 h		
Frequent PAC	3	300									1	2
Frequent PAC	4	300							1			2
c̄ PAT		600									1	
Frequent PAC c̄ A.flut. or A.fib.	2	600										2
Junctional	4	300									1	
extrasystoles		600		3								
Frequent	36	300		10	2		3				1	
PVC		600	6	6	2	1	2	1		1	1	
Transient PVT	2	300									2	
W-P-W.	2	300					1					1
Totals	53		6	19	4	1	6	1	1	1	7	7

PAC, premature atrial contraction; PAT, paroxysmal atrial tachycardia; PVC, premature ventricular contraction; PVT, paroxysmal ventricular tachycardia; W-P-W, Wolff-Parkinson-White syndrome

Table 3. Long-term therapeutic effect of oral Rytmonorm in 51 cases

Diagnosed Arrhythmias	No. of cases	Therapeutic effect		
		Marked effect	Effective	Ineffective
SVT	4	4		
VT	3	1	2	
Atrial arrhythmia (PAC, PAC c̄ A.flut. or A.fib)	7		1	6
W-P-W c̄ A.fib.	2	1	1	
PJC	2		2	
PVC	33	32	1	
Totals	51	38	7	6

SVT, supraventricular tachycordia; VT, ventricular tachycardia; PAC, premature atrial contraction; A.flut., atrial flutter; A.fib., atrial fibrillation;W-P-W, Wolff-Parkinson-White syndrome; PJC, premature junetional contraction; PVC, premature ventricular contraction; PVT, paroxysmal ventricular tachycardia; PAT, paroxysmal atrial tachycardia

Side Effects of Rytmonorm

Along with the immediate antiarrhythmic effect of oral Rytmonorm a temporary drop in blood pressure was observed in 14 patients, dizziness in 26, nausea in 12, vomiting in 5, and dryness of mouth in 19. These side effects were dose-related and usually appeared in those patients receiving 600 mg Rytmonorm orally. Dizziness also occurred occasionally among those on maintenance dosage and disappeared as the doses were reduced. No definite sign of toxicity was seen in any of the patients observed.

Duration of Therapeutic Effects of Rytmonorm

Among patients who received Rytmonorm orally, PVCs sometimes reappeared 8 h after a single dose. In the long-term follow-up cases the arrhythmias might recur on the 2nd or 3rd day after discontinuation of the maintenance dose. When an attack of tachycardia was controlled by intravenous Rytmonorm, a long-term maintenance dose was neccessary to keep the attack from recurring.

Discussion

Effect on the Sinoatrial Node

Rytmonorm did not show depressive effect on sinus rhythm as other antiarrhythmic drugs. No sinus bradycardia occur during the single dose test, nor was it seen in the long-term therapy. During the i.v. conversion of tachy-rhythmias two cases had abnormally long pauses of 2.44 and 2.66 s before the sinus rhythm resumed. However, both of these instances occurred in patients suffering from coronary heart disease and the longer pauses might be attributable to the ischemia of the sinoatrial region rather than to the effect of Rytmonorm.

Effect on Intra-atrial Conduction

There was a noticeable slowing of intra-atrial conduction after administration of a relatively large single dose of Rytmonorm, either intravenously or per os. This inhibitory effect was manifested in several ways: First, the P waves widened gradually by a average of 30% after a single dose. The prolonged atrial depolarization reached its maximum at 4–5 h following an oral dose. Second, in cases of atrial fibrillation treated with intravenous Rytmonorm, the fibrillary waves first changed to F waves, and then the F-F interval gradually lengthened, signifiying a slowing of the conduction along the intra-atrial pathways. Although the reentry conduction was slowed down, total blockade was rare, since only five of 13 cases of atrial fibrillation resumed the sinoauricular rate. Among these five one could not rule out the possibility that blockage may have taken place in the AV node. In any case, Rytmonorm can be listed as one of the drugs useful in slowing the ventricular rate in atrial fibrillation, despite the fact that its therapeutic effects on atrial arrhythmias were not as satisfactory as those it had on the SVT (probably junctional), ventricular tachycardia, and ventricular premature systoles.

Effect on the AV Junctional Tissue

It was observed that the P-R intervals were invariably prolonged after Rytmonorm treatment. This prolongation was due to (a) slowing down of intraatrial conduction as reflected by the widening of P waves, and (b) slowing of the AV junctional conductivity, estimated by the elongation of the P-R segment. This lengthening appeared rather early, reaching its maximum 2–3 h after an oral dose. It was evident that Rytmonorm did induce prolongation of P-R intervals but no partial or complete heart block was observed in any of our cases. Three of 15 cases had a prolongation of the P-R interval, ranging from 0.21 to 0.24 2–6 h after a 300-mg oral dose of Rytmonorm, while a 600-mg dose induced a prolongation ranging from 0.21 to 0.26 seconds in 12 of 22 cases. The maximal lengthening of P-R interval was reached 1–5 h following oral medication.

Effect on the AV Accessory Bundle

The phenomenon of preexcitation disappeared in eight of the ten cases following administration of Rytmonorm, indicating a marked blocking effect on the conduction of impulse along the AV accessory bundle. This action explains the efficacy of Rytmonorm in the treatment of tachyarrhythmias associated with preexcitation syndrome.

Effect on Bundle of His

It was found that the QRS interval gradually widened after oral administration of Rytmonorm, reaching a maximum at the 3rd h. In seven cases the QRS interval was over 0.12 s and in one case up to 0.16 s. In other patients the QRS interval was widened, but still within normal limits. Widened QRS intervals were seen either as a result of overdosage or in patients with organic heart disease.

Temporary fascicular hemiblock occured in four cases as soon as therapeutic effects were achieved.

Effect on Q-T Interval

Along with the immediate effect of Rytmonorm, prolonged Q-T intervals ranging from 0.41 to 0.51 s were found in 12 cases. This phenomenon occurred only within 6 h following administration of Rytmonorm, indicating that the inhibitory effect upon the myocardial cell was temporary. Among the long-term follwo-up cases such prolongation of the Q-T interval was not seen. This suggests that there is no cumulative toxic effect of Rytmonorm.

Summary

Rytmonorm was used as an antiarrhythmic drug in 102 trials on 96 patients. Its therapeutic effects with intravenous and oral administration were observed. It was shown that the drug was most efficient in the control of junctional and ventricular tachycardia as well as of junctional and ventricular premature beats and in the Wolff-Parkinson-White syndrome. For these arrythmias the efficacy of Rytmonorm was up to 100%. Among cases of atrial fibrillation 38% were controlled by this drug. Rythmonorm was least effective in the treatment of atrial arrythmias, i.e. atrial premature beats, atrial flutter, and atrial paroxysmal tachycardia.

The characteristics of Rytmonorm were that (a) its therapeutic effect appeared rather promptly, (b) it lasted for 5–6 hours only and (c) there was no cumulative effect. Clinically, it proved useful in the treatment of junctional and ventricular tachyarrhythmias. It may also be tried in the therapy of paroxysmal atrial fibrillation.

Comparative Study of the Therapeutic Effect of Propafenone and Disopyramide in the Oral Treatment of Chronic Ventricular Premature Beats

J. Clementy, M. Dallocchio and H. Bricaud

The aim of this study was to test the efficacy and tolerability of propafenone and disopyramide (Rhythmodan) in the treatment of ventricular premature beats (VPBs) in a double-blind experiment.

Methods

Choice of Patients

All patients treated in this study presented the same arrhythmias: VPBs. Only those patients who had at least one VPB per min were included, however. Frequency was determined by a 24-h ECG. Patients with the following conditions were excluded:
1. Atrioventricular block
2. Irreversible cardiac insufficiency
3. Severe renal insufficiency
4. Recent infarction
5. Glaucoma

Also excluded were patients who were receiving other antiarrhythmic treatment.

Ten patients, four women and six men, ranging in age from 35 to 67 years (mean age 52.5) took part in the experiment. In three cases (patients 2, 4, and 7) the VPBs appeared during treatment for hypertensive cardiopathy. In two cases (patients 1 and 8) they were of an idiopathic nature. In two cases (patients 3 and 9) they were observed in patients who exhibited ischemic cardiopathy. In patients 5 and 6 they appeared concomitantly with myocardiopathy. In patient 10 they appeared suddenly with a mitral valve prolapse.

Treatment

The agents being tested – propafenone (P) and disopyramide (D) – were administered in two successive periods, with a so-called wash-out interval in between. The patients and the medications were chosen at random: During the first treatment period patients 2, 3, 4, 5, and 10 received P in a dose of 450 mg/day (three tablets of 150 mg each) for 5 days; during the same period patients 1, 6, 7, 8, and 9 received D in a dose of 300 mg/day (three capsules of 100 mg each). During the 5-day "wash-out" interval all patients received three placebo tablets (LP3) daily. In the second treatment period patients 2, 3, 4,

5, and 10 received D in the daily dose of 300 mg as above, and patients 1, 6, 7, 8, and 9 received P in the daily dose of 450 mg, also as above. This period also lasted 5 days.

At the end of each treatment period, those patients who did not exhibit a sufficient decrease in frequency of VPBs, measured against the frequency recorded at the beginning of the periods (i.e., for the first period of therapy, the beginning average, for the second period of therapy, the average during the wash-out period), received a double dose over the next 5 days: 900 mg/day (three tablets of 300 mg each) for the patients who had been taking propafenone, with the exception of patient 7, and 600 mg/day (six capsules of 100 mg each) for those who had been taking disopyramide, except for patients 1, 3, and 4. Patient 7 demonstrated a 99.9% decrease in VPB frequency while taking three tablets of propafenone daily during the first 5 days of the second period of therapy. Patient 1 had a 99.8% reduction in VPB frequency with three capsules of disopyramide daily during the first 5 days of the second period of therapy. Patients 3 and 4 experienced side effects which did not permit of further use of D in higher doses.

Criteria of Evaluation

Efficacy

The main criterion for the evaluation of the experiment and the results was the hourly absolute frequency of VPBs, which was monitored continuously by a Holter apparatus for 24 h.

An additional criterion was the number of atrial complexes on the ECG (or the systoles) which served as a measure of the time dependency of the treatment.

Six recordings were made for each patient:

1. Before the first treatment (H0)
2. At the end of the low dose in the first period, i.e., 3 × 150 mg P, or 3 × 100 mg D (H1)
3. After the first high dose, i.e., 3 × 300 mg P, or 6 × 100 mg D (H1′)
4. At the end of the wash-out period (H0′)
5. After the low dose in the second period (H2)
6. After the high dose in the second period (H2′)

Patients 1, 3, 4, and 7 were recorded only five times, for reasons already mentioned.

The final aim of this statistical analysis was to put the efficacy of the treatment to the test; the changing conditions of the experiment were meant to show various results, namely the consequences of sequence, of the individual medications, of the day/night rhythm, and of dose.

The individual effects and their possible combination were evaluated as a whole from case to case using differential analysis, as well as *t*-tests of the mean obtained in paired series and nonparametric tests, in order to examine the effect of dose. The method used for each effect studied is here explained in detail, justified, and documented.

Tolerability

Clinical tolerability was tested by questioning the patients and by clinical examination following each period of therapy. Biological tolerability was judged by comparing the following parameters prior to and after treatment:

1. Blood count
2. Composition of blood
3. Potassium content
4. Urea content in blood
5. Creatine content
6. Blood sugar
7. Transaminases
8. Alkaline phosphatases
9. Bilirubin

Results and Discussion

Analysis of the Chief Evaluative Criterion: Number of VPBs

Study of the Correlation Between Treatment and Sequence

The two effects – treatment as such and sequence of medication – were studied by factor analysis. Before each of these effects can be evaluated, the possible correlation between them must be studied. The investigative method used is a simplification of the one recently introduced by Hills and Armitage [1]. The mean VPB frequency is ascertained for each patient in connection with treatment. If no correlation exists between treatment and sequence, the mean for the group that received first P and then D (414.10) should be no different from the mean for the other group, which received first D and then P (228.08). The difference between these means is subjected to a Student's t-test, whereby a weighted variant from each group is taken as the common variant:

$$t_8 = \frac{414.10 - 228.08}{\sqrt{2\left(\frac{78047.17}{5}\right)}} = 1.05$$

This is not a significant difference; it implies no correlation between treatment itself and sequence of medication. Therefore, the analysis concerning the two periods of treatment can be continued.

Effect of Treatment (Low Dose): The effect of the treatment was studied by means of differential analysis of complete, weighted blocks [2], in which the chief variable was the treatment factor; there are four treatment factors – H0, H1, H0′, and H2. Additional influencing variables are the patients, divided into ten blocks, and each of 24 iterations which represent the hourly VPB values during the day/night rhythm, recorded from 9 a.m. to 8 a.m. on the following day. Table 1 shows the results of these studies.

The correlation between treatment and patient is significant, i.e., the patients did not all react to the various treatments in the same way. This means, for example, that their reaction to propafenone or to disopyramide is not proportional to the number of VPBs before the first treatment or to the number of VPBs during the wash-out period.

However, this does not hamper the interpretation of the significance of the effect of treatment, particularly when this effect is evaluated with a t-test, for which the differen-

Table 1. Analysis of the efficacy of treatment by complete weighted blocks

Origin of fluctuation	ddj	Estimate of variance	F_{920}	*P*
Treatment	3	11557600	147.3	< 0.001
Patient	9	8986560	114.5	< 0.001
Correlation between treatment and patient	27	1653050	21.07	< 0.001
Residual	920	78448	–	–

tial used is the residual differential resulting from the analysis [3]. The *t*-test for determining the difference of the mean hourly VPBs following propafenone (274.74) and disopyramide (367.34) is highly significant ($P < 0.001$):

$$t_{920} \simeq \varepsilon = \frac{274.74 - 367.34}{\sqrt{2\left(\frac{78448}{240}\right)}} = -3.62$$

There are considerably fewer VPBs with the use of P than there are with the use of D.

In the same way, the effect of the wash-out period was obtained by testing the mean hourly VPBs, that is the difference of the value before any therapy and that after wash-out, which is:

$$t_{920} \simeq \varepsilon = \frac{707.4 - 656.8}{\sqrt{2\left(\frac{78448}{240}\right)}} = 1.98$$

This is a test with borderline significance ($P \cong 0.05$). Thus, there is probably a residual effect from the first treatment at the end of the wash-out period. Nevertheless, this residual effect does not influence the analysis, since the two treatment periods with P and D are symmetrically distributed on either side of the wash-out interval. In any case, the analysis can be continued as if there were no effect of sequence.

Effect of Sequence (Low Dose): The effect of the sequence of administration was studied in a similar manner, by means of a differential analysis with complete, weighted blocks, in which the most important variable was the sequence factor (H1 or H2); the additional variable was the patient factor, as well as the series of test values (iterations) representing the absolute number of hourly VPBs over the day/night rhythm.

Here the correlation between sequence and patients is still significant ($P < 0.001$). The patients do not react in the same way to the first and second treatments (whether with propafenone or with disopyramide); in a certain sense there is an "individual" effect of sequence. The analysis of the overall effect of sequence can follow, using the calculation of a corresponding F; however, not the residual differential, but the differential of the correlation according to Table 2 [4] is used, which is a consequence of the "individual" effect of sequence.

$$F_9^1 = \frac{3204110}{701827} = 4.57 \text{ (NS)}$$

Table 2. Estimated differentials from the analysis of the effect of sequence in complete weighted blocks

Origin of fluctuation	ddl	Estimate of variance
Sequence	1	3204110
Patients	9	3788790
Correlation between sequence and patients	9	701827
Residual	460	60647

There is no significant difference between treatment periods H1 and H2; an overall effect of sequence cannot be proven.

Effect of Day/Night Rhythm (Low Dose): The effect of the day/night rhythm, i.e., the study of the variation of the mean number of VPBs – here considered the mean hourly value, or the mean of the three treatment periods over 8 h – is analysed using differential analysis of complete, weighted blocks, in which the chief variable is the day/night rhythm, the second being the patient factor. If one considers every hour of the daily routine, or if the mean is reckoned over an 8-h period, there is no iteration; if one examines each individual hour of the 8-h period, there are eight iterations.

The effect of the day/night rhythm was evaluated before the treatment (H0 and H0′): hour by hour without iteration through an $F^{23}_{207} = 0.59$, or through 8-h periods, in which case one considers each of the 8 h of the three periods (eight iterations), $F^{2}_{210} = 2.75$, or the mean of the three periods of 8 h each (without iteration) $F^{2}_{18} = 0.51$. In no case is there a significant difference; a day/night effect cannot be proved if one studies it hour by hour or in 8-h periods. Apparently, the lack of a clearly proven overall day/night effect is due to the strong (individual) correlation between day- or nighttime and patient, in that the individual patients exhibit strong variations from person to person in their day/night reactions.

Under propafenone there is a strong (individual) correlation between day- or nighttime and patient, if one examines the three 8-h periods (with eight iterations): $F^{2}_{210} = 7$ ($P < 0.001$); changes during the day/night cycle are different from one patient to the next. Therefore, one cannot infer a significant difference between the three 8-h periods: $F^{2}_{210} = 6.04$. The results are the same as if one examines the day/night effect hour by hour (without iterations). All of these conclusions are equally applicable for disopyramide in low doses.

Influence of Dose (Low and High)

The dose effect was tested by a Student's *t*-test in paired series. The reduction in the number of VPBs with increased dose (double dose) is clear in those patients in whom the expected effect had not appeared before – the nine who had received propafenone and the seven who had received disopyramide; however, in the latter case the effect is not as great:

With propafenone $t_8 = 2.89$ ($P = 0.02$)
With disopyramide $t_6 = 2.75$ ($P < 0.05$)

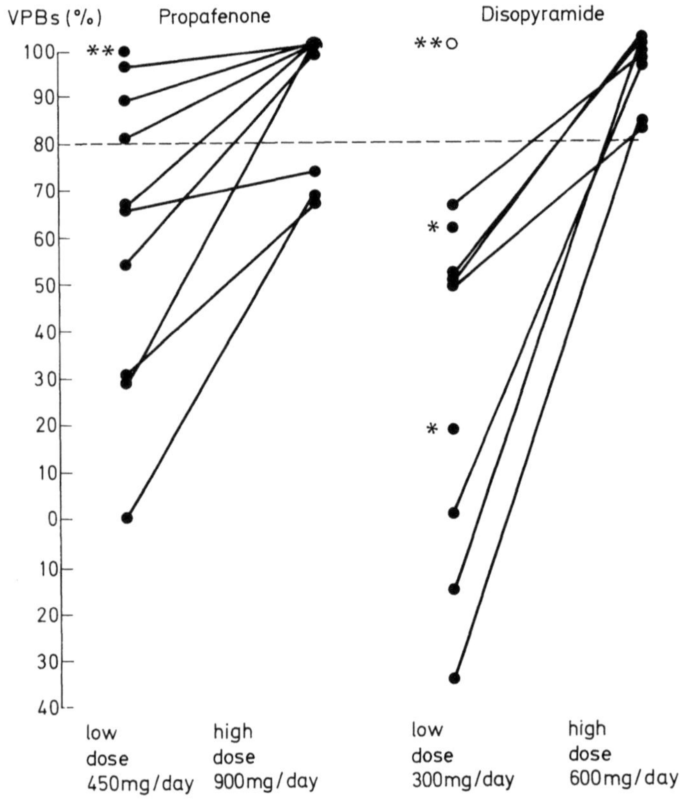

Fig. 1. Decrease in VPBs related to administered dose, shown as percentage of the number of VPBs at the beginning (before the first treatment for the first period, during the wash-out interval for the second). *, side effects; **, efficacy

The decrease in VPBs as a function of the administered dose is shown in Fig 1. Relative to a threshold value of 80% reduction in VPBs – this is considered an acceptable minimum because antiarrhythmic treatment is regarded as effective at that level – we can state the following: Of the ten patients who were treated with P in low doses, four exceeded this threshold, i.e., patients 1, 3, 5, and 7 (the last showed a very good response with a low dose right from the beginning of therapy). In comparison, only one patient of the ten who received the low doses of D exceeded this threshold; this was patient 1, who showed a very good response from the beginning, in spite of the low dose.

A comparison of the efficacy of the total treatment – high dose following low dose – between P and D was made with the patients above and below the 80% threshold. Those patients who exceeded the 80% threshold with the high dose as well were, with P, patients 1, 2, 3, 5, 9, and 10, and with D, patients 2, 5, 6, 7, 8, 9, and 10. There is no significant difference between the number of patients in the P group (six) and that in the D group (7); a test with paired series gives F=0.52 (NS). The exact comparison of the efficacy of P and D in high doses was made with a Rang test – a nonparametric U test after Mann and Whitney [5]. The results are shown in Fig. 2:

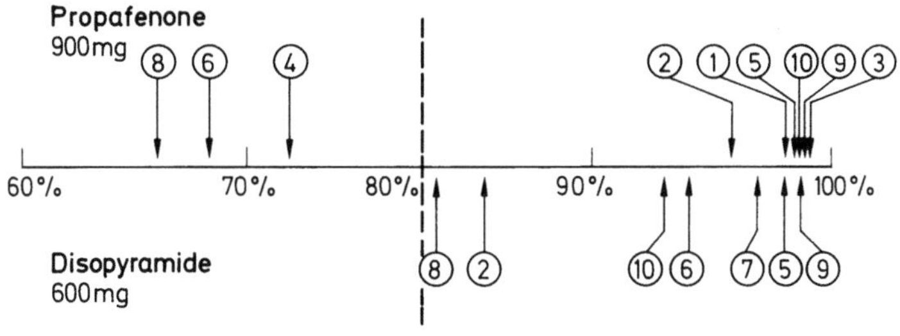

Fig. 2. Reduction in VPBs shown as percentage of beginning value

$$U_{D<P}=36.5\ (n_P+n_D=6+7=13 \text{ and } n_P\times n_D=42)$$

$$=\frac{36.5-\frac{1}{2}\times 42}{\sqrt{42\times\frac{13+1}{12}}}=2.21\ (P<0.03)$$

There is a significant difference between the results with P (which are much higher) and those with D. At an effective dose the efficacy of propafenone is clearly stronger than that of disopyramide.

Analysis of the Additional Criterion: Number of QRS Complexes (Systoles)

We did a differential analysis of occasionally appearing chronotropic effects for each of the treatments, with weighted complete blocks [2] over two factors. The first factor was the "period" without iteration (the resulting number for each of the three periods was the mean of the 8 h), the second was the "patient" (ten persons).

Without any Treatment

There is a significant change in the number of systoles in connection with the period, $F^2_{18}=23.15$ ($P<0.001$). The number of systoles during the night is smaller than those observed by day.

Treatment with Propafenone and Disopyramide

At low doses there is a very considerable mean decrease in the number of systoles per h (209) under propafenone. The *t*-test in paired series shows

$$t_{239}=6.10\ (P\ll 0.001)$$

The result is a negative chronotropic effect of propafenone.

There is a similar, considerable reduction in systoles per h (358) with disopyramide, a negative chronotropic effect of D.

With high doses (for the seven patients who received high doses of each medication) the negative chronotropic effects of P and D remain clearly the same: 210 instead of 209 for P, and 325 instead of 358 for D.

Table 3. Analysis of the negative chronotropic effect in complete weighted blocks – comparison of P and D

Origin of fluctuation	ddl	Estimate of variance	F_{40}	*P*
Negative chronotropic effect, P vs D	1	30858	0.60	NS
Patients	9	434027	8.42	<0.001
Correlation between treatment and patient	9	61168	1.19	NS
Residual	40	51556	–	–

Comparison of Decrease in the Number of Systoles with Propafenone and Disopyramide

At low doses there is no noticeable difference in the decrease in the number of systoles between P and D. The negative chronotropic effect ("treatment" effect) which was observed with both P and D was analyzed differentially according to two factors; the one is the reduction in VPBs on each treatment with P and D – relative to the corresponding values without therapy – and the other is the patient factor, as shown in Table 3: $F^{1}_{40} = 0.60$ (NS)

Thus, with low doses there was no difference between the negative chronotropic effect using P and that using D. However, as always, there was a "patient" effect with $F^{9}_{40} = 8.42$ ($P < 0.001$), although there was no correlation between treatment and "patients".

The difference between propafenone and disopyramide was studied in the same way with high doses; the results are similar. No difference could be proven between the negative chronotropic effect with P and that with D:

$$F^{1}_{28} = 2.79 \text{ (NS)}$$

Statistical Interpretation

This therapeutic study, set up so that the patient was his own observer and could judge the efficacy of the two antiarrhythmics on VPBs himself, had the following results:

1. A "treatment" effect: At all doses, the reduction in VPBs caused by propafenone is much more significant than that caused by disopyramide.
2. A "dose" effect: The reduction in VPBs after an increase in the dose of propafenone is significantly greater than the reduction seen after a dose increase with disopyramide, if the 80% threshold for decrease of VPBs – taken as the measure of efficacy – is exceeded.
3. A negative chronotropic effect without significant differences between the two therapies.

There was no correlation between the type of therapy (P or D) and the sequence of administration, just as there was no effect of sequence and no day/night effect. In this connection it should be noted that the day/night effect was checked hourly, namely during three 8-h periods, which is the usual method described in the literature [6]. On a statistical level, these results illustrate the importance of factor analysis, whereby the pa-

Table 4. Side effects observed during therapy with disopyramide and propafenone

Therapy	No. of observed patient	Dose (mg/day)	Side effect
Disopyramide	3[a]	300	Pyrosis
		600	Pyrosis
			Dizziness
			Double vision
			Urinary dysfunction
	4[a]	600	Urinary tract disorders
	6	600	Urinary tract disorders
	8	600	Dizziness
	9	600	Pyrosis
	10	600	Double vision
			Pyrosis
Propafenone	5	450	Pyrosis
	6	900	Pyrosis

[a] Side effects led to cessation of therapy

tient is his or her own observer and undergoes a large number of recordings. On a medical/therapeutic level, they show the superiority of propafenone over disopyramide at effective doses.

Tolerability

Clinical

Table 4 lists the side effects which were observed. During therapy with disopyramide, relatively numerous and intensive side effects appeared in six of ten patients, as opposed to two of ten during propafenone therapy. In two cases (patients 3 and 4) they were sufficiently serious to lead to the cessation of therapy, while in no case was propafenone therapy suspended.

Biological

Biological tolerability of both propafenone and disopyramide was excellent. No significant difference was found between the values of the parameters analyzed before and after therapy (Table 5 and 6).

Table 5. Biological tolerability of propafenone ($n = 10$)

Parameter	Before therapy		After therapy		"t"	Significance
	Mean	SD	Mean	SD		
Erythrocytes (/mm³)	4760000	500000	4700000	260000	0.50	NS
Leukocytes (/mm³)	5380	680	5720	1390	1.21	NS
Neutrophils (%)	58.99	5.41	59.82	4.93	0.87	NS
Eosinophils (%)	2.46	0.95	2.31	0.90	0.53	NS
Basophils (%)	0.92	0.50	0.82	0.34	0.62	NS
Lymphocytes (%)	31.11	4.76	31.43	5.58	0.49	NS
Monocytes (%)	6.12	3.51	5.88	2.36	0.29	NS
Potassium (mEq/l)	4.30	0.18	4.32	0.24	0.21	NS
Transaminases						
SGPT (IU/l)	17.20	8.73	18.20	9.05	0.87	NS
SGOT (IU/l)	15.10	2.51	15.50	3.64	0.33	NS
Blood sugar (g/l)	0.89	0.09	0.91	0.09	1.07	NS
Urea (g/l)	0.38	0.10	0.36	0.09	0.62	NS
Creatine (mg/l)	11.14	1.24	11.04	0.95	0.23	NS
Bilirubin (mg/l)	6.90	1.87	6.56	1.75	0.37	NS
Alkaline phosphatases (IU/l)	52.20	14.70	52.40	12.90	0.07	NS

Table 6. Biological tolerability of disopyramide ($n = 10$)

Parameter	Before therapy		After therapy		"t"	Significance
	Mean	SD	Mean	SD		
Erythrocytes (/mm³)	4760000	500000	4840000	410000	0.63	NS
Leukocytes (/mm³)	5380	680	5690	890	1.83	NS
Neutrophils (%)	58.99	5.41	59.24	5.28	0.50	NS
Eosinophils (%)	2.46	0.95	2.48	1.27	0.04	NS
Basophils (%)	0.92	0.50	0.82	0.34	0.62	NS
Lymphocytes (%)	31.11	4.76	31.40	4.33	0.39	NS
Monocytes (%)	6.12	3.51	5.88	2.36	0.29	NS
Potassium (mEq/l)	4.30	0.18	4.32	0.24	0.21	NS
Transaminases						
SGPT (IU/l)	17.20	8.73	16.90	6.74	0.19	NS
SGOT (IU/l)	15.10	2.51	15.50	3.54	0.33	NS
Blood sugar (g/l)	0.89	0.09	0.87	0.10	0.64	NS
Urea (g/l)	0.38	0.10	0.29	0.11	0.29	NS
Creatine (mg/l)	11.14	1.24	10.88	0.74	0.49	NS
Bilirubin (mg/l)	6.90	1.87	7.77	3.52	0.71	NS
Alkaline phosphatases (IU/l)	52.20	14.70	57.00	15.97	1.83	NS

General Conclusions

In this quantitative study, in which the patient was his own observer, we have proven the therapeutic superiority of propafenone over disopyramide in the treatment of VPBs.

The sequence of administration of P and D was established by having the patients draw lots. A pretreatment period of 2 days served as the basis for evaluation, after which each period of therapy lasted 10 days. An interval of 5 days, during which the patients received placebos, served as "wash-out".

Two different doses of a drug were administered, one after the other for 5 days each, in the course of a therapy period. For propafenone, these were 150 mg three times daily for 5 days, then 300 mg three times daily for the following 5 days. For disopyramide, the doses were 100 mg three times daily for the first 5 days, then 100 mg six times daily for the following 5 days.

Efficacy was checked with a 24-h ECG before each treatment, after the wash-out period, and after each dose during each treatment period. The fixed criterion of efficacy was the reduction of VPBs by 80%, relative to the number registered per h before treatment.

The statistical interpretation of the results showed a much clearer and more lasting reduction in VPBs with the administration of propafenone than with disopyramide, and this at all doses given. Moreover, the reduction in VPBs was much closer to 100% at a high dose of propafenone than it was at a high dose of disopyramide. Both preparations showed negative chronotropic effects.

In general, the minimal therapeutically effective dose of propafenone is between 450 and 900 mg/day, depending on the individual case.

Clinical tolerability of propafenone was very good at all doses studied. In contrast, side effects – urinary dysfunction and gastric trouble – were observed at a 600-mg daily dose of disopyramide, leading in two cases to cessation of therapy. Biological tolerability was very good with both drugs.

In conclusion, propafenone is the more effective and more tolerable of the two drugs, and is the antiarrhythmic of choice in the treatment of ventricular premature beats.

Propafenone, Flecainide and Mexiletine in the Treatment of Stable Ventricular Premature Beats

H.-W. Klempt and A. Nayebagha

Materials and Methods

The antiarrhythmic effects of oral doses of propafenone (P), flecainide (F), and mexiletine (M) were compared with one another in 12 patients with coronary heart disease and ventricular premature beats (VPBs) requiring treatment.

The patients were men ranging in age from 40 to 67 years (mean = 55.6 years) and in weight from 67.5 to 100.5 kg (mean = 80.4 kg). In all patients the arrhythmia developed as a sequel to a transmural myocardial infarction, and in one the arrhythmia followed a prosthetic mitral valve replacement and aortocoronary bypass to the RCA.

The study began with a 3-day pretreatment phase, followed by alternating phases of 4 days on drug therapy and 3 days on placebo (Table 1). The duration of the study was 24 days. The antiarrhythmic drugs were administered according to a single-blind scheme, and the sequence of administration was determined by random criteria.

The daily doses were 900 mg P, 400 mg F, and 600 mg M. F was administered twice daily at 12-h intervals, and M and P three times daily at 8-h intervals.

Electrocardiograms were recorded on a Lown drum for 1 h each day between 12:30 and 1:30 p.m. At the end of the pretreatment phase and at the end of each drug and placebo phase a 24-h tape-storage ECG record was obtained. A total of 24 drum ECG records and seven tape-storage ECG records were made for each patient.

The counting and classification of VPBs was done by three experienced assistants who knew the patients but not the therapy. The VPBs were individually counted on the large screen of the Camscan video analyzer, which can display all cardiac actions within a given 60-s interval. The tape being analyzed can be advanced in exact 1-min intervals, thus dividing a continuous 24-h trace into 1440 segments that can be manually evaluated individually.

Unless otherwise indicated, the paired *t*-test was used for all statistical computations.

Table 1. Design of study

	Day						
	1 2 3	4 5 6 7	8 9 10	11 12 13 14	15 16 17	18 19 20 21	22 23 24
	Pretreatment	Test I	Placebo	Test II	Placebo	Test III	Placebo
Standard ECG	X	X	X	X	X	X	X
1-h ECG	XXX	XXXX	XXX	X X X X	X X X	X X X X	X X X
24-h ECG tape	X	X	X	X	X	X	X
Plasma level	X	XXXX	XXX	X X X X	X X X	X X X X	X X X
Laboratory tests	X	X	X	X	X	X	X

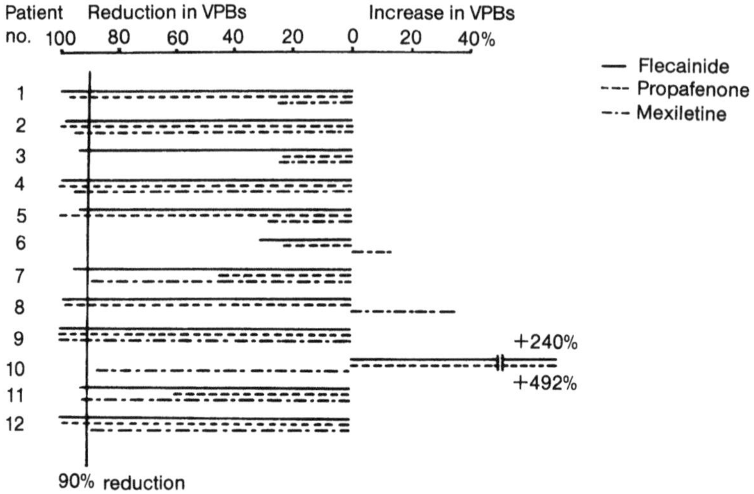

Fig. 1. Percentage changes in VPBs during antiarrhythmic therapy. The results of the 24-h ECG are shown

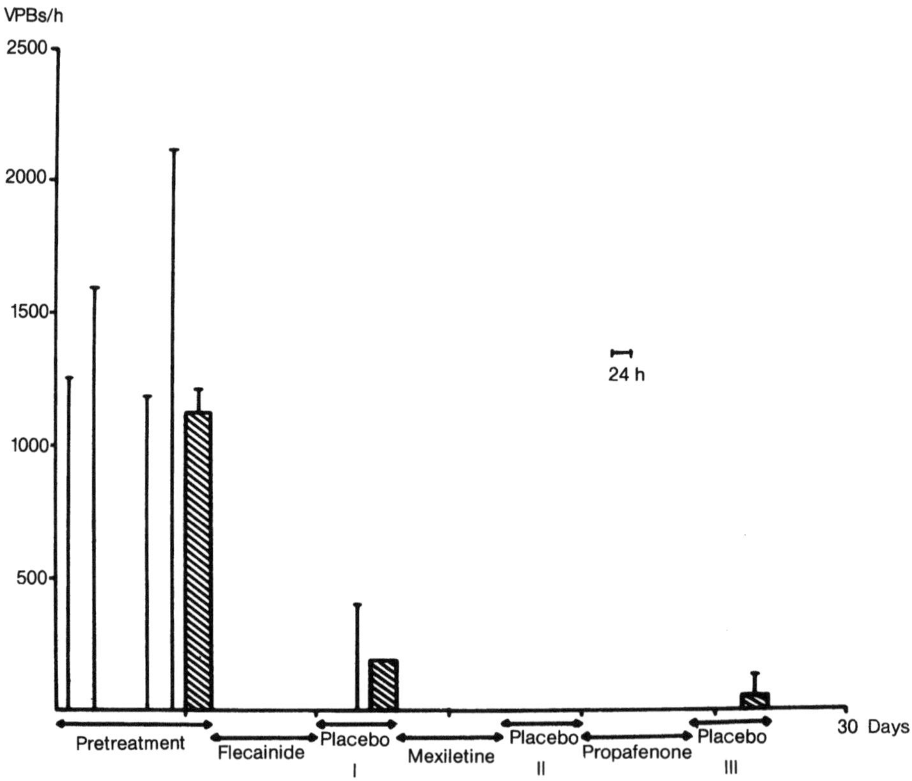

Fig. 2. Strong suspicion of spontaneous cessation of VPBs in a 50-year-old patient with arrhythmia following a posterior myocardial infarction. *Lines,* 1-h ECG; *cross-hatched bars,* 24-h ECG

Results

Figure 1 shows the percentage changes in VPBs during treatment with the three antiarrhythmic drugs as compared with the pretreatment phase. A rhythmogenic effect of F and P is evident in patient no. 10, while M leads to a reasonably satisfactory reduction of VPBs. In patient no. 6, none of the three drugs exerts a significant antiarrhythmic action. The best apparent antiarrhythmic effect is seen in patient no. 9. However, as Fig. 2 indicates, the massive VPBs observed in this patient during the pretreatment phase terminate abruptly when F is started and remain at low levels during the remainder of the study. Thus, despite the relative constancy of the VPBs during the pretreatment phase, it appears likely that the cessation of premature beats was a spontaneous phenomenon; therefore, data from this patient were excluded from our statistical evaluation.

The behavior of the VPBs in the remaining 11 patients is illustrated in Fig. 3. It must be emphasized that this diagram does not correspond to the chronologic course of the study, for only four patients received F as their first antiarrhythmic drug, while four others began the study with P or M. Compared with the pretreatment phase, F leads to a 94.2% reduction of VPBs ($P < 0.001$), P to an 80.2% reduction ($P = 0.005$–0.001) and M to a 52.8% reduction ($P = 0.02$–0.01). Thus, all three drugs exert a significant antiarrhythmic effect.

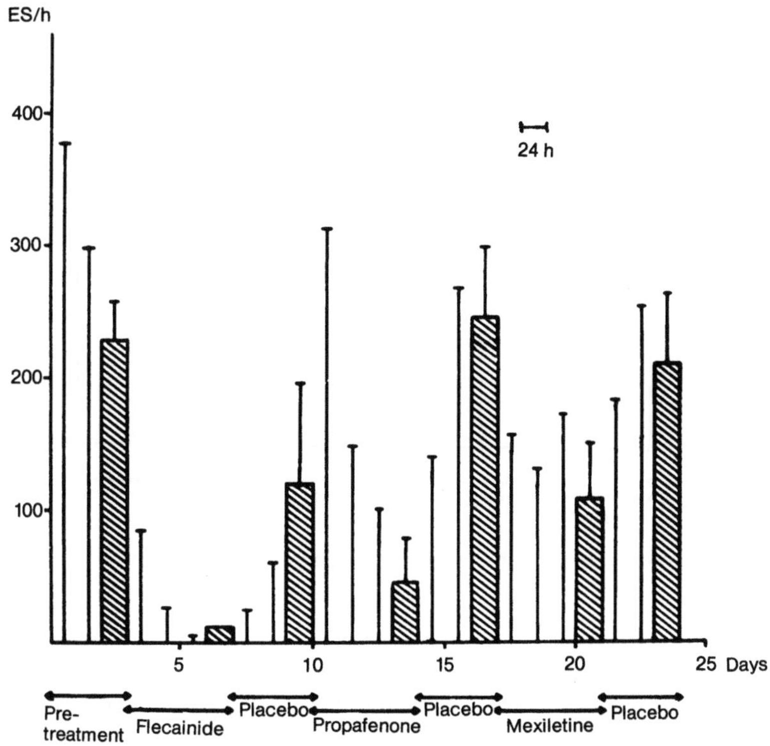

Fig. 3. Behavior of VPBs in 11 patients. The results of the 1-h, daily ECG (*lines*) and the 24-h ECG are shown

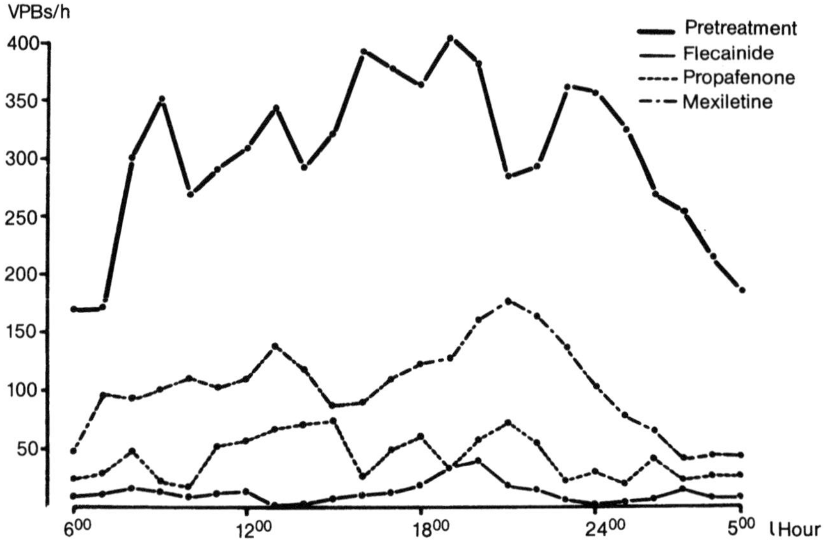

Fig. 4. A 24-h profile of VPBs during the pretreatment phase and during antiarrhythmic therapy

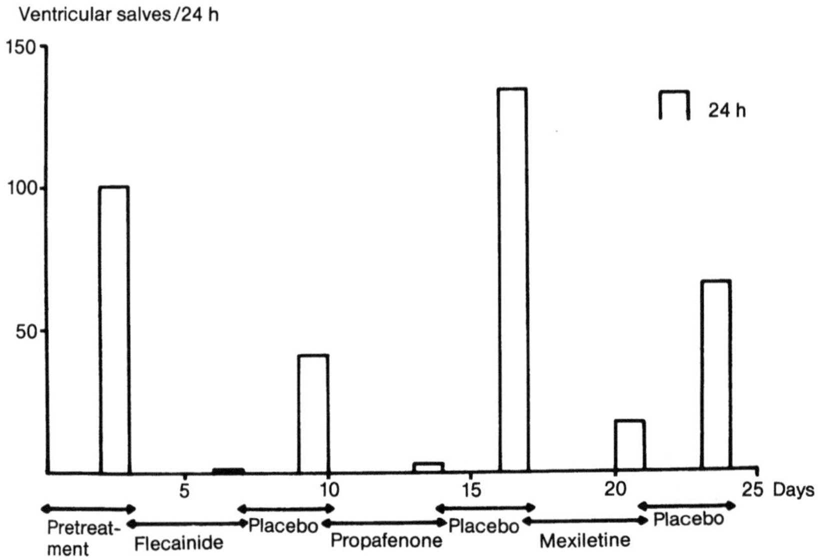

Fig. 5. Behavior of ventricular salvos in nine patients

It is interesting to note that 3 days after the discontinuance of F, the number of VPBs is still below the initial level, the difference being statistically significant ($P = 0.025–0.02$). This is attributable to the long half-life of F, which in our patients had a mean value of 19.0 h (13.5–29.9). The half-life was calculated from the exponential fall of the plasma concentration following discontinuance of the drug, which requires that at least three measurements be made at different times. The half-life of P was measured in only three of eight patients and amounted to 6, 9, and 12 h. That of M was measured in three of 12 patients, and the plasma concentration showed an exponential change in only one, in whom an 11-h half-life was measured.

Figure 4 shows the variations over a period of 23 h in the frequency of VPBs. The marked overall decrease in frequency at night is evident even during treatment with M. No increase in VPB frequency is observed prior to the times at which the various drugs were taken – 8:00 a.m. and 8:00 p.m. for F and 6:00 a.m., 2:00 p.m., and 10:00 p.m. for both P and M. This indicates that all three antiarrhythmic drugs remain active for 24 h at the doses and schedules employed.

The three drugs lead to a significant reduction in the frequency of ventricular salvos (Fig. 5). This reduction amounts to 98.5% with F, 96.8% with P and 83.3% with M. The reduction could be statistically confirmed with the Wilcox-Rank test ($P = 0.05–0.005$).

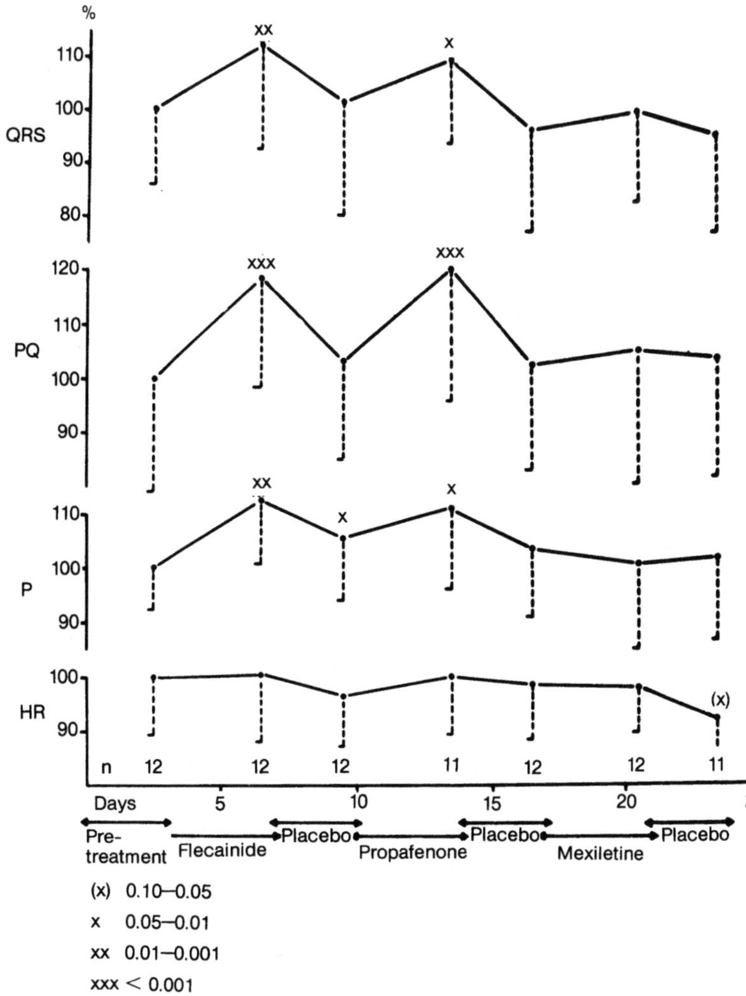

Fig. 6. Behavior of heart rate (*HR*) and P, PQ, and QRS intervals during the study

Nine of the 12 patients had grade-4A or -4B VPBs according to the Lown grading system, although only five of the 12 had more than 24 salvos in 24 h during the pretreatment phase (43–798 couplets or salvos per 24 h, mean = 163). F led to a complete suppression of salvo-like events in four to these five patients, P in three of five, and M in only one of five.

A complete suppression of all premature beats was achieved only in isolated cases. Disregarding a patient in whom the cessation of VPBs was presumably spontaneous, complete suppression of VPBs was achieved in only one patient on F, while another patient on P had only premature beat in 24 h.

Figure 6 shows the changes in certain ECG intervals during the course of the study. Both F and P led to a marked increase in P-wave width, PQ interval, and QRS width, the lengthening of the PQ interval being more pronounced than the widening of the P wave. It may be concluded from this that both the atrial and the atrioventricular conduction times are increased during treatment with F and P. In contrast to these drugs, M has no effect on the ECG intervals mentioned. The frequency-corrected QT interval, not shown in Fig. 6, and the heart rate are not altered by any of the three antiarrhythmic drugs.

Side Effects

The side effects are summarized in Table 2. Patient no. 2 and patient no. 9 had such severe subjective side effects from P and M respectively that prolonged treatment with these drugs would not have been possible. Patient no. 6 complained of severe constipation during medication with P, but this could be adequately controlled with a mild laxative.

Conclusions

A 24-day study was done to objectively compare the effects of three modern antiarrhythmic drugs. Dosages were determined in accordance with manufacturers' recommendations. The doses of P and F were approximately maximal, while considerably higher doses of M have frequently been used since our study was done.

F and P, taken in respective doses of 400 and 900 mg/day, appear to be similar in the potency of their antiarrhythmic action, F showing perhaps a slight superiority in this regard. P and F exert a markedly stronger antiarrhythmic action than M taken in a daily dose of 600 mg, although the differences among the drugs are not statistically significant. M, in fact, proved to be the only effective drug in one patient. Of course it cannot be concluded from our findings that higher doses of M would be more effective than the 600 mg dose selected for the study. On the whole, however, our results support the findings of Bethge and Lichtlen (1981), who, using different methods, found that P was clearly superior to M in its antiarrhythmic action.

Table 2. Subjective side effects of antiarrhythmic drugs

Patient no.	Flecainide	Placebo	Propafenone	Placebo	Mexiletine	Placebo
1	–	–	–	–	–	–
2	Dizziness on days 3 and 4	–	Days 2–4: severe headache and depression; took tablets only to be cooperative	–	–	–
3	–	–	–	–	Slight nausea on day 1	–
4	–	–	–	–	–	–
5	–	–	Annoying pressure in head	–	–	–
6	–	–	Severe constipation	–	–	–
7	Dizziness on days 1–4	Dizziness on day 3	Dizziness on days 1–3; strong nausea on day 4, skipped evening dose	Dizziness, fatigue day 3	Dizziness, hand tremors, days 1 and 2	Did not take place
8	–	–	–	–	–	–
9	–	–	–	–	Severe stomach pain after first dose, improvement after laxative; laterm, dizziness and nausea	–
10	–	–	–	–	–	–
11	–	–	–	–	–	–
12	–	–	–	–	–	–

The effects of antiarrhythmic agents on ECG intervals are of considerable practical importance. While we found no changes in these parameters during treatment with M – thus confirming the findings of other authors (Seipel and Breithardt 1978) – 900 mg P and 400 mg F produced almost identical prolongations of the P wave, PQ interval, and QRS complex. In some cases these changes may prevent necessary dose increases or may preclude the use of P and F altogether.

As mentioned, F taken at 12-h intervals at the administered doses produced an antiarrhythmic action lasting 24 h, as did P and M taken at 8-h intervals. This twice-daily dosing of F represents a simplification of the regimen. On the other hand, the long half-life of F (up to 30 h) raises the possibility of accumulation.

The great variability in the half-life of F probably explains why it is more difficult to ascertain the necessary individual dose for this drug than for P or M. Among our patients, for example, the daily dose of F varies between 100 and 500 mg. We have observed no similar variability for P or M.

References

Bethge K-P, Lichtlen PR (1981) Die Beurteilung der antiarrhythmischen Therapie durch Langzeitelektrokardiographie. In: Luederitz B (ed) Ventrikulaere Herzrhythmusstörungen. Springer, Berlin Heidelberg New York p 170

Seipel L, Breithardt G (1978) Electrophysiological effects of mexiletine in man: Influence on stimulus-induced ventricular arrhythmias. In: Sandøe E, Julian DG, Bell JW (eds) Management of ventricular tachycardia – role of mexiletine. Excerpta Medica, Amsterdam p 219

Long-term Prognosis for Patients with Complex Ventricular Arrhythmias of Lown Grades IVa and IVb

F. Theisen, K. Theisen and H. Jahrmärker

It is generally thought that complex ventricular arrhythmias in patients with cardiac disease, especially coronary heart disease, constitute an increased risk of sudden death [5, 7]. There is no agreement in the literature, however, on the definition of complex ventricular arrhythmias. Many authors regard Lown grades III (multiform ventricular premature beats), IVa (couplets), and IVb (ventricular tachycardias) as complex ventricular arrhythmias. The prognostic value of this classification, however, is still uncertain, especially for long-term prognosis and with regard to therapeutic response.

We therefore undertook to investigate the long-term prognosis and the course of antiarrhythmic therapy in patients with ventricular arrhythmias of Lown grades IVa and IVb.

Patients and Methods

We examined 28 patients (18 male and 10 female) with a mean age of 57 (18–72) years.

Eight patients had coronary heart disease, seven valvular heart disease, four dilative cardiomyopathy, two hypertensive heart disease, one a mitral valve prolapse syndrome, and six cardiac arrhythmias of obscure origin.

Within our series, 19 patients suffered from cardiac failure (NYHA classes II–IV). Twenty patients underwent cardiac catheterization; their mean ejection fraction was $38 \pm 11\%$ SD. In four patients ventricular fibrillation had been eliminated by successful resuscitation; in one of these patients arrhythmias were observed, although no other heart disease could be detected.

Long-term ECG recordings were made using a Reynolds Pathfinder II system with semiautomatic evaluation. In each case recording was done over a period of 24 h.

At the beginning of the study the course of therapy was analyzed on the basis of existing medical records (all patients were already receiving antiarrhythmic therapy). The aim of the first 24-h ECG check was to monitor the success of the antiarrhythmic therapy being used. Successful therapy was defined as disappearance of Lown grades IVa or IVb during a 24-h ECG.

Where successful therapy was demonstrated, the antiarrhythmic therapy was continued, and for further follow-up 24-h ECGs were carried out at 6-month intervals. In case of treatment failure, further therapeutic attempts were initiated. The therapeutic efficacy of each trial was also checked by 24-h ECG.

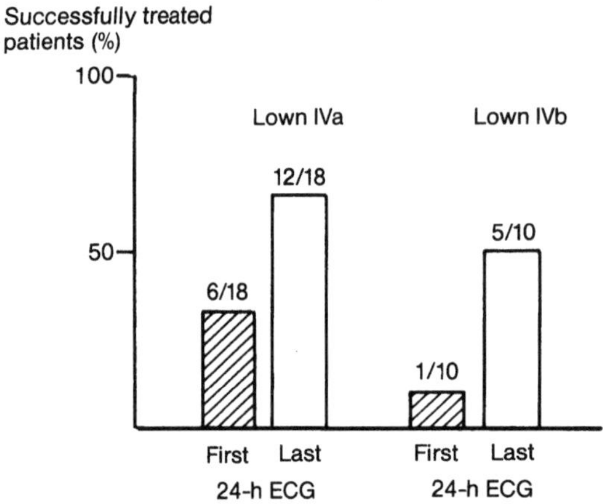

Fig. 1. Long-term therapeutic success in patients with Lown IVa and IVb. *Hatched column*, therapeutic success of antiarrhythmic therapy at the beginning of the study, checked by the first 24-h ECG. On the basis of the criteria applied at the time (rest ECG, rhythm strips, stress ECG, 4-hour telemetry), all of the patients were thought to have already been successfully treated. *open column*, therapeutic success as assessed in the last 24-h ECG, which was performed at the end of the study after further therapeutic attempts had been made on the patients who had not been successfully treated at the beginning of the study

Results

The mean follow-up period was 5.1 (1–12) years. Three of the 28 patients died. One, suffering from arrhythmias of Lown grade IVb, succumbed to sudden death after a year of unsuccessful antiarrhythmic therapy; one died as a result of an acute myocardial infarction, which was verified by autopsy (observation period, 3 years); and one died of terminal myocardial failure (observation period, 12 years).

Results of the first and last 24-h ECG checks are shown in Fig. 1. Only seven of 28 patients – six of the 18 with Lown IVa and one of the ten with Lown IVb – were treated with success, according to the first check. Yet all of the 28 had been classified previously as having been successfully treated on the basis of other types of therapeutic checks (resting ECG, rhythm strips, stress ECG, and telemetry recordings over about 4 h).

The last check showed that 17 of the 28 patients – 12 of the 18 with Lown IVa, and five of the ten with Lown IVb – had now been successfully treated. For the patients with Lown IVa, and average of 5.3 (2–15) therapeutic attempts with various antiarrhythmic drugs and combinations were required to achieve success; for those with Lown IVb, an average of 8.6 (5–11) attempts were needed.

Seven of the eight patients with coronary heart disease and five of the six with cardiac arrhythmias of unknown origin were successfully treated (Fig. 2). However, success was attained in only one of the four patients with cardiomyopathy and in four of the seven with valvular heart disease.

To achieve success, an average of 6.3 (2–15) therapeutic attempts were necessary in the patients with coronary heart disease, 6.2 (3–18) attempts in the patients with arrhyth-

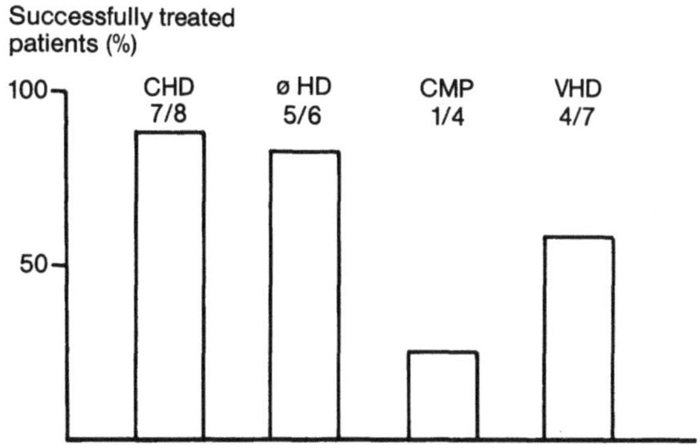

Fig. 2. Therapeutic success in patients with coronary heart disease *(CHD)*, heart disease of indeterminable origin *(HD)*, cardiomyopathy *(CMP)* and valvular heart disease *(VHD)*

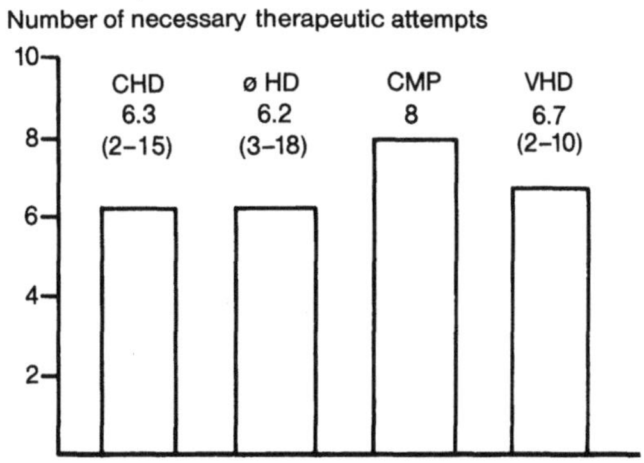

Fig. 3. Mean number of therapeutic attempts necessary to achieve success in patients with coronary heart disease *(CHD)*, heart disease of indeterminable genesis *(HD)*, cardiomyopathy *(CMP)* and valvular heart disease *(VHD)*

mias of unknown origin and 6.7 (2–10) attempts in the patients with valvular heart disease (Fig. 3). The one patient with cardiomyopathy who was successfully treated required eight attempts. One of the two patients with hypertensive heart disease required four attempts. By contrast, the second patient had not been successfully treated after the eighth attempt, nor the patient with a mitral valve prolapse syndrome after nine attempts.

An average of 8.6 (8–15) attempts were made in those 11 patients who were not treated successfully.

Table 1 shows the successfully administered antiarrhythmic drugs and combinations.

Discussion

The unfavorable prognostic significance of complex ventricular arrhythmias in patients after myocardial infarction appears to be established [5, 7]. For patients with other myocardial diseases, or for patients with arrhythmias of indeterminable origin, the prognosis remains the subject of discussion [1, 9, 11]. Prophylactic antiarrhythmic therapy in com-

Table 1. Successfully used antiarrhythmic drugs and antiarrhythmic combinations

Drug	Dosage	Times used	Times successful
Propafenone	600–900 mg	20	5
Ajmaline tartrate	60 mg	21	2
Amiodarone	200–600 mg	7	3
Quinidine	1 g	7	1
Propafenone with propranolol	750 mg 60 mg	8	1
Mexiletine with propranolol	600 mg 60 mg	3	1
Tocainide with amiodarone	800–1200 mg 200–600 mg	3	2
Ajmaline tartrate with propranolol	60 mg 80 mg	10	1
Tocainide with propranolol	800–1200 mg 120 mg	1	1

plex ventricular arrhythmias is also still controversial [8]. A preventive effect against sudden death has so far been demonstrated only for the beta-adrenergic blockade following myocardial infarction [10]. The mechanism of action underlying this prophylaxis is unknown. Studies using prophylactic antiarrhythmic therapy are contradictory and fail, in part, to reveal a preventive effect [8]. On the other hand, for patients with ventricular tachycardias and recurrent ventricular fibrillation, the prognosis has been significantly improved by means of systematic therapeutic titration with antiarrhythmics [6].

For our group of patients with various cardiac diagnoses and arrhythmias of Lown grades IVa and IVb, the prognosis was relatively good over a mean follow-up period of 5.1 years. Only one of the 28 patients suffered sudden death. Other authors studying similar patients have found markedly higher mortality during observation periods of 12 and 19 months [2, 9]. However, either these patients were not treated at all with antiarrhythmic drugs, or treatment was not consistent.

It should therefore be considered whether the good prognosis with respect to sudden death for our group was due to the antiarrhythmic therapy being carried out consistently throughout the entire observation period, even though this therapy did not result in complete suppression of the arrhythmias in a large portion of the patients. At the end of the study 40% of the patients still manifested arrhythmias of Lown grades IVa and IVb, although an average of 8.6 therapeutic attempts had been made. On the whole, cardiac arrhythmias proved extremely difficult to treat.

Myerberg et al. [6] also found a significantly improved prognosis in patients with recurrent ventricular tachycardias who received antiarrhythmic therapy in the therapeutic plasma level range, although the arrhythmias were not completely abolished by the therapy. It is therefore conceivable that antiarrhythmic therapy, without leading to complete suppression of complex arrhythmias, improves prognosis with regard to sudden death by directly influencing the myocardium or by blocking autonomic mechanisms [4], thus preventing the fatal progression of arrhythmias into ventricular fibrillation.

Summary

Twenty-eight patients with ventricular arrhythmias of Lown grades IVa and IVb were examined in a long-term study, carried out partly retrospectively and partly prospectively over an average observation period of 5.1 years. Therapy was monitored by means of 24-h ECG recordings. Therapeutic success was defined as disappearance of Lown IVa or IVb in a 24-h ECG. At the beginning of the study all 28 patients were thought – on the basis of the therapy monitoring criteria available at the time (resting ECG, rhythm strips, ergometry, and approximately 4-h ambulatory telemetry) – to have already been successfully treated. According to the first 24-h ECG, however, only seven of the 28 patients had been successfully treated. Following further antiarrhythmic therapy attempts, each monitored by a 24-h ECG, the therapeutic success increased to 17 of 28 patients at the end of the study. To achieve this, an average of 6.3 therapeutic attempts were needed. Of the 28 patients, 11 (40%) could not be successfully treated, despite an average of 8.6 therapeutic attempts. Three of the 28 patients died, only one of sudden death. In light of these findings, arrhythmias of Lown grades IVa and IVb appear to be extremely difficult to treat. Yet the prognosis for our patients was relatively good. Perhaps antiarrhythmic therapy, without leading to complete suppression of complex arrhythmias, improves prognosis with regard to sudden death by directly influencing the myocardium or by blocking autonomic mechanisms, thus preventing the fatal progression of arrhythmias into ventricular fibrillation.

References

1. Brisse B, Bender F (1982) Herzrhythmusstörungen bei Koronargesunden. MMW 124 No 15: 373–376
2. Follansbee WP, Michelson L, Morgenroth J (1980) Nonsustained ventricular tachycardia in ambulatory patients: Characteristics and association with sudden cardiac death. Ann Intern Med 92: 741
3. Lown B, Graboys TB (1977) Management of patients with malignant ventricular arrhythmias. Am J Cardiol 39: 910–918
4. Lown B (1980) Neural and psychologic factors in sudden death. Verh Dtsch Ges Herz Kreislaufforsch 46: 28
5. Moss AJ, David HT, DeCamilla J, Bayer LW (1979) Ventricular ectopic beats and their relation to sudden death after myocardial infarction. Circulation 60 No 5: 998–1003
6. Myerburg RJ, Conde C, Sheps DS, Appel RA, Kiem I, Sung RJ, Castellanos A (1979) Antiarrhythmic drug therapy in survivors of prehospital cardiac arrest: Comparison of effects in chronic ventricular arrhythmias and recurrent cardiac arrest. Circulation 59: 855–863
7. Ruberman W, Weinblatt E, Goldberg JD, Frank CW, Chaudhary BS, Shapiro S (1981) Ventricular premature complexes and sudden death after myocardial infarction. Circulation 64 No 2: 297–305
8. Seipel L, Breithardt G (1980) Indikation zur Therapie tachykarder Rhythmusstörungen. Pharmakotherapie 3 No 6: 251–257
9. Spielberg C, von Leitner ER, Andresen D, Schröder R (1982) Prognostische Bedeutung komplexer tachykarder ventrikulärer Rhythmusstörungen im 24-Stunden-Langzeit-EKG. Z Kardiol 71: 271–277

10. The Norwegian Multicenter Study Group (1981) Timolol-induced reduction in mortality and reinfarction in patients surviving acute myocardial infarction. New Engl J Med 304: 801–807
11. Winkle RA (1980) Detection of patients at high risk for sudden death: The rule of electrocardiographic monotoring. In: Kulbertus HE, Wellens HJJ (eds) Sudden death. Developments in cardiovascular medicine, vol 4. Martinus Nijhoff, The Hague pp 275–296

Experience with Propafenone in the Treatment of Arrhythmias in Pediatric Patients*

H. Weber, G. Eigster and H. Wesselhoeft

Introduction

Numerous reports have been published on cardiac arrhythmias in the pediatric age group that are serious enough to warrant treatment (Landtman 1947; Rutkowski et al. 1973). Especially in infants, arrhythmias can lead to severe heart failure and cardiogenic shock. Unless the arrhythmia is effectively treated, sudden cardiac death is a danger.

Propafenone is a drug that is included in the class of antiarrhythmic agents with membrane-stabilizing action. Its effect on fast action potentials appears to be similar to that of lidocaine and quinidine. In addition, there is evidence that propafenone inhibits slow action potentials and possesses β-blocking properties (Scholz 1981).

Patients and Methods

From July, 1978 to May, 1982, 66 patients ranging in age from 2 days to 23 years (six younger than 9 months and 13 older than 14 years; mean = 8 years, 4 months), comprising 37 males (56%) and 29 females (44%), were treated with propafenone for significant abnormalities of cardiac rhythm. Sixteen of the arrhythmia patients (24.2%) had a congenital heart defect; 21 (31.8%) had already been treated with various other antiarrhythmic drugs as either in- or outpatients before being admitted to our hospital; 19 (28.8%) presented as emergency cases during arrhythmic episodes; and nine others (13.6%) had spells of syncope and dizziness.

Except for the emergency cases, all patients underwent long-term ECG monitoring over a period of 20–48 h before antiarrhythmic treatment with propafenone was started. Cardioversion was done in three of the emergency patients, and in 11 others rapid intracardiac pacing was used to establish a sinus rhythm. Each of 42 arrhythmic patients received an intravenous injection of propafenone in the catheterization laboratory, during which time continuous atrial, His-bundle, and ventricular electrograms were recorded, in addition to a three-lead surface ECG (V_2, I, aVF). Of these patients, 18 were arrhythmic when they presented for cardiac catheterization; in the remaining 24, arrhythmia was induced by intracardiac stimulation. The propafenone was injected at a rate of 1 mg/kg per 5 min until a sinus rhythm was established. This was followed by high-frequency atrial stimulation at increasing frequencies until an atrioventricular block was induced, followed in turn by programmed stimulation of the right atrium and right ventri-

* Supported by the *Deutsche Forschungsgemeinschaft* SFB 89 *Kardiologie,* Göttingen

cle using a pulse width of 2 ms and twice the measured threshold current intensity. Arrhythmias could still be elicited in 11 of the 42 patients following intravenous administration of propafenone. Seven of these cases went on to spontaneous remission, but in four a sinus rhythm could be restored by rapid atrial pacing.

Following the invasive studies the patients were placed on monitors, and an ECG was recorded hourly, or as needed. On the next day oral propafenone therapy was started in a dose equal to ten times the effective intravenous dose as determined previously. This was administered in divided doses, three to four times daily. Concurrent, continuous ECG recordings were made for periods ranging from 20 to 48 h.

Laboratory tests for the early detection of possible side effects were performed before the start of treatment, 1 and 3 weeks afterwards, and at more frequent intervals if deemed necessary.

Serum levels of propafenone were determined for 32 patients by drawing blood 20–50 min after the intravenous propafenone injection and once daily during the subsequent 5-day course of oral propafenone, in the morning, before the first tablet was swallowed. Two additional checks of the serum propafenone level were made after the patients were discharged, at 14 days and at 3 months after the start of treatment. In the remaining 34 patients, one to five checks of serum propafenone levels were carried out at varying intervals. Only the serum levels of patients who had taken their tablets on a regular basis were recorded for evaluation. All serum concentrations were determined in the laboratories of the firm Knoll AG, which also furnished us, free of charge, with propafenone ampules and children's tablets of 5, 10, and 50 mg.

Results

Arrhythmias

The types and prevalence of the cardiac arrhythmias in our study population are shown in Table 1. In the majority of cases (66.6%) the arrhythmia was caused by a reentry cir-

Table 1. Incidence of various types of arrhythmias in 66 patients

Arrhythmia	No. of patients
Paroxysmal supraventricular tachycardia	
Accessory atrioventricular pathway	33
AV nodal tachycardia	4
Atrial flutter	4
Ventricular arrhythmias	
Ventricular tachycardia	9
Ventricular premature beats	5
Combined arrhythmias	
Accessory pathway with atrial flutter	6
Accessory pathway with ventricular premature beats	5

cuit involving an accessory atrioventricular or atriofascicular conduction pathway. Only eight of the affected patients showed constant or intermittent signs of WPW- or LGL-type preexcitation in their ECGs.

Propafenone Dose

According to our findings the active intravenous dose of propafenone was between 11.5 and 63.8 mg/m^2, body surface area, mean = 39.7 mg/m^2. The active oral dose was between 200 and 605 mg/m^2 body surface area per day, mean = 308.5 mg/m^2 per day.

These doses showed no specificity to age group from infancy through young adulthood.

Action

The patients were observed for periods ranging from 36 days to 3 years, 10 months (mean = 1 year, 8 months). During this time 44 patients (66.6%) were free of arrhythmias and complaints from the start of therapy, and 11 other patients (16.6%) experienced significant improvement or a significant decrease in the number and duration of arrhythmic episodes. In four cases (6%) the response was rated as unsatisfactory, and seven cases (10.6%) were ultimately rated as failures. The response to therapy according to arrhythmia type is presented in Table 2. While good results were obtained in patients with accessory pathways, response was less satisfactory in patients with combined arrhythmia types.

The observed effects of propafenone on sinus node function and intracardiac impulse conduction at the aforementioned doses were investigated in 23 patients and are presented in Table 3. Only slight conduction delays were noted in the AV node and His-Purkinje systems. No effect on either sinus node function or the threshold of myocardial activation was apparent at the doses administered.

It is noteworthy, however, that in patients with reentry excitation via an accessory pathway the arrhythmic episode could invariably be terminated by inhibiting the conduction of impulses via this accessory pathway.

Table 2. Results of treatment

Arrhythmia	Response			
	++	+	○	–
Accessory pathway	22	7	1	3
Ventricular tachycardia	8	1		
Ventricular premature beats	4		1	
Congenital atrial flutter	3			1
AV nodal tachycardia	3			1
Accessory pathway with atrial flutter	2	2	1	1
Accessory pathway with VPBs	2	1	1	1

VPB, ventricular premature beat; ++, free of arrhythmia from start of therapy; +, significant improvement; ○, unsatisfactory; –, failures

Table 3. Electrophysiologic effects of propafenone at mean i.v. dose of 39.7 mg/m² body surface area; change measured in ms

Effect on	Deviation of mean ($n = 23$) after propafenone (%)
Cycle length during Spontaneous sinus rhythm	+9.1
Frequency-corrected sinus node recovery time	+1.0
Functional refractory period, AV node	+11.8
Effective refractory period, AV node	+14.1

Table 4. Side effects related to propafenone therapy, observed in 31 of 66 patients

Symptom	No. of patients	(%)
Nausea	17	25.7
Vomiting	5	7.6
Anorexia	5	7.6
Fatigue	5	7.6
Insomnia	4	6.0
Dizziness	3	4.5
SGOT elevation	2	3.0
γ-GT elevation	1	1.5

Propafenone therapy could be discontinued in nine patients who had been free of arrhythmias for more than a year; four of these continued free of arrhythmias, while the remaining five experienced recurrences and had to be placed on at least an intermittent regimen of propafenone therapy.

Side Effects

As Table 4 illustrates, 31 patients (46.9%), displayed clinical symptoms during the observation period that were referable to the propafenone therapy. These involved mainly gastrointestinal and orthostatic complaints. In no case were signs of acute intoxication observed. Laboratory tests showed an elevation of the γ-GT in one infant that was markedly above the age-normal level, and a transitory elevation of the SGOT in two other patients. Side effects were never severe enough to warrant a discontinuance of therapy, however, and both the subjective complaints and abnormal laboratory findings disappeared within 1–3 weeks after the start of treatment.

Three patients given higher propafenone doses showed a significant increase in atrioventricular conduction time (PQ interval in the ECG); however, this interval normalized during exercise on the bicycle ergometer, and no arrhythmias occurred.

Serum Levels

From 20 to 50 min after intravenous administration, the serum level of propafenone was between 236 and 1500 ng/ml. After 24 h the level was at or below detectable limits.

With the start of oral dosing, the serum propafenone level rose until the 4th day, at that time assuming a mean value of 447 ng/ml with isolated extreme values (112–2706 ng/ml). No relation was found between high serum propafenone levels and the observed side effects. However, arrhythmic relapses occurred in patients whose serum levels were below 150 ng/ml; patient noncompliance with the oral dosing regimen was often a factor in such cases.

Discussion

Except for four patients whose arrhythmias were thought to be sequelae of myocarditis, all the arrhythmias in the study population were congenital in nature. A pressure or volume load could be ruled out in all but three of the 16 patients with congenital heart defects, for their defects were either well corrected or hemodynamically insignificant.

Three of the four patients with suspected postmyocarditic arrhythmias and two with volume load due to a severe congenital cardiac lesion were among the "therapeutic failures," and in these cases propafenone therapy was discontinued 4 weeks to 3 years after treatment had commenced.

Three patients with unsatisfactory therapeutic results were repeatedly found to have low ($<$ 50 ng/ml) or undetectable serum propafenone levels, due mostly to noncompliance with oral dosing. There was only one case in which the antiarrhythmic therapy failed despite an adequate plasma concentration of propafenone (200 ng/ml). After repeated, unsuccessful attempts at treatment, including trials with other antiarrhythmic agents, all antiarrhythmic drug therapy was discontinued, after which the patient was free of arrhythmia.

Intravenous digitalization of arrhythmic newborns and infants with heart failure is still the treatment of choice in the majority of pediatric cardiology centers. It is also recommended after cardioversion for the prevention of arrhythmias (Gilette 1981). This lends special importance to our observation of four newborns who presented as emergency cases with severe heart failure and signs of cardiogenic shock despite adequate digitalization. Even adequate digitalization was incapable of relieving either the heart failure or the arrhythmia in these patients. This emphasizes the need for a potent antiarrhythmic drug with minimal side effects and good tolerability even in patients of the neonatal age group.

Techniques for intracardiac ECG recording in infants and children have made it possible to investigate the mechanism of occurrence of various arrhythmias in these age groups (Brodsky et al. 1971). The most frequent arrhythmia is paroxysmal supraventricular tachycardia involving a reentry mechanism. Antiarrhythmic drugs of the membrane-stabilizing group are especially well suited for the treatment of these disorders.

Our experience with pediatric patients indicates that propafenone is a highly effective membrane-stabilizing antiarrhythmic drug with relatively good tolerability and minimal side effects when administered in the doses indicated.

References

Brodsky SJ, Mirowsky M, Krowetz LJ, Rowe RD (1971) Recordings of His bundle and other conduction time potentials in children. J Pediatr 79: 61–67
Gilette PC (1981) Dysrhythmias in infants and children. In: Engle MA (ed) Pediatric cardiovascular disease. Davis, Philadelphia pp 79–95
Landtman B (1947) Heart arrhythmias in children. Acta Paediatr [Suppl] 34: 1–107
Rutkowski MM, Doyle EF, Cohen SN (1973) Drug therapy of heart disease in pediatric patients. III. The therapeutic challenge of supraventricular tachyarrhythmias in infants and children. Am Heart J 86: 562–568
Scholz H (1981) Therapie der Arrhythmien. Neue Antiarrhythmika. Z Kardiol 70: 255

Electrophysiologic Effects and Antiarrhythmic Efficacy of Rytmonorm Evaluated with Programmed Electrical Stimulation of the Heart in Patients with Recurrent Reentrant Supraventricular Tachycardia

A. Waleffe and H. Kulbertus

Introduction

Propafenone has previously been observed to have a marked antiarrhythmic activity intravenously and/or orally [1, 4]. The initial studies of the drug indicated that this effect resulted from a local anesthetic membrane-stabilizing property [5]. The fast inward current of sodium and to a smaller extent the slow calcium current are depressed [6]. In this study we investigated the electrophysiologic effects of propafenone administered intravenously in 12 patients, of whom 11 had paroxysmal supraventricular arrhythmias which could reproducibly be initiated in the laboratory. The antiarrhythmic properties were reevaluated after chronic oral administration of the drug in five patients.

Patients and Methods

Twelve patients (five male, seven female) with disabling recurrent attacks of electrocardiographically documented supraventricular tachycardia were studied (Table 1). They ranged in age from 19 to 72 years. Five of them had, at least intermittently, electrocardiographic evidence of Wolff-Parkinson-White syndrome. In patients 1–5, the electrophysiologic investigations revealed that atrial activation during tachycardia occurred simultaneously with ventricular activation. In addition, ventricular premature complexes introduced with increasing prematurity during paced ventricular rhythm were followed by a gradual increase in VA conduction time and by the appearance of a retrograde His-bundle spike with a H-LRA interval compatible with conduction through the AV node. These patients were considered to have intranodal reentrant tachycardia. Four of the five subjects with Wolff-Parkinson-White syndrome were shown to have circus movement tachycardia. In patient 11 left atrial activation during ventricular pacing and tachycardia preceded low right atrial septal activation recorded in the His-bundle electrogram, thus indicating the presence of a left-sided accessory pathway for retrograde conduction. Finally, in patient 10 high right atrial activation preceded low right atrial septal activation during tachycardia; this patient was considered to have a right-sided concealed accessory pathway.

Table 1. Description of patients

Case	Age	Sex	Type of arrhythmia	Previous antiarrhythmic treatment
1	27	F	AVNT	Quinidine bisulfate 1 500 mg/day, propranolol 120 mg/day, verapamil 240 mg/day
2	45	F	AVNT	Quinidine bisulfate 1 500 mg/day, disopyramide 600 mg/day, desacétyl lanatoside C 0.50 mg/day
3	51	M	AVNT	Propranolol 320 mg/day, quinidine bisulfate 1 500 mg/day, verapamil 120 mg/day
4	26	F	AVNT	Propranolol 120 mg/day, metoprolol 200 mg/day, mexiletine hydrochloride 400 mg/day
5	32	F	AVNT	Quinidine bisulfate 1 000 mg/day, verapamil 200 mg/day
6	19	M	WPW B; CMT	Propranolol 160 mg/day, disopyramide 600 mg/day
7	22	M	WPW B; atrial fibrillation and flutter	Disopyramide 600 mg/day, quinidine bisulfate 1 500 mg/day, désacétyl lanatoside C 0.50 mg/day
8	20	M	WPW B; CMT	Several drugs, details unknown
9	58	F	WPW A; CMT	Quinidine bisulfate 1 500 mg/day, procainamide 1 000 mg/day, ajmaline 300 mg/day
10	72	F	Right concealed accessory pathway; CMT	Quinidine bisulfate 1 500 mg/day, ajmaline 300 mg/day, procainamide 1 000 mg/day, aprinidine 100 mg/day, amiodarone 300 mg/day 3 weeks per month
11	36	F	Left concealed accessory pathway	Amiodarone 300 mg/day 3 weeks per month
12	24	M	Intermittent WPW; CMT	Disopyramide 600 mg/day, verapamil 80 mg/day

Abbreviations: AVNT, atrioventricular nodal tachycardia; WPW, Wolff-Parkinson-White syndrome (type A or B); CMT, circus movement tachycardia

Electrophysiologic Study

All patients gave informed consent. Cardioactive drugs were discontinued 72 h prior to the procedure. Patients 10 and 11, who had received amiodarone and had developed clinical and biological signs of hyperthyroidism, had been off the drug for 6 weeks at the time of the investigation.

The protocol, the apparatus, and the definition used in this investigation have been described previously [7]. The electrophysiological parameters were measured before and 10 min after the end of an intravenous injection of 2 mg/kg propafenone administered over a 10 min period. In five patients [2, 6, 8, 9, and 11] who accepted a second invasive study the complete protocol of stimulation was repeated after 3 days treatment with oral propafenone (300 mg tds) and 2 h after the last dose administered. The protocol did not include investigations and follow-up during long-term oral use. Plasma levels of propafenone were determined by liquid chromatography under pressure.

Results

Electrophysiologic Effects of Propafenone

Effects on Basic Electrophysiologic Measurements

No systematic change of spontaneous cycle length was observed after propafenone. During atrial pacing, the AH interval increased in 9 of the 11 patients in whom it could be measured. The increase ranged from 84 ± 30 ms to 99 ± 32 ms ($p < 0.001$). Propafenone failed to have statistically significant effects on the functional refractory period of the AV node. The right atrial pacing cycle length required to produce second-degree atrioventricular block did not change significantly after drug administration.

The His-Purkinje conduction time (HV interval) increased significantly from 37 ± 5 ms to 43 ± 7 ms ($P < 0.05$). Before drug administration, VA conduction over the AV node could be measured in eight instances. After propafenone, VA conduction was blocked in two patients and lengthened in five (variations of 60–250 ms). The right ventricular pacing cycle length inducing a VA block increased in all cases.

The effective refractory period of the right atrium increased from 198 ± 28 ms to 220 ± 37 ms ($p < 0.05$). No systematic effect on the refractory periods of the right ventricular muscle was noted.

Effects on Accessory Pathways

The effects of propafenone on the effective refractory period of accessory pathways with anterograde conduction could be assessed in cases 6–9. In the two subjects whose accessory pathways had a relatively short effective refractory period (250 ms and < 260 ms), the increase was 30 ms and > 60 ms respectively. In the other two the administration of propafenone was followed by a 50-ms prolongation of the effective refractory period or by total blockade of conduction along the accessory pathway.

The effective refractory period of the bypass in retrograde conduction could be assessed in six instances. After propafenone it increased in four cases by 30–50 ms, but did not change in the remaining two cases. On the whole, the increase of the retrograde effective refractory period of the accessory pathway was statistically significant ($p < 0.05$).

Effects of Propafenone on Reentrant Tachycardias

In ten patients, administration of propafenone during episodes of tachycardia resulted in return to sinus rhythm. In each case, the length of time during which the tachycardia was sustained before administration of propafenone was longer than the interval required for termination by the drug. It should be noted that in patients 5, 6, and 8 tachycardia stopped during the perfusion of propafenone, but after and because of the appearance of spontaneous ventricular premature beats which had not been recorded in these patients either during the control period or during previous routine electrocardiograms.

AV Nodal Reentrant Tachycardia

Propafenone was administered in patients 1–5 during an episode of AV nodal tachycardia. In the first four patients, tachycardia stopped as a result of blockade of the fast retrograde pathway. In patients 1, 2, and 4 AV nodal reentrant tachycardia could not be reinitiated after the drug. In case 3, tachycardia could still be reinitiated but was slow and unsustained. In patient 5, the tachycardia cycle length showed only a very small increase (20 ms) after administration of the drug.

Circus Movement Tachycardia Incorporating an Accessory Pathway

In six patients, appropriately timed ventricular and/or atrial stimuli during the control period startet episodes of circus movement tachycardia. Propafenone injected during such episodes resulted in interruption of the tachycardia circuit, three times as a result of retrograde blockade of the accessory pathway (cases 10–12) and twice after the occurence of spontaneous ventricular premature beats which had not previously been observed in these patients. In patient 9, at the end of the perfusion the tachycardia cycle length had increased by 160 ms and the arrhythmic was interrupted by two induced atrial premature beats. After propafenone tachycardia could be reinitiated in five patients, but the cycle length of the tachycardia had increased in every case due to prolongation of both the AH interval and the VA conduction time through the bypass.

Effects of Chronic Oral Propafenone Administration

In five patients (2, 6, 8–10), the effect of chronic oral propafenone could be tested. The values of the refractory periods were of the same magnitude as after acute administration. In patient 2, with AV nodal tachycardia, no tachycardia could be elicited during the repeated investigation. Among the four patients with circus movement tachycardia no initiation was possible in patient 11, but tachycardia was still elicitable in the other three cases. However, the tachycardia cycle length was as great as (patient 8) or even greater than during the acute administration (increase of cycle length of 50 ms in patient 9 and 100 ms.

Drug Plasma Levels

Due to technical difficulties, plasma levels were not available in all patients and no mean peak value could be calculated for the whole group. A typical curve of the plasma levels observed after intravenous perfusion of the drug at a dose of 2 mg/kg over 10 min is shown in Fig. 1.

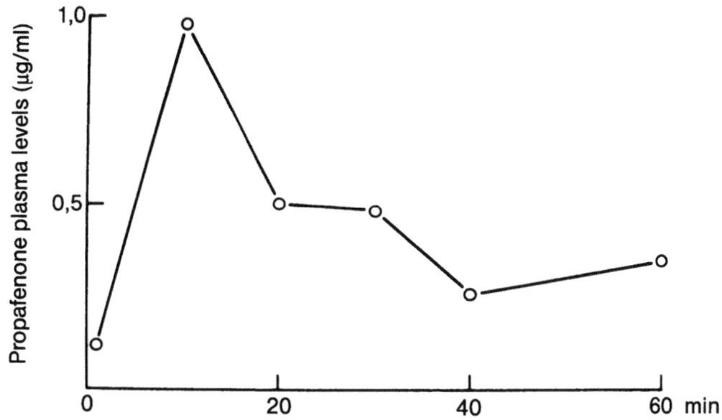

Fig. 1. Typical curve of propafenone plasma levels after intravenous injection of the drug at a dose of 2 mg/kg over 10 min

Side Effects

No Side Effects were Observed During this Study

Discussion

The objective of an antiarrhythmic drug therapy is to prevent the recurrence of arrhythmias inducing symptoms or associated with electrical or hemodynamic hazards. Reliable methods for reproducible initiation of tachycardia (i.e., programmed electrical stimulation of the heart) as well as reliable methods for evaluation of the patient's response to therapy (i.e., attempts to reinitiate the tachycardia after therapy) have recently been introduced. They allow a better understandig of the mode of action of antiarrhythmic agents and permit the selection of the agent best suited to the needs of the individual patient.

Electrophysiologic Effects of Propafenone

In Purkinje and myocardial fibers, propafenone mainly reduces the maximum rate of rise of the action potential, the response of Purkinje fibers being markedly more pronounced than that of common myocardial fibers. The effective refractory period is only slightly lengthended [5, 6]. Propafenone thus appears to share the properties of class I agents.

In our series propafenone showed a definite action on the AH and HV intervals, the effective refractory period of the right atrium, and the time needed for VA conduction along the AV nodal pathway. In spite of the lengthening of transnodal conduction time, the other functional properties of the AV node in the anterograde direction did not show statistically significant alterations after propafenone. This observation is in accordance with the moderate effect of the drug on the slow calcium inward flux, with the absence of systematic changes of sinus rhythm in our patients, and with the mode of termination of AV nodal reentrant tachycardias as discussed below.

Effects of Propafenone on Accessory Pathways

Propafenone either lengthened the refractory period or produced complete blockade of accessory pathways used in the anterograde direction. It prolonged retrograde refractoriness of the bypass in four of six patients. By depressing anterograde conduction in the accessory pathway as well as in the normal pathway, propafenone offers protection against rapid ventricular rates during circus movement tachycardia, atrial fibrillation, or atrial flutter. Although we agree with Wellens et al. [8] that the length of the refractory period of an accessory pathway during the control period often correlates with the magnitude of the change it undergoes under the influence of most conventional antiarrhythmic agents, our data on propafenone contrast with this general observation. The same was previously observed with moxaprindine [9]. It is possible that these new pharmacological agents might provide a better coverage for patients having a preexcitation syndrome and bypasses with short anterograde refractory periods.

Effects of Propafenone on Tachycardia

Infused intravenously during sustained episodes of AV nodal reentrant tachycardia, propafenone was seen to interrupt the rhythm disorder in four of six patients as a result of blockade of the fast retrograde pathway. This adds further support to the concept that the fast retrograde nodal pathway possesses Purkinje-like functional properties [10].

Among patients who have circus movement tachycardia with retrograde conduction over an accessory pathway, propafenone prevents reinitiation of the tachycardia only in those in whom retrograde conduction along the accessory pathway is profoundly affected. This can easily be explained. Propafenone delays anterograde conduction over the normal pathway (AH and/or HV intervals). Therefore when it does not prolong retrograde refractoriness of the bypass, it may widen the zone of the cardiac cycle during which paroxysmal supraventricular tachycardia can be initiated and also render more difficult the termination of this tachycardia [11–14]. These considerations probably explain the ease with which reinitiation of tachycardia could be achieved after propafenone in five of six patients with preexcitation. In the group with AV nodal tachycardia, reinitiation was possible in only one of five cases.

Investigations performed after the acute administration of a drug have obvious limitations. In this study, however, we have demonstrated that the favorable results obtained with propafenone in acute condition could be extrapolated to chronic oral use. Similar findings have recently been made with other agents [15, 16].

Conclusions

Our results indicate that propafenone is a useful antiarrhythmic agent for the treatment of patients with paroxysmal supraventricular tachycardia. The properties of the drug are such that under its influence patients suffering from AV nodal tachycardia may expect protection against recurrence of tachycardic episodes.

On the other hand, the drug is less likely to prevent attacks of circus movement tachycardia using an accessory pathway, and might even increase their frequency. In these conditions, however, propafenone may be expected to slow the rate of tachycardia when it develops and thus to make it more tolerable or even not perceptible to the patient. In addition, it may offer protection against high ventricular rates in the presence of atrial flutter or fibrillation, even in individuals whose accessory pathways spontaneously have a relatively short refractory period.

References

1. Beck OA, Kräuer KD, Wolfe R, Müller A, Hochrein H (1975) Propafenone: a new antiarrhythmic drug for treating tachycardia and extrasystolic arrhythmias. Med Klin 70: 95–101
2. Beck OA, Abdulla S, Hochrein H (1975) Clinical studies on the oral activity of the antiarrhythmic drug propafenone. Med Klin 70: 1713–1716
3. Fill WD, Kühn P, Probst P, Zilcher H (1977) Anwendung von Propafenon am Menschen. In: Hochrein, H, Hapke HJ, Beck OA (eds) Fortschritte in der Pharmakotherapie von Herzrhythmusstörungen. Fischer, Stuttgart, pp 71–79
4. Fischer G, Seipel L (1977) Klinische Erfahrungen mit der oralen Propafenon-Therapie. In: Hochrein H, Hapke HJ, Beck OA (eds) Fortschritte in der Pharmakotherapie von Herzrhythmusstörungen. Fischer, Stuttgart, pp 109–114
5. Bergmann M, Bolte HD (1977) Elektrophysiologische Untersuchungen mit Propafenon an myokardialen Einzelfasern. In: Hochrein EH, Hapke HJ, Beck OA (eds) Fortschritte in der Pharmakotherapie von Herzrhythmusstörungen. Fischer, Stuttgart, pp 29–34
6. Kohlhardt M (1977) Der Einfluß von Propafenon auf der transmembranären Na^{+} und Ca^{++} – Strom der Warmblütler Myokardfasermembran. In: Hochrein H, Hapke HJ, Beck OA (eds) Fortschritte in der Pharmakotherapie von Herzrhythmusstörungen. Fischer, Stuttgart, pp 35–38
7. Waleffe A, Bruninx P, Mary-Rabine L, Kulbertus HE (1979) Effects of tocainide studied with programmed electrical stimulation of the heart in patients with reentrant tachyarrhythmias. Am J Cardiol 43: 292–299
8. Wellens HJJ, Bar FW, Gorgels AP (1978) Effects of drugs in WPW syndrome. Importance of initial length of effective refractory period of accessory pathway (abst). Am J Cardiol [Abstr] 41: 372
9. Waleffe A, Mary-Rabine L, Kulbertus HE (1980) Study of moxaprindine with programmed electrical stimulation of the heart in patients with reentrant tachyarrhythmias. Am J Cardiol 45: 640–647
10. Rosen KM, Bauernfeind RA, Wyndham CR, Dhingra RC (1979) Retrograde properties of the fast pathway in patients with paroxysmal atrioventricular nodal reentrant tachycardia. Am J Cardiol 43: 863–865
11. Spurrell RAJ, Krikler DM, Sowton E (1974) Effects of verapamil on electrophysiological properties of anomalous atrioventricular connection in Wolff-Parkinson-White syndrome. Br Heart J 36: 256–264
12. Wellens HJJ, Dürer DR, Liem KL, Lie KI (1975) Effect of digitalis in patients with paroxysmal atrioventricular nodal tachycardia. Circulation 52: 779–788

13. Denes P, Cunnings JM, Simpson R, Wu D, Amat-Y-Leon F, Dhingra RC, Rosen KM (1978) Effects of propranolol on anomalous pathway refractoriness and circus movement tachycardias in patient with preexcitation. Am J Cardiol 41: 1061–1067
14. Waleffe A, Bordalo A, Bruninx P, Wellens HJJ, Kulbertus HE (1979) Electrophysiologic effects of L 9394 (benzoylindolizine) in man. Br Heart J 41: 89–98
15. Wu D, Wyndham CR, Denes P, Amat-y-Leon F, Miller RH, Dhingra RC, Rosen KM (1977) Chronic electrophysiologic study in patients with recurrent paroxysmal tachycardia: A new method for developing successful oral antiarrhythmic therapy. in: Kulbertus HE. Reentrant arrhythmias: mechanism and treatment. Lancaster, MTP Press, pp 144–152
16. Fisher JD, Cohen HL, Mehra R, Altschuler H, Escher DJW, Furman S (1977) Cardiac pacing and pacemakers. II Serial electrophysiologic-pharmacologic testing for control of recurrent tachyarrhythmias. Am Heart J 93: 658–68

Antiarrhythmic Effect and Study of Segmentary Contractility Following the Administration of Propafenone in Coronary Patients with Ventricular Arrhythmias

J. L. Palma, A. Bayés de Luna, M. Fiol, P. Yuste, V. Aza, J. Sadurni, C. E. R. y Cajal, R. Son Dureta and H. San Pablo

Introduction

Propafenone hydrochloride (2′-(2-hydroxy-3-propylamino-propoxy)-3-phenylpropiophenone) is a synthetic product developed in West Germany, and recently introduced into Spain for the treatment of cardiac arrhythmias of varying origin. Numerous studies on this new antiarrhythmic have appeared over the past 5 years and have made it possible to establish its pharmacological (Davis and Tempte 1968; Keller et al. 1978; Kohlhardt 1977; Ledda et al. 1980; Tritthart et al. 1971; van Rossum 1963; von Hapke and Prigge 1976); electrophysiological (Bergmann and Bolte 1977; Disertoni et al. 1980; Fill et al. 1977; Seipel et al. 1975; Seipel et al. 1977; Waleffe et al. 1981), and antiarrhythmic (Durante et al. 1980; Lüderitz 1978; Meyer-Estorff et al. 1978; Rutsch 1978; Seipel and Breithardt 1980; Vergara et al. 1980; Wiebrinhaus et al. 1978; Wieser et al. 1979) properties, as well as its toxicity. The drug may be administered either orally or intravenously. With oral administration the absorption is approximately 50% and plasma concentration is at its highest 2 h later. The mean half-life is 3–6 h. A high percentage of the drug is bound to the plasma proteins and is eliminated almost totally by the urinary tract within 24 h, although its antiarrhythmic properties decrease considerably 6–8 h after administration. The effective oral dose varies between 450 and 900 mg/day, according to patient. For intravenous administration, 1–2 mg/kg should be injected within a period of 5 min keeping a strict ECG control simultaneously.

From an electrophysiological point of view it has been shown that propafenone produces a block of the fast sodium channels, and to a lesser degree of the calcium channels. It reduces the amplitude of the action potential without modifying the resting potential. Intravenously, 2-mg/kg a dose has been shown to increase the ventricular fibrillation threshold, an effect similar to that produced by an equal i. v. dose of lidocaine; it also produces an antiarrhythmic effect following acute coronary occlusion in anesthetized animals. At equal doses a lengthening of the conduction velocity at Hisian, His-Purkinje, and muscle-Purkinje levels has been observed, as well as a depressor effect on sinusal automatism and sinoatrial conduction.

It has also been seen that with an i. v. dose of 2 mg/kg there is a slight decrease of arterial pressure, secondary to a reduction of maximum dp/dt. Cardiac index is slighty lowered and the telediastolic pressure of the left ventricle is slightly increased. All these hemodynamic effects suggest that the drug may have a negative inotropic effect.

Between 20% and 50% of patients treated with propafenone have some side effect – either a clinical type or an electrocardiographic alteration. Among the most common are vertigo, nausea, constipation, diarrhea, sickness, taste alterations, and cutaneous eruptions. With respect to the ECG, nearly all reports mention greater or lesser lengthening of AV and intraventricular conduction, as well as of the Q-T interval, although this does not usually lead to withdrawal of treatment.

In this paper we analyze the antiarrhythmic value of propafenone for coronary patients with severe ventricular arrhythmias and study possible changes due to the drug in segmentary contractility, with two-dimensional echocardiography.

Material and Methods

Group A

A group of 17 coronary patients (14 males and 3 females) aged between 44 and 69 years (mean ± 16) were submitted to an ambulatory electrocardiographic study over a 24-h period outside the hospital, and were selected for this study on the basis of the arrhythmias found in their first Holter ECG (H-ECG). All patients were separated, according to the number and severity of the arrhythmias, into the 3rd or 4th grade of Lown's classification (Table 1), although all had over 600 P.V.C. in 24 h. Lown's 5th grade was not studied, as our Holter system is unable to detect its presence. Of the 17 patients, 15 had suffered myocardial infarction between 3 and 49 months earlier, and two suffered from effort angina. Of the 15 patients with myocardial infarction, nine presented with anterior and eight posterior-inferior localization. None of these showed signs or symptoms of cardiac insufficiency superior to class II of the NYHA. The examination of the long-term electrocardiographic tapes was done with an Avionics 660 A electrocardioanalyzer with Data Terminal 680 DCG. The analysis of the tape was made both manually and automatically.

Before beginning treatment, nine patients were subjected to two-dimensional echocardiography using digitalized ATL-500 equipment. The M-technique was derived from the longitudinal and transverse planes. Each patient was then given 900 mg propafenone daily in three administrations of 300 mg. The dosage was continued over a period of 5–7 days, after which H-ECG and two-dimensional echocardiograms (ECHO-2D) were again recorded and a clinical evaluation and anamnesis were made.

Table 1. Lown's classification

Grade	Type of arrhythmia
0	Without PVCs
1	Less than 30 PVCs/h
2	More than 30 PVCs/h
3	Polymorphic
4 A	Pairs
4 B	Ventricular tachycardia
5	R on T

PVC, premature ventricular contraction

Following this period, patients received daily dose of three tablets (one every 8 h) of a placebo substance (lactose – similar in appearance to propafenone) for 4–6 days, after which they were again subjected to H-ECG and ECHO-2 D.

The following parameters, before and after propafenone and after placebo, were then analyzed from the H-ECG:

1. Maximum, minimum, and mean cardial frequency
2. Number of supraventricular ectopic beats
3. Number of premature ventricular complexes (PVC) – morphology and characteristics
4. Classification of the PVC according to Lown's criteria (Table 1)
5. PR interval (maximum recorded) in accordance with hourly samples
6. QRS duration (maximum recorded) in accordance with hourly samples
7. QT duration (maximum recorded) in accordance with hourly samples

Only the cases which presented a number of PVCs similar to the control recording ($\pm 20\%$) were included in the study.

The following parameters were studied from the ECHO-2 D in nine cases: the systolic and diastolic measurements, the shortening of the axis, and the first measurement of the shortening determined on the paper recording. The two-dimensional segmentary analysis included the study of nine segments (Kisslo et al. 1977) utilizing the transverse planes at the mitral valve and papillary levels, as well as the four-chamber and two-chamber planes from the apex (Fig. 1). A series of recordings before, during, and after treatment were obtained.

After each period the patient was questioned about tolerance to the drug, following a standard questionnaire, to evaluate possible secondary effects.

χ^2-method was used for statistical evaluation.

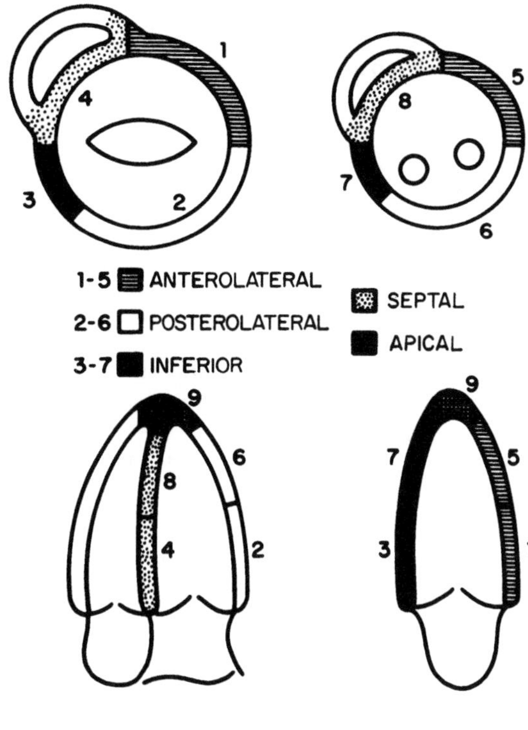

Fig. 1. Nine segments in nine cases studied by ECHO-2

Group B

Twelve patients were studied, 11 male and 1 female, aged between 38 and 71 years (mean 55 ± 18). Five presented with posteroinferior necrosis, five with anterior necrosis, and two with unstable angina. At the time of the study 11 of these patients with ischemic cardiopathy were hemodynamically in Killip class I, and one was in Killip class II. Six patients had antecedents of arterial hypertension, and three showed moderate signs of left cardiac failure.

Patients with acute edema of the lung, cardiogenic shock, electrolitic disturbances, and those taking vasoactive drugs were excluded from the study.

The electrocardiographic control was carried out by means of a computerized system of arrhythmias, HP 78 220 A (SCA).

The indications for administering propafenone were Lown's 4th grade ventricular arrhythmias in ten cases (three with pairs and seven with runs of ventricular tachycardia, VT), grade 5 in one case, and over 10 PVC per minute in the last case. The i. V. doses used were 1 mg/kg in two cases, 1,5 mg/kg in seven cases and 2 mg/kg in three cases.

The following controls were carried out:

1. Immediately prior to the beginning of the study, an evaluation was made of the number and morphology of the premature ventricular complexes (PVC), pairs of PVCs, and runs of ventricular tachycardia from the histograms and automatic recording of the SCA. Cardiac frequency, arterial tension and electrocardiographic intervals (P, PR, QRS, QT) were measured.
2. Cardiac frequency and arterial pressure were measured 5, 10, 15, 20, and 30 min after the administration of propafenone.
3. ECG parameters were taken again after 30 min.
4. The presence of arrhythmias in the 120-min period following the administration of propafenone and the presence of secondary effects were checked.

The variations in the number of PVCs within periods of 30 and 90 min were evaluated for the group as a whole.

Results

Group A

The maximum, minimum, and mean cardiac frequency in the control phase, after the administration of propafenone and placebo, was analyzed by the Data Terminal of the H-ECG. The results can be seen in Fig. 2. Lower frequency values were obtained with propafenone, the mean being 62.1 ± 10. In the control phase, the mean result was 66.9 ± 14, and after placebo 67.2 ± 12. The statistical differences among these data were not significant.

In Fig. 3, the data corresponding to the evaluation of the PR and QT intervals in the three phases of the study, i.e., in the control stage, following propafenone, and after placebo, can be seen. With respect to the PR interval, the measurement of control type was 0.168 s ± 0.017, but was 0.21 s ± 0.030 after propafenone and 0.172 s ± 0.015 after placebo ($P < 0.005$). Two patients showed a basal PR in the limit (0.20 s) and both developed AV block (one being first degree and the other Wenckebach second degree). The

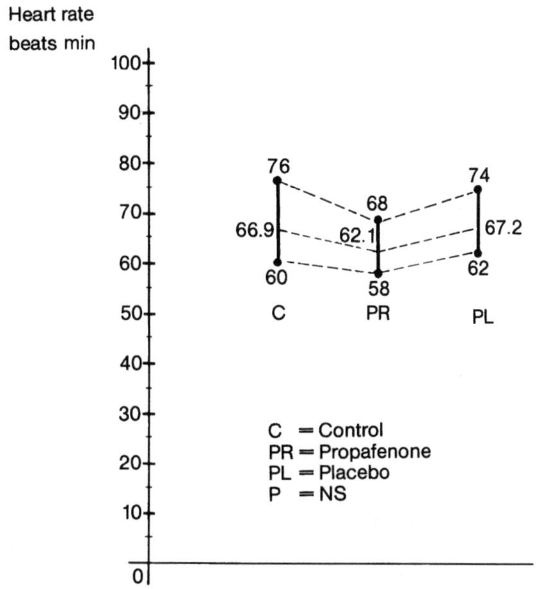

Fig. 2. Maximum, minimum, and mean heart rate in control, after propafenone and after placebo recordings

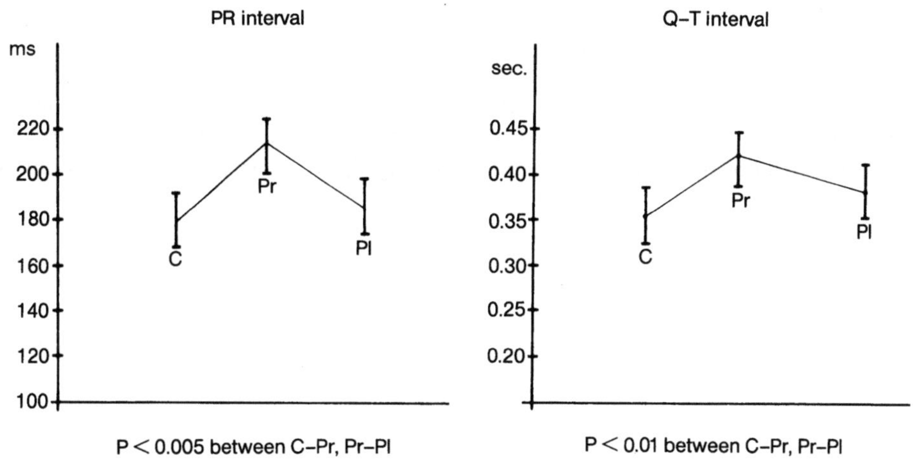

Fig. 3. Mean value and standard deviation of PR intervals *(left)* and QT intervals *(right)* in control, post-propafenone, and post-placebo recordings

rest of the patients but one showed lengthenings of the PR between 0.02 and 0.08 s due to the effect of propafenone, and five of them showed PRs of O.22 s or more. Three cases also presented long pauses. It is necessary to point out that the most common conduction disturbances resulting from the drug always appeared except in a case of SA block) during sleep.

Five patients showed widening of the QRS between 0.01 and 0.02 s, while another who in a basal situation showed incomplete right-branch block (QRS = 0.10 s) developed advanced transitory right-branch block (QRS = 0.14 s). However, the comparison of the mean duration of the QRS before and after propafenone was not statistically significant.

The control QT interval had a mean of 0.35 ± 0.021 s; after propafenone it was 0.40 ± 0.04 s, and after placebo 0.36 ± 0.03 s ($P < 0.01$). There was no relation between the lengthening of the QT and greater antiarrhythmic efficacy.

In analyzing the percentage relation of the total number of PVCs after propafenone in relation to the control and placebo recordings the following data was obtained: In ten cases (59%) the result was considered excellent, as a reduction of over 80% in the total number of PVCs in respect to the control and placebo was obtained (Morganroth et al. 1978). An acceptable result (reduction of over 60% but less than 80%) was found in three cases (17.5%), while in four patients (23.5%) the result was considered unsatisfactory (reductions of 12% and 20% in two cases, and increases of 16% and 20% in another two).

Before taking propafenone, 12 patients were classified as Lown's grade 4 (eight 4 A and four 4 B) and five were classified in grade 3 as they had polymorphic PVCs. The H-ECG carried out after propafenone showed that nine patients were Lown's grade 1, two grade 2, and three grade 3, while another three had remained in grade 4 (two 4 A, one 4 B) (Fig. 4, left). Before propafenone there were no cases with Lown's grades 1 or 2, while 64% passed to these groups following the drug. Following placebo all the cases were in Lown's grades 3 or 4.

Analyzing the results in more detail, we can see that of the four patients with Lown's grade 4 B, one remained in the same grade after administration of the drug, as he presented runs of ventricular tachycardia composed of five complexes with a frequency of 136x′. However, in this case the percentage reduction of the total number of ventricular extrasystoles was 78%. Two cases with the same grade 4 B changed to grade 2, and one to 1. The eight patients initially classified in 4 A were divided, after 900 mg/day propafenone, in the following way: two remained unchanged, two passed to grade 3 and four to

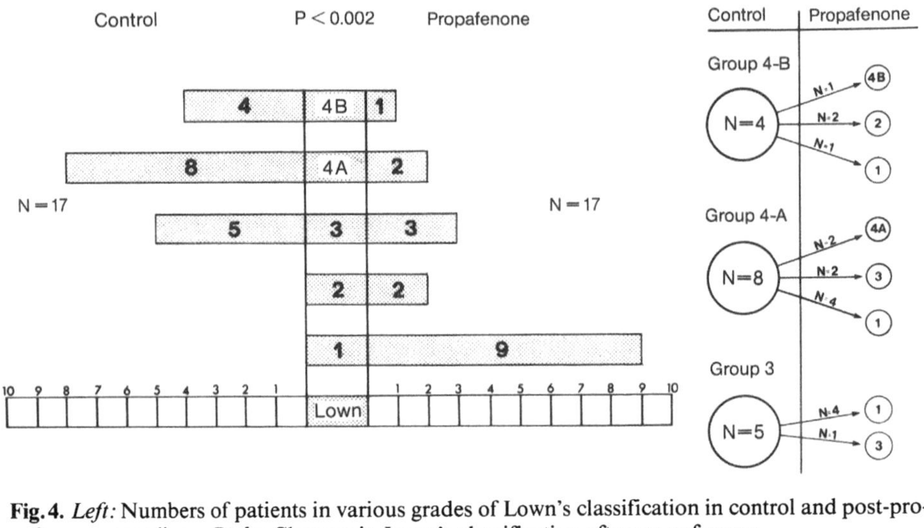

Fig. 4. *Left:* Numbers of patients in various grades of Lown's classification in control and post-propafenone recordings. *Right:* Changes in Lown's classification after propafenone

grade 1. Finally, of the five patients with grade 3, only one remained the same, while the other four passed to grade 1. After placebo all the cases showed Lown's grade 3 or 4.

From an echocardiographic point of view no changes appeared in the study of segmentary contractility after propafenone in the seven patients with abnormalities of wall motion (all with abnormalities of more than one segment) and in the two patients without abnormalities of wall motion in control ECHO-2D.

With respect to the clinical type of secondary effects attributable to the drug, it must be said that six patients (35%) complained of nausea or vertigo (two of these very marked), and one patient presented taste changes of little importance, and complained of gastric disorders and pyrosis. Three cases (17%) were later withdrawn from the drug due to the secondary effects.

Group B

A reduction of more than 80% in the number of PVCs was observed in five patients (42%), of 60%–80% in two (17%) and of less than 60% in five (41%); in three cases (24%) there was no reduction (Fig. 5). In Fig. 6 we see trends of arrhythmias in the computerized system.

Evaluating all the patients together, a reduction of 79% in the number of PVCs was seen studying 30-min periods, and of 92% studying periods of 90 min. On the other hand, a global reduction of 74% was seen in the number of ventricular tachycardias and of 58% in the number of PVC pairs. The total disappearance of repetitive phenomena (VT and pairs) was achieved in 42% of the patients.

An increase in the duration of the PR, QRS, and QT intervals was seen, but was not statistically significant. However, a significant drop ($P < 0.01$) was observed in the value of mean systolic arterial pressure 5 min after injection (Fig. 7), lasting 30 min.

Some secondary effect was observed in 50% of the patients (Fig. 8): nausea and dry

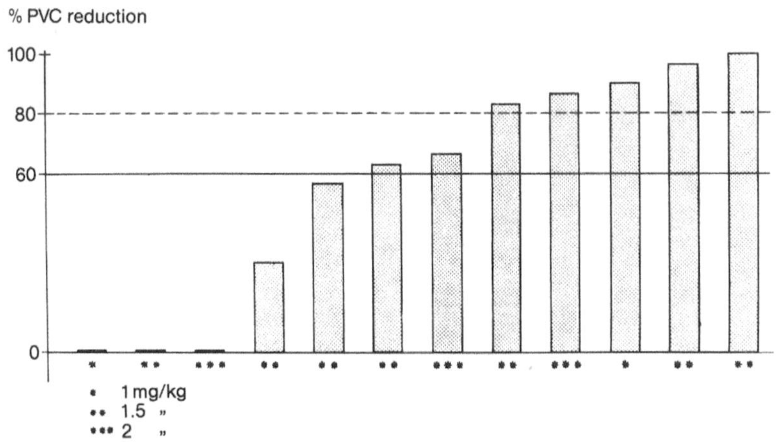

Fig. 5. Reduction in the number of PVCs (%) after intravenous administration of various doses of propafenone

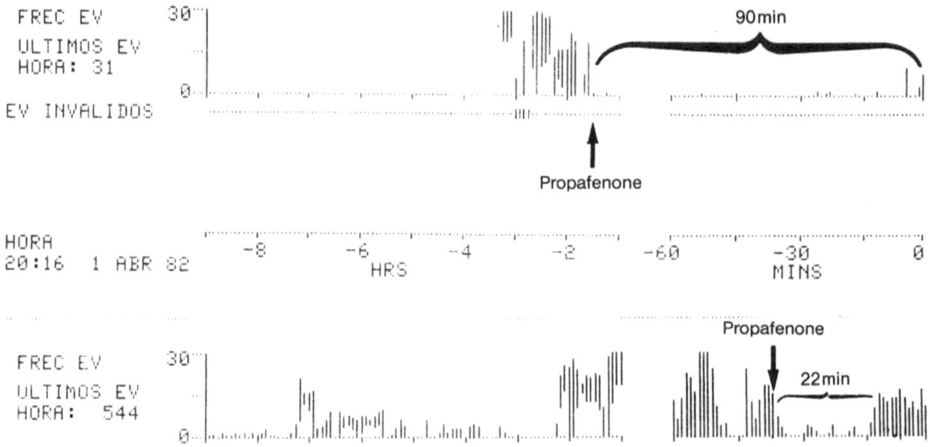

Fig. 6. Two trends of the computerized system showing how the duration of the effect of i.v. propafenone oscillates between 22 min and 90 min

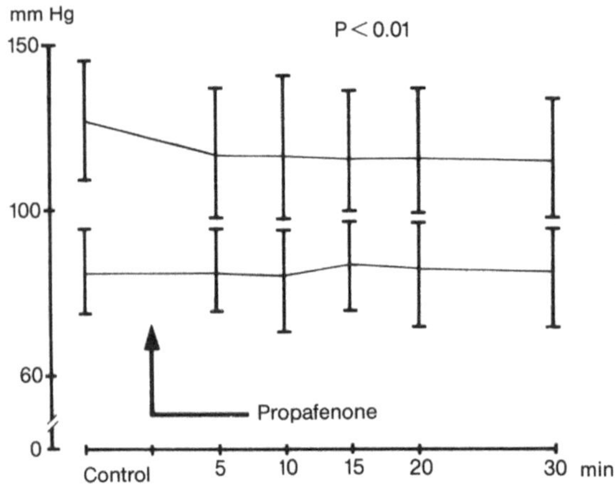

Fig. 7. Significant reduction in mean value of systolic arterial pressure after i.v. propafenone

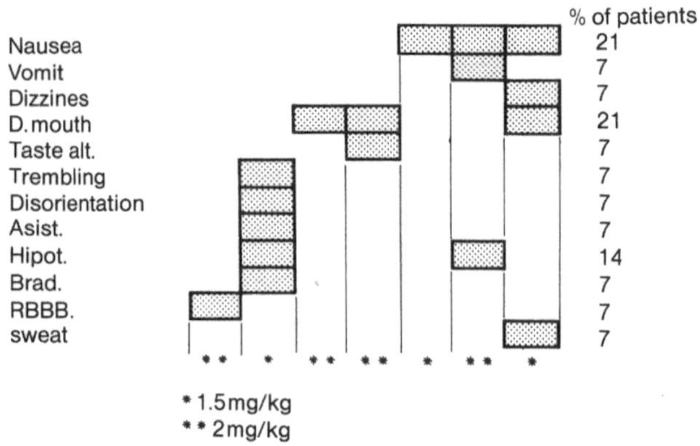

Fig. 8. Secondary effects in group B patients

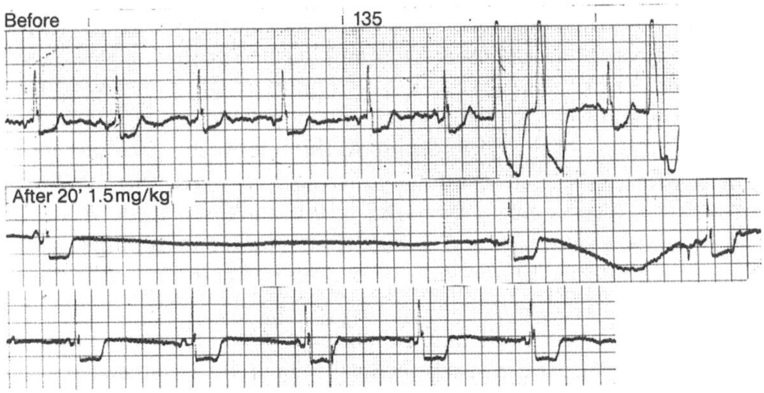

Fig. 9. Pause of 5 s appeared 20 min after i. v. injection of 1.5 mg/kg propafenone

mouth in three (21%); marked hypotension in two (14%); vomiting, dizziness, taste alterations, trembling, disorientation, sinusal bradycardia, first degree right branch block, sweating, and marked depression of automatism (Fig. 9) in one (7%).

Discussion

Numerous studies have previously described the efficacy of propafenone in reducing PVCs of diverse origin. Our study confirms that the drug is efficient in prevention and control of rhythmic disturbances in patients with ischemic heart disease as in nearly two-thirds of cases (59%) the result was excellent, in 17.8% acceptable, and in 23.5% unsatisfactory. We did not observe any correlation between the failure of the drug and the severity of the cardiopathy. We administered 900 mg/day in three doses, as this has been suggested by many authors as an evidently efficient dose and because in our experience the dose of (150 × 3) 450 mg/day was often not sufficient to obtain a satisfactory reduction of the PVCs. However, in some cases we have had good results with doses of 450 or 600 mg (150 + 300 + 150), and we have shown that, once the therapeutic effect is obtained it is sometimes maintained with doses smaller than those used initially (600 mg/day instead of 900, for example). The cause-effect relation (drug-arrhythmia) in our series has also been evident, as in the placebo phase an increase in the rhythm disturbances with characteristics similar to those of the control phase could be seen.

The secondary effects appearing in the ECG which are provoked by the propafenone action are quite evident. Three of our patients in Group A developed long pauses, probably due to sinoatrial block. The depressor effect on both AV and intraventricular conduction was evident although in neither case it was severe. However, if a satisfactory antiarrhythmic effect is not achieved with a dose that produces lengthening of the PR interval or other conduction alteration, an increase in dose is not indicated. Other experiences have also shown that the degree of block appearing after propafenone does not usually modify, even after months of treatment (Baedeker et al. 1979).

It must be noted that the presence of first or second degree AV block during sleep is relatively frequent in healthy subjects and in cardiopathic patients when they are monitored with H-ECG. These events are not important when the vagal tone plays a preponderant role, and when they are isolated phenomena (Gras et al. 1981).

The widening of the QRS (Group A) did not exceed 0.02 s except in one case. One patient with partial right bundle-branch system block (0.10 s) developed advanced RBBsB (0.14 s) remaining with a QRS of 0.12 s in the placebo stage. This same patient was examined 1 week later and the QRS had returned to its initial value. The QT lengthening which affected all the patients was more significant, although this disappeared when medication was stopped.

We observed neither alterations in arterial pressure nor presence of clinical signs of cardiac insufficiency owing to the action of the orally administered drug. In the patients in our intravenous series we have not been able to detect any clinical sign of negative inotropic effect. In our oral series, ECHO-2D findings suggested the absence of an effect on myocardial function affectation. We have found only one small reference to this in an article by Fazzini et al. (1980), affirming that no variations of the ventricular kinetics or ventricular diameters were found by ECHO. To confirm these findings it will be necessary to use isotopic gated equilibrium techniques. We were surprised by the high number of patients presenting extracardial secondary effects from both oral and intravenous administration. These symptoms would have disappeared with a lower dose. In another series with lower doses the percentage of extracardial secondary effects was lower. In no case were evident hematic alterations detected (Baedeker et al. 1979). With these results in mind it seems advisable to begin treatment whenever possible with a dose of 450 mg/daily and to slowly increase the dose, observing both clinical and electrocardiographic tolerance and therapeutic efficacy.

From our study we deduce that propafenone is a potent antiarrhythmic agent, above all useful orally. This must be kept in mind when choosing an efficient drug for control of the arrhythmias that coronary patients suffer and which are often responsible for sudden death. We do not, however, have any arguments for considering propafenone the drug of first choice to treat grave ventricular arrhythmias. In its favor is the fact that the oral dose used by us does not alter segmentary contractility although the study of cardiac function should probably be done with the isotopic gated equilibrium technique. Although it is necessary to watch the effects on AV and intraventricular conduction during treatment, because with the dose in which propafenone is evidently useful the incidence of conduction disorders is quite high, it does not seem that the conduction delay of the stimulus that appears at the beginning of treatment increases in the following months (Baedeker et al. 1979).

In cases such as severe ventricular arrhythmias in which there is no drug which is an authentic solution, the appearance of propafenone in cardiac therapy must be welcomed.

Conclusions

Orally: In a dose of 900 mg/day propafenone significantly reduces the number of PVCs (> 80%) in 60% of cases, and 64% of patients pass to Lown's grades 1 or 2. It does not alter the segmentary contractility and it produces a significant lengthening of the PR and QT intervals; there are secondary clinical effects in 53% of cases.

Intravenously: In a dose of 1–2 mg/kg daily propafenone eliminates the repetitive phenomena (VT or pairs) in 42% of cases. In over 40% of cases it significantly reduces the number of PVCs (> 80%). It causes a transitory but significant drop in systolic arterial pressure, and produces clinical-type secondary effects in 33% of patients.

References

Baedeker W, Klein G, Ertl G (1979) Tratamiento prolongado de las alteraciones del ritmo ventricular con propafenona. Z Kardiol Angiol 11: 330–335

Bergmann M, Bolte HD (1977) Elektrophysiologische Untersuchungen mit Propafenon an myokardialen Einzelfasern. In: Hochrein H, Hapke HJ, Beck OA (eds) Fortschritte in der Pharmakotherapie von Herzrhythmusstörungen. Fischer, Stuttgart pp 29–34

Davis LD, Tempte JV (1968) Effects of propanolol on the transmembrane potentials of ventricular muscle and Purkinje fibers of the dog. Circ Res 22: 661–667

Disertoni M, Vergara G, Dal Fondo P, Inema G, Furlanello F (1980) Profilo di un nuovo antiarritmico: Il propafenone. Tipicizzanione elettrofisiologica. In: Furlanello F, Disertoni M, Vergara G, Bettini R (eds) Le nuove frontiere delle arritmie. Piccin, Padova pp 213–220

Durante G, Del Forno P, Vergara G, Frisanco L, Furlanello F (1980) Utilization of propafenone for the prophilaxis of ventricular hyperkinetic arrhythmias in mitral valve prolapse syndrome. In: Fifth International Seminar on Cardiology, Abstracts Book pp 98–99

Fazzini P, Marchi F, Santoro G, Pucci P, Zambaldi G (1980) Profilo di un nuovo antiarritmico: Il propafenone: Aspect farmacologica. In: Furlanello F, Disertoni M, Vergara G, Bettini R (eds) Le nuove frontiere delle arritmie. Piccin, Padova pp 243–247

Fill WD, Kuhn P, Probst P, Zilcher H (1977) Anwendung von Propafenon am Menschen. In: Hochrein H, Hapke HJ, Beck OA (eds) Fortschritte in der Pharmakotherapie von Herzrhythmusstörungen. Fischer, Stuttgart pp 71–79

Gras X, Bayes de Luna A, Oter R, Ange J (1981) Second degree heart block in healthy men. Padua F, McFarlane P (eds) New frontiers of electrocardiology. Pitman Medical, London

Keller K, Meyer-Estorff G, Beck OA, Hochrein H (1978) Correlation between serum concentration and pharmacological effect on atrioventricular conduction time of the antiarrhythmic drug propafenone. Eur J Clin Pharmacol 13: 17–20

Kisslo I, Robertson D, Gilbert B, von Rem O, Benhar V (1977) Comparison of real time, two-dimension echocardiography and cineangiography in detecting left ventricular asynergy. Circulation 55: 134–141

Kohlhardt M (1977) Der Einfluß von Propafenon auf der transmembranären Na^{+} und Ca^{++} Strom der Warmblütler Myokardfaser membrana. In: Hochrein H, Hapke HJ, Beck OA (eds) Fortschritte in der Pharmakotherapie von Herzrhythmusstörungen. Fischer, Stuttgart pp 35–38

Ledda F, Mantelli L, Migelli A (1980) Profilo di un nuovo antiarritmico: Il propafenone. Aspetto farmacologico. In: Furlanello F, Disertoni M, Vergara G, Bettini R (eds) Le nuove frontiere delle arritmie. Piccin, Padova pp 207–211

Lüderitz B (1978) Fortschritte in der medikamentösen Arrhythmiebehandlung. Herzkreisl 10: 99–106

Meyer-Estorff G, Keller K, Beck OA, Hochrein H (1978) Antiarrhythmische Wirksamkeit von Propafenon in Abhängigkeit von Serumkonzentration und Erregungsleitungshemmung. Z Kardiol 67: 332–356

Morganroth J, Michelson E, Horowitz LN, Josephson ME, Perelman AS (1978) Limitations of routine long-term ECG monitoring to assess ventricular ectopic frequency. Circulation 58: 408–414

Rutsch W (1978) Beeinflussung der ventrikulären Extrasystolie durch Propafenon. Herzkreisl 10: 183–186

Seipel L, Breithardt G (1980) Propafenone – A new antiarrhythmic drug. Eur Heart J 1: 309–313

Seipel L, Both A, Breithardt G, Loogen F (1975) Die Wirkung neuer Antiarrhythmika (Aprindin, Propafenon CI 661) auf die intrakardiale Erregungsleitung und die Sinusknoten Automatie beim Menschen. In: Seipel L, Loogen F, Both A, Schattauer FK (eds) His-Buendel-Elektrographie. Fischer, Stuttgart pp 191–197

Seipel L, Breithardt G, Both A, Wiebrinhaus E (1977) Wirkung von Propafenon auf den Sinusknoten und die intrakardiale Erregungsleitung beim Menschen. In: Hochrein H, Hypke HJ, Beck OA (eds) Fortschritte in der Pharmakotherapie von Herzrhythmusstörungen. Fischer, Stuttgart pp 45–55

Tritthart H, Fleckenstein B, Fleckenstein A (1971) Sone fundamental actions of antiarrhythmic drugs on the excitability and the contractility of single myocardial fibers. Naunyn Schmiedebergs Arch Pharmacol 269: 212–219

Van Rossum JM (1963) Cumulative dose-response curves. Technique for the making of dose-response curves in isolated organs and the evaluation of drug parameters. Arch Int Pharmacodyn Ther 143: 299–330

Vergara G, Disertoni M, Del Forno P, Stefenelli C, Furlanello F (1980) Profilo di un nuovo antiarritmico: Il propafenone. Esperienza clinica. In: Furlanello F, Disertoni M, Vergara G, Bettini R (eds) Le nuove frontiere delle arritmie. Piccin, Padova pp 225–231

Von Hapke HS, Prigge E (1976) Zur Pharmakologie von 2′-(2-Hydroxy-3-propylaminopropoxy)-3-phenylpropiophenon (Propafenon, SA 79)-hydrochlorid. Arzneimittelforsch 26: 1849–1857

Waleffe A, Mary-Rabine L, De Rijbel R, Soyeno O, Legrend V, Kulbertus HE (1981) Electrophysiologic effects of propafenone studied with programmed electrical stimulation of the heart in patients with recurrent paroxysmal supraventricular tachycardia. Eur Heart J 2: 345–352

Wiebrinhaus E, Seipel L, Breithardt G, Loogen G (1978) Langzeitergebnisse mit dem neue Antiarrhythmikum Propafenon unter Berücksichtigung der Plasmaspiegel. Z Kardiol 66: 625–632

Wieser H, Philippi M, Schuler CF (1979) Die antiarrhythmische Wirkung von Propafenon bei stabiler ventrikulärer Extrasystolie (Ergebnisse einer überkreuzten Doppelblindstudie mit Propafenonhydrochlorid gegen Plazebo). Herzkreisl 11: 71–76

Propafenone in Office Use: Results of an Open, Multicenter Study

H.-F. Spies and F. Sesto

Clinical studies have demonstrated the therapeutic efficacy of propafenone (Rytmonorm) [1–10]. The question of tolerance, however, is especially important when an antiarrhythmic drug is administered daily to outpatients. This question can best be resolved in an open, multicenter study involving a large patient population. Moreover, the participation of many practicing physicians is needed if a study of this magnitude is to be completed successfully and on schedule. It is hoped that the results of such a study presented here will further our understanding of the therapeutic efficacy of propafenone as well as of its cardiac and extracardiac side effects.

A total of 161 physicians participated in the study – 116 internists and 45 general practitioners. The period of the study was from November, 1979 to October, 1980. Indication, dosage, laboratory findings, side effects, and response to treatment were recorded for a total of 793 patients. Because a portion of the questionnaires were not filled out completely, results for the total patient population are not available for some of the points covered in the study.

The patients consisted of 416 men and 377 women, with an average age of 58.6 and 59.2 years respectively. All of the patients studied had supraventricular or ventricular arrhythmias. None had suffered a myocardial infarction within at least 8 weeks prior to enrollment in the study. The most frequent arrhythmias are listed in Table 1; ventricular arrhythmias were the most common, occurring in over 65% of patients.

The need for antiarrhythmic therapy was determined solely by the attending physician. As a result, indications varied considerably from one case to the next, so we are unable to categorize the patients according to the degree of severity of their arrhythmias. In the great majority of cases coronary artery disease and/or heart failure, especially when associated with hypertension, was identified as the underlying cause of the arrhythmia.

Table 2 shows the length of observation and treatment, which was less than 3 months in the majority of cases.

Table 1. Treated cardiac arrhythmias

	Tatal	Male	Females
Ventricular premature beats (VPBs)	419	226	193
Atrial fibrillation with absolute arrhythmia	106	55	51
Supraventricular premature beats	66	31	35
Ventricular tachycardia and VPBs	45	18	27
Concomitant ventricular and supraventricular VPBs	33	20	13
Paroxysmal supraventricular tachycardia	29	10	19
Absolute arrhythmia with VPBs	26	16	10
Wolff-Parkinson-White syndrome	12	5	7
Atrial flutter	10	6	4

Table 2. Duration of treatment

Time	*n*
14–30 days	146
1–3 months	224
3–6 months	95
>6 months	35

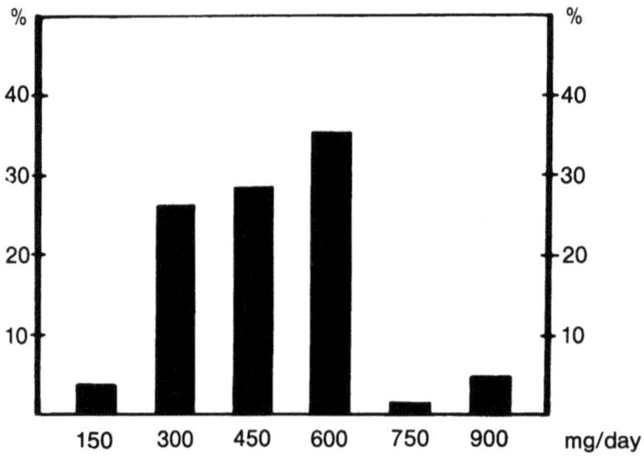

Fig. 1. Propafenone dosages in 729 patients

Figure 1 shows the daily doses that were used. Twenty-six percent received 300 mg, 28.7% 450 mg, and 35% 600 mg/day. These dose levels are somewhat lower than those used in clinical trials.

The diagnostic facilities of the participating physicians varied greatly. Optimum diagnosis and monitoring through the use of long-term ECGs were practiced in only a few cases. But this method is not yet widely available in outpatient practice, and had we made it a criterion for enrollment, the size of our study population would have been significantly smaller.

The response to treatment was rated „good" by the attending physician if the arrhythmia disappeared, if the number of premature beats decreased by about 80%, or if there was an adequate lowering of the heart rate.

Based on these criteria, a good response was achieved in 87% of patients (Fig. 2). Side effects occurred in 4.6%, and only 3.4% showed no response. Treatment was consequently discontinued in 13% of cases.

Of particular significance is the effect of propafenone on AV conduction time and intraventricular impulse spread, according to the site of action of the drug [11, 12].

In 285 cases, a daily dose of 300–600 mg resulted in a prolongation of the P–Q interval of up to 25% compared with initial recordings. In 250 cases the AV conduction time remained unchanged. Prolongations of up to 10% were recorded in 33 cases within a dose range of 450–900 mg/day, and in one case with a dose of 150 mg/day. In 25 patients a prolonged P–Q interval was already evident in the initial ECG. In five of these patients there was an additional slight lengthening of AV conduction time during treatment, but this was too mild to warrant discontinuance. In six cases the P–Q interval re-

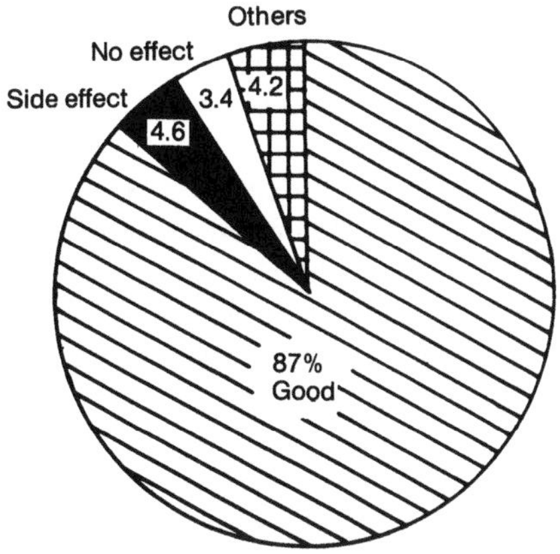

Fig. 2. Therapeutic efficacy of propafenone

Table 3. Laboratory findings before and after 14 days' treatment with propafenone

	Leukocyte count		SGOT		Alkaline phosphatase		Serum potassium level	
	Before	Day 14	Before	Day 14	Before	Day 14	Before	Day 14
Median	6400	6200	14	14.2	120	120	4.3	4.3
Lower confidence limit of median (95%)	6300	6100	13	14	116	116	4.2	4.2
Upper confidence limit of median (95%)	6600	6300	14	15	123	122	4.3	4.3
Lowest value	3500	2800	4	4	52	50	3.2	3.4
Highest value	14100	12500	62	50	295	340	6.7	6.72
No. of values	611		605		479		597	

mained unchanged, and a shortening or normalization of the P–Q interval was even observed in a few cases.

Treatment had to be discontinued in three patients because of side effects with severe SA or AV block. In 570 cases the width of the QRS complex was measured before and after 14 days' medication. In 196 cases (34%) the QRS interval was prolonged by up to 20% compared with the initial value; in 188 cases this occurred at a daily dose between 300 and 900 mg. In 374 cases no change in QRS width was observed [13]. The Q–T interval was unaffected by propafenone.

Table 3 shows the laboratory parameters measured in the study population before and after 14 days' treatment. No significant difference is seen in the leukocyte count, SGOT, alkaline phosphatase, or serum potassium. The only noticeable change is a slight decline in the leukocyte count. In one patient the leukocyte count fell from 11000 to 2800. This change reversed completely after the drug was withdrawn, and resumption of propafenone therapy did not produce a recurrence. This suggests that other causes may have been responsible for the leukocyte change observed in this patient.

In one case the alkaline phosphatase and SGOT were elevated to pathologic levels. The change was reversible.

The 42 cases of observed extracardiac side effects are listed in Table 4 according to the nature of the complaint. Of particular interest, besides the high incidence of gastrointestinal complaints, is the occurrence of dizziness and vision impairment. One case of urticaria was reported.

The cardiac side effects associated with propafenone are listed in Table 5. It is apparent that these involve specific effects of an antiarrhythmic agent. The sinoatrial and atrioventricular blocks and sinus bradycardia are attributable to the essentially desirable affect of the drug on the impulse-forming and -conducting tissue. The single Stokes-Adams attack that occurred during treatment was probably also associated with a bradycardiac disturbance. An increase in ventricular premature beats and the ventricular tachycardia observed in one case are uncommon. In some circumstances they can be attributed to the known paradoxic effect of antiarrhythmic agents. Changes in blood pressure are attributable to the negative inotropic effect of any antiarrhythmic drug.

In summary, the physicians taking part in the study rated the therapeutic efficacy of propafenone as "good" in the great majority of patients tested. This 87% positive rating is disproportionately high when compared with clinical studies. We believe this can be explained by two circumstances. First, it is possible that ambulatory patients have a less severe underlying disease than hospitalized patients. Second, as most of the physicians did not employ long-term ECGs for examination and monitoring, the response to treatment may have been overrated in some cases.

The present study shows that propafenone is very well tolerated when used in the customary daily doses of 300–600 mg. In particular, the incidence of extracardiac side

Table 4. Extracardiac side effects

	No. of cases
Dizziness	10
Gastrointestinal complaints	26
Dry mouth	6
Headache	3
Vision impairment	2
Loss of appetite	1
Urticaria	1
Elevation of AP and gamma-GT to pathologic levels	1

Table 5. Cardiac side effects

	No. of cases
SA block, 2nd-degree Wenckebach type	1
AV block, 2nd-degree	2
Sinus bradycardia	3
Stokes-Adams attack	1
Fall of blood pressure topoint of collapse	1
Orthostatic circulatory complaints	3
Polytopic VPBs	1
Ventricular tachycardia	1

effects (4.3%) is relatively low for a potent antiarrhythmic drug. Serious cardiac side effects were observed in only 13 of a total of more than 800 patients.

Even if we acknowledge the inherent inadequacies of a study involving more than 800 patients and 161 physicians, we must conclude that propafenone – in the dosages used in this study – is a well-tolerated antiarrhythmic drug that rarely causes cardiac and extracardiac side effects. On close inspection, these results do not contradict the findings presented by Neuss and others, if the higher daily doses used by the latter are taken into consideration.

Nevertheless, there remains a need for further systematic assessment of the relation between the therapeutic benefit of the drug and its possible side effects. Particularly with high-risk patients, it is essential that responses be monitored electrocardiographically, special note being taken of sinus rhythm, AV conduction time, and QRS width. This should be combined with a concurrent check of laboratory parameters with respect to leukocyte counts and liver values.

References

1. Bachour G, Hochrein H (1977) In: Hochrein H, Hapke, Beck OA (eds) Fortschritte in der Pharmakotherapie von Herzrhythmusstörungen. Fischer, Stuttgart NewYork, pp 39–44
2. Seipel L et al. (1977) In: Hochrein H, Hapke, Beck OA (eds) Fortschritte in der Pharmakotherapie von Herzrhythmusstörungen. Fischer, Stuttgart New York, pp 45–55
3. Fill WD et al. (1977) In: Hochrein H, Hapke, Beck OA (eds) Fortschritte in der Pharmakotherapie von Herzrhythmusstörungen. Fischer, Stuttgart New York, pp 71–79
4. Koch R (1977) In: Hochrein H, Hapke, Beck OA (eds) Fortschritte in der Pharmakotherapie von Herzrhythmusstörungen. Fischer, Stuttgart New York, pp 84–89
5. Fischer G, Seipel L (1977) In: Hochrein H, Hapke, Beck OA (eds) Fortschritte in der Pharmakotherapie von Herzrhythmusstörungen. Fischer, Stuttgart New York, pp 109–114
6. Schulze PR (1977) In: Hochrein H, Hapke, Beck OA (eds) Fortschritte in der Pharmakotherapie von Herzrhythmusstörungen. Fischer, Stuttgart New York, pp 120–130
7. Beck OA, Hochrein H (1978) Dtsch Med Wochenschr 103: 1261–1265
8. Wieser H et al. (1979) Herz Kreisl 11: 71–76
9. Petri H, Rudolph W (1979) Herz 4: 344–358
10. Lüderitz B (1979. 1981) Therapie der Herzrhythmusstörungen, Leitfaden für Klinik und Praxis. Springer, Berlin Heidelberg New York 1981
11. Neuss H, Buss J (1978) Internist 19: 234–240
12. Kohlhardt M (1977) In: Hochrein H, Hapke, Beck OA (eds) Fortschritte in der Pharmakotherapie von Herzrhythmusstörungen. Fischer, Stuttgart New York, pp 35–44
13. Meyer-Estorf G et al. (1978) L Kardiol 67: 352–356

The Safety and Efficacy of Propafenone in Suppressing Ventricular Ectopy

N. deSoyza, M. Murphy, M. Sakhaii and L. Treat

Propafenone is a potent antiarrhythmic agent with a strong membrane-stabilizing effect (Fill et al. 1977; Zeiler et al. 1981) which has been commercially available in Europe since 1977 under the trade name Rytmonorm. Clinical studies have indicated effectiveness in suppressing chronic recurrent supraventricular and ventricular tachyarrhythmias and ectopic beats (Aldor and Haeger 1977; Baedeker et al. 1977; Harlin 1976; Koch 1977).

The purpose of our study was to determine the safety and efficacy of propafenone in the suppression of ventricular ectopy in patients with organic heart disease and significant ventricular arrhythmias.

Methods

We studied 30 male patients with an average age of 62 years, ranging in age from 48 to 75. Of these patients, 23 were diagnosed as having coronary artery disease, four had valvular heart disease, and two had hypertensive cardiovascular disease; one patient with severe ventricular arrhythmias had no documented organic heart disease.

All 30 patients had a history of clinically significant ventricular arrhythmias defined as $\geq$30 PVC/hr as recorded by a 48-h Holter monitor. These recordings were performed after all antiarrhythmic medication had been discontinued for at least 48 h. Patients were excluded from the study if they demonstrated any of the following: symptoms of heart failure; evidence or suspicion of digitalis toxicity; clinically significant renal failure; clinically significant hepatic failure; a history of myocardial infarction within the last 2 months; or a stroke within the last 3 months.

This 12-week study included three phases: a placebo run-in phase; a dose titration phase; and a double-blind, placebo-crossover phase. During the first week of the study, a placebo was administered while appropriate baseline data were obtained. The dose titration phase of the study lasted 1–4 weeks, depending upon the individual patient's response. The initial propafenone dose was 150 mg b. i. d.; it was increased to 150 mg t. i. d., 300 mg b. i. d., and then 300 mg t. i. d. at weekly intervals unless complete ventricular ectopy suppression occurred at a lower dose. Weekly 24-h Holter recordings done at each dose level were analyzed to evaluate drug efficacy. Not all of the 30 patients have completed the double-blind, placebo-crossover phase of the study.

For statistical analysis, the paired *t*-test was used.

Table 1. Effect of propafenone on ventricular ectopy in 30 patients

	Baseline	150 mg b.i.d.	150 mg t.i.d.	300 mg b.i.d. (n=29)	300 mg t.i.d. (n=27)
Single VE/hour (mean ± SD)	550 ± 87	389 ± 71	253 ± 38	162 ± 41	58 ± 19
No. of patients with paired VE	29	24	24	17	11
No. of patients with V-T	23	6	5	5	0

VE, ventricular ectopy; VT, ventricular tachycardia

Results

Total Group

At baseline, the VE/h was 550 ± 87 (mean ± SD) for the 30 patients (Table 1). On maximum dose, this was reduced to a mean VE/h of 58 ± 19. At baseline, there were 23 patients with episodes of ventricular tachycardia (VT); however, on maximum propafenone therapy, none of the patients demonstrated VT. At baseline there were 29 patients with paired ventricular ectopy (VE), Yet on the maximum dose of propafenone there were only 11 patients with paired VE. While taking the maximum propafenone dose, ten patients had 100% VE reduction from baseline, 11 had greater than 95% reduction, and only five had less than 80% reduction.

Plasma propafenone levels of the first 16 patients while on maximum dose showed a mean drug level of 1261 ng/ml. The range was 404–3653 ng/ml. These blood samples were drawn 2–5 hours postmedication.

Effects on Electrocardiographic Measurements

Some significant electrocardiographic interval changes were observed while the patients were receiving propafenone. A PR interval of ≥ 0.20 s was observed in one patient at baseline and in 13 patients while on maximum therapy. A prolonged QRS of ≥ 0.12 s was observed in two patients at baseline and in nine patients while on maximum therapy. New left-bundle-branch block appeared during therapy in two of these patients. A prolongation of the QT interval beyond 0.40 s was noted in four patients at baseline and in five at maximum dose. However, no bradyarrhythmias, symptomatic or otherwise, were observed.

Side Effects

Baseline chest roentgenograms compared to those taken while the patients were on maximum propafenone therapy showed no significant change in cardiac size, and none of the patients developed symptoms or signs of congestive heart failure during therapy. Seven patients reported an abnormal taste in the mouth and one reported dizziness but no gastrointestinal disturbances were noted. While no patient developed a positive antinuclear antibody titer on therapy, one patient with a positive ANA titer at baseline did have a rising titer while on therapy, without developing any symptoms. No ocular side effects were observed in any of the patients.

One patient who had a past history of two myocardial infarctions died suddenly while taking 300 mg propafenone t.i.d. The autopsy findings, while demonstrating severe multivessel coronary atherosclerosis and remote myocardial infarction, were inconclusive as to the exact cause of death. The patient had experienced an increase in frequency of angina in the 2 weeks prior to death. His weekly 24-h monitors showed significantly decreasing ventricular ectopy in response to propafenone up until his death; the last tape recorded showed a 59% reduction from baseline.

Conclusions

We feel that propafenone is a safe and highly effective drug for the suppression of ventricular ectopy. It appears to be generally well tolerated. Propafenone seems to prolong certain electrocardiographic parameters without causing symptoms or bradyarrhythmias. Confirmation of these favorable findings during the double-blind crossover phase is awaited at this time. Thus, propafenone appears to be a safe and effective antiarrhythmic for the patient with severe ventricular arrhythmias.

References

Aldor E, Haeger H (1977) Clinical experiences with propafenone. Drug Dev Eval 1: 115–119

Baedeker W, Wirtzfeld A, Sack D (1977) The antiarrhythmic effect of propafenone in ventricular tachycardias. Herz/Kreisl 9: 348–352

Fill WD, Kuehn P, Probst P (1977) Use of propafenone in man. Clinical results on the effects on electrophysiological and hemodynamic parameters. Drug Dev Eval 1: 71–79

Harlin M (1976) Propafenone in therapy-resistant arrhythmias. Medical Tribune 2: 40–41

Koch R (1977) Action of propafenone in ventricular arrhythmia. Drug Dev Eval 1: 84–89

Zeiler RH, Gough WB, Sung R (1981) Electrophysiologic effects of propafenone on canine ischemic cardiac cells. Am J Cardiol 47: 483

Dose-Response Effect of Propafenone in Patients with Ventricular Arrhythmias

P. Larochelle, L. Belanger, F. Lemire, D. Phaneuf and R. Huot

Propafenone has electrophysiologic properties which permit its classification as a class I antiarrhythmic agent (agents in this class have characteristics similar to quinidine and procainamide). These properties were reviewed in many presentations at an international symposium (Hochrein et al. 1977). In animal studies, propafenone increased both the ventricular fibrillation threshold and the functional refractory period in the isolated guinea pig atrium. In Purkinje and myocardial fibres, the compound reduced mainly the rate of rise of the action potential (Bergmann and Bolte 1977). In human studies, propafenone induced a relatively uniform slowing of the conduction rate of all sections of the heart (Seipel et al. 1975) and the delay in the atrioventricular node was markedly dose-dependent (Keller et al. 1978). In initial clinical studies propafenone was found to be effective in ventricular and supraventricular arrhythmias (Ivancic and Goldner 1977; Rutsch 1978; Wieser et al. 1979).

The pharmacokinetic half-life was found to be between 2.5 and 4.0 h, and the drug itself to be extensively metabolized (Knoll AG, unpublished data. The plasma concentration reaches its peak in 2–3 h. There is still a prolongation of the conduction time and antiarrhythmic effect of propafenone 8 h after 300-mg oral doses have been administered. The drug has been marketed in some countries since 1977 and clinical studies have confirmed its effectiveness in ventricular arrhythmias.

This study was designed as a single-blind evaluation of the efficacy of propafenone in a group of patients with ventricular arrhythmias.

Methods

Twenty-two patients, 16 women and 6 men, with a mean age of 50 years (range 26 to 70), were admitted to the study. The criteria for inclusion were persistent high-grade ventricular irritability and chronic ventricular arrhythmia. Twelve of the patients admitted were unresponsive to other antiarrhythmic agents or were symptomatic due to their treatment. All patients signed an informed consent. Patients were excluded from this trial if they had had a myocardial infarction within the past 3 months, or if they had congestive heart failure, bradycardia of less than 50 beats/min, conduction disorder, obstructive pulmonary disease, electrolytic imbalance or evidence of renal or hepatic failure.

The study consisted of four phases. The first was a placebo period of 10 days' maximum duration. This phase could be conducted in hospital if the physician felt the patient might be at risk from withdrawal of his other antiarrhythmic medication. Patients received a placebo similar to propafenone three times a day.

The second phase consisted in the administration of 450 mg propafenone, the third phase of 600 mg and the fourth phase of 900 mg. Patients were asked to take the drug with equal intervals between doses. The dose of propafenone was increased if they showed less than 80% reduction in arrhythmias or if they did not develop significant adverse effects, such as marked atrial ventricular conduction delays or prolongation of the QRS duration by more than 25%. Each phase was of 10 days' maximum duration. At the end of each phase, the patient had a 24-h ambulatory electrocardiogram (Holter monitoring) recording and was tested while exercising on a treadmill. Blood pressure, heart rate and physical examinations were done after the 3rd day of each phase and at the end of each phase. An SMA 20 (systemic multiple analysis), a haemogram, platelets and ANA (antinuclear antibody) were also recorded at the end of each period. Adverse effects were recorded at the end of each phase; they were voluntarily reported by the patients and no specific questions were asked.

Ambulatory Electrocardiographic Recordings

Ambulatory ECGs were recorded with a two-channel Electrocardiorecorder from Del Mar Avionics. The tapes were analyzed by the same observer (R. H.) at the Montreal Heart Institute on a Del Mar Avionics no. 660A. Results were reported, indicating the number of heart beats/24 h, the number of isolated PVCs and a combination of PVCs. Premature atrial contractions were also reported. Heart rate over a 24-h period was calculated from the Holter monitoring.

Exercise Electrocardiograms

An exercise electrocardiogram was made while the patient was on a treadmill, according to the Bruce method. Tests were performed by the same observers and ended with the appearance of symptoms or when the patients reached 85% of their maximal heart rate capacity. A trained technician recorded PVCs during the exercise test and the recuperation phase. They were classified as numerous, present, or absent.

Data Analysis

Results are reported as the mean ± standard deviation of the mean. They were analyzed when necessary using a two-way analysis of variance (ANOVAR) and a Student's *t*-test.

Results

The results from the tests of 19 of 22 patients admitted to the study were used for evaluation of the drug. Three patients were excluded because they did not fulfill the admission criteria after Holter analysis.

Response of PVCs

Of the 19 patients studied, three received a maximal dose of 450 mg (Group 1), four received a maximal dose of 600 mg (Group 2) and 12 received a maximal dose of 900 mg (Group 3).

Group 1: These three patients received a dose of 450 mg each throughout the study. The number of PVCs recorded by Holter monitoring and the percentage reduction in PVCs are summarized in Tables 1 and 2. Patient no. 2 had a few PVCs which did not improve on treatment at 450 mg; however, the dose of propafenone was not increased because the patient developed a first-degree atrioventricular block and some sinus arrests. Patient no. 12 had a reduction of less than 50% in the number of her PVCs. Her dose was not increased because she had a widening of her QRS. Patient no. 21 had a marked reduction in the number of PVCs (98%), and the patient decided not to have her dose increased; for technical reasons her last Holter monitoring could not be analyzed.

Group 2: These four patients each received a maximal dose of 600 mg. The results are summarized in Tables 3 and 4. Patient no. 3 asked to be withdrawn from the trial because

Table 1. Number of premature ventricular contractions during 24-h Holter monitoring in patients who received 450 mg propafenone

Patient no.	With placebo	With propafenone		
		450 mg	450 mg	450 mg
21	40504	5009	744	NI
12	33055	17519	NI	19413
2	500	442	179	689

NI, Holter not interpretable

Table 2. Percentage reduction in premature ventricular contractions at each phase in patients who received 450 mg propafenone

Patient no.	With placebo (no. of PVCs)	With propafenone		
		450 mg	450 mg	450 mg
21	40504	88%	98%	NI
12	33055	47%	NI	41%
2	500	12%	65%	(137)

NI, Holter not interpretable

Table 3. Number of premature ventricular contractions during 24-h Holter monitoring in patients who received 600 mg propafenone

Patient no.	With placebo	With propafenone		
		450 mg	600 mg	600 mg
20	24090	3485	16936	*
5	16985	1931	0	2900
3	12722	20014	11498	*
6	1076	17	43	70

* Did not complete the fourth phase of the study

Table 4. Percentage reduction in premature ventricular contractions in patients who received 600 mg propafenone

Patient no.	With placebo (no. of PVCs)	With propafenone		
		450 mg	600 mg	600 mg
20	24090	85 %	30%	*
5	16985	88 %	100%	83%
3	12722	57 %	10%	*
6	1076	98,4%	96%	93%

* Did not complete fourth phase of the study

of adverse effects, mainly trouble with her vision, dizziness, palpitations, and pollakiuria. Except for the difficulty of accommodation of her vision, she had complained of these effects during the placebo period as well. Patient no. 5 was stopped at the 600-mg dose of propafenone because of dyspnea during her exercise ECG; an echocardiogram showed an increase in the size of the left ventricle, and it was decided not to increase the dose since she already had a 100% reduction in her PVCs at 600 mg. Patient no. 6 had an almost complete reduction in her PVCs at 600 mg and complained of dizziness. Patient no. 20, who had had previous attacks of ventricular tachycardia had responded poorly to other agents. Although there was an improvement in the number of PVCs at 450 mg, he had a further episode of ventricular tachycardia and fibrillation at 600 mg. He was successfully reanimated and taken off the drug at that point.

Group 3: Twelve patients received all three doses of propafenone (Tables 5 and 6). All 12 had more than an 80% reduction in their PVCs and 11 of them had more than an 87% reduction. The average reduction at 900 mg was 95% ± 7% (Fig. 1). Therefore, 15 of the 19 patients evaluated had more than an 80% reduction in the number of PVCs during the 40 or so days of the trial and four were treatment failures three owing to adverse reactions and one to lack of efficacy.

The 24-h Holter monitoring also permitted an evaluation of the type of PVCs recorded and the conduction charges. Of the 19 patients, two developed a first-degree AV block and one patient temporarily developed a second-degree AV block, type 2. It is also significant to note that at the highest dose, PVCs were recorded as unifocal and isolated, except in four cases where they were recorded at two sites. There were no recorded episodes of bigeminy or trigeminy at 900 mg propafenone.

Table 5. Number of premature ventricular contractions during 24-h Holter monitoring of 12 patients with each dose of propafenone

Patient no.	With placebo	With propafenone		
		450 mg	600 mg	900 mg
22	74081	23055	24915	23
10	23972	1623	44	0
17	20125	13979	10430	3920
1	13601	2149	33	177
14	9527	25	192	47
9	8081	4024	2538	64
16	7712	910	500	650
15	6520	1840	1	430
8	2995	7182	1530	62
13	2492	260	862	195
7	1800	1948	816	214
4	1459	200	100	0
$\bar{X}$	14363	4766	3497	513
SD	±20125	±6989	±7343	±1108

Table 6. Percentage reduction in premature ventricular contractions in 12 patients with each dose of propafenone

Patient no.	With placebo (no. of PVCs during 24-h Holter)	With propafenone		
		450 mg	600 mg	900 mg
22	74081	69%	66%	99%
10	23972	93%	99%	100%
17	20125	30%	48%	80%
1	13601	84%	99%	99%
14	9527	99%	98%	99%
9	8081	50%	69%	99%
16	7712	88%	94%	87%
15	6520	72%	100%	94%
8	2995	+139%	49%	98%
13	2492	90%	65%	92%
7	1800	+ 8%	55%	87%
4	1459	86%	93%	100%
$\bar{X}$	14363	51%	78%	95%
SD	±20125	±67	±21	±7

Exercise Electrocardiogram

Exercise electrocardiograms up to 85% of maximal capacity were done for all patients. The 12 patients of group 3 who received all three doses of propafenone each had four exercise electrocardiograms. The number of PVCs was evaluted by a technician as numerous, present, or absent. During the placebo phase the patients demonstrated PVCs either during the test or in the recuperation period (Table 7). At 600 mg of propafenone

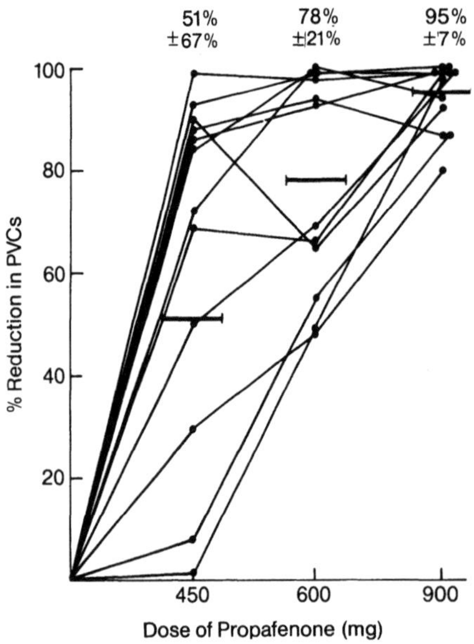

Fig. 1. Percentage reduction in PVCs with each dose of propafenone for 12 patients, mean reduction at a given dose

Table 7. Exercise electrocardiograms – premature ventricular contractions recorded during test and recuperation periods in 12 patients on propafenone

Patient no.		With placebo	With propafenone		
			450 mg	600 mg	900 mg
22	Test	+ +	0	0	0
	Post.	+ +	+ +	0	0
10	Test	+	0	0	0
	Post.	+	0	0	0
17	Test	+ +	–	0	0
	Post.	+ +	–	0	0
1	Test	+ +	+	+	0
	Post.	+ +		+	0
14	Test	0	0	0	0
	Post.	0	0	0	0
9	Test	+	0	0	0
	Post.	+	0	0	0
16	Test	0	0	–	0
	Post.	+	+	–	0
15	Test	+ +	0	0	0
	Post.	+	0	0	0
8	Test	–	+	+	0
	Post.	–	+	+	0
13	Test	+ +	0	0	0
	Post.	+ +	0	0	0
7	Test	+ +	+ +	0	0
	Post.	+ +	+ +	+	0
4	Test	+	0	0	0
	Post.	+	+ +	0	0

+ +, Numerous PVCs; +, presence of PVCs; 0, no arrhythmia recorded

eight of these patients did not have PVCs, and at 900 mg none of them had any PVCs during either the test or the recuperation phase.

Of the four patients in group 2, one was unable to sustain an exercise ECG, two showed definite improvement with complete disappearance of PVCs, and one showed temporary improvement.

Heart Rate

Heart rate was evaluated in this group of patients by dividing the number of heart beats during a Holter monitoring period by the duration of the period in minutes (Table 8). There were no significant changes in heart rate among the four phases.

Blood Pressure

Blood pressure was measured at each of the patients' visits (Table 9). There were no reductions in blood pressure, although there was a tendency toward an increase in the systolic standing pressure at the highest dose.

Table 8. Heart rate of patients who received all three doses of propafenone (beats/min)

Patient no.	With placebo	With propafenone		
		450 mg	600 mg	900 mg
22	90	73	73	72
10	81	98	78	74
17	81	67	76	69
1	73	73	77	73
14	74	79	78	79
9	56	59	63	58
16	78	61	91	77
15	61	68	74	72
8	83	84	78	80
13	88	80	83	74
7	70	67	61	61
4	76	79	80	
$\overline{X}$	76	74	76	72
SD	±9	±11	±8	±7

Table 9. Blood pressure of 11 patients who received all doses of proprafenone (mean ± SD)

	With placebo	With propafenone		
		450 mg	600 mg	900 mg
Supine	*130 ± 21*	*130 ± 22*	*128 ± 21*	*133 ± 20*
(mmHg)	82 ± 10	82 ± 12	82 ± 10	83 ± 8
Standing	*121 ± 17*	*121 ± 17*	*123 ± 21*	*129 ± 16*
(mmHg)	76 ± 9	78 ± 11	79 ± 1	79 ± 10

Table 10. Adverse effects spontaneously reported by 19 patients during the trial with each dose

	With placebo	With propafenone			Total no. of patients
		450 mg	600 mg	900 mg	
Palpitations	12	8	3	4	14
Dryness of mouth	3	4	4	3	7
Blurred vision	1	3	3	3	6
Dizziness	2	6	6	4	9
Headache	7	5	5	5	7
Constipation	3	3	5	3	5
Fatigue	2	4	5	2	5
Pollakiuria	1	3	–	–	3
Nausea	2	2	1	3	3

Adverse Effects

Adverse effects reported by the patients at the end of each phase are summarized in Table 10. Owing to the small number of patients in the study, although nine complained of dizziness, seven of dryness of mouth and seven of headaches, no obvious pattern of adverse effects could be demonstrated.

Laboratory

No significant changes were observed from the laboratory examinations performed – SMA 20, urine analysis or complete blood count. Antinuclear antibody was measured in 16 patients; two of them developed positive ANA which they had not had during placebo treatment.

Discussion

Propafenone is an antiarrhythmic agent which has been investigated for many years in Germany. It has been shown to reduce the irritability of the human ventricle with a maximum effectiveness of between 150 and 300 min (Diewitz and Anton 1977). It also slows down both atrioventricular and intraventricular conduction and produces a statistically significant prolongation of the AH interval (Beck et al. 1975). Simultaneously, it causes a delay of intraventricular spread of excitation and a slowing down distal from the His bridge, and therefore possesses properties also observed in procainamide. Measurement of the cell membrane characteristics shows a reduction in the maximum rate of rise of the action potential with low degree prolongation of the action potential and the effective refractory period (Beck et al. 1975).

Haemodynamic studies have demonstrated that propafenone has a moderately negative inotropic effect. This was evidenced by an increase in the pulmonary capillary pressure and a reduction in the cardiac output. There was a brief hypotension reaction which was secondary to the rapidity of the parenteral injection of the drug (Bachour and Hochrein 1977).

Clinical studies published in the first international studies on propafenone have reported its effectiveness in the treatment of arrhythmias, whether ventricular or supraventricular.

Our study was a single-blind evaluation with a placebo of 19 patients with significant premature ventricular contractions. Our results demonstrate that the drug was well tolerated by 15 of the patients with a more than 90% reduction in PVCs in 12 of them. It is very interesting to note that in the 12 patients who received 900 mg of propafenone, exercise electrocardiograms normalized entirely. There was also a dose-response effect with nine of the 15 patients who had more than a 90% reduction in PVCs at 600 mg propafenone. There was no significant effect on either heart rate or blood pressure, although it has been reported that it lowers heart rate in acute studies.

Adverse effects were well tolerated by the patients, if one considers their underlying disease and the symptomatic improvement they felt from reduction in PVCs. However, there were three cases of treatment failure associated with the impossibility of increasing the dose due to some of the adverse effects reported, and one case of treatment failure associated with an episode of ventricular tachycardia. The significance of two patients developing a positive ANA is limited, in view of the lack of adequate controls over a similar period of time.

The lack of data regarding plasma serum concentration does not permit us to draw a conclusion on the presence of a plasma concentration dose-effect response curve. In a previous study, Blank et al. (1979) were able to demonstrate a correlation between propafenone plasma concentration and frequency of ectopic beats. They also demonstrated a pronounced interindividual variation.

Still, we can conclude that in this limited drug study, propafenone proved to be an effective antiarrhythmic agent.

Acknowledgements: We wish to acknowledge the help of Miss France Boulianne, R. N. and Mrs. Martine Bouchard, R. N. and to thank Miss Isabelle Morin for graphics, and Mrs. Marie Bernier for secretarial work.

References

Bachour G, Hochrein H (1977) Hemodynamic responses to propafenone. Drug Dev Eval 1: 39–44

Beck OA, Witt E, Hochrein H (1975) Effect of the antiarrhythmic agent propafenone on cardiac conduction. Z Kardiol 64: 179–187

Bergmann M, Bolte HD (1977) Electrophysiological studies of propafenone in individual myocardial fibers. Drug Dev Eval 1: 29–34

Blanke H, Aschbrenner B, Karsch KR, Kreuzer H (1979) Plasma level, effectiveness, and organ distribution of propafenone. Dtsch Med Wochenschr 104: 587–591

Diewitz M, Anton D (1977) Effects of intravenous and oral propafenone hydrochloride on the myocardial threshold stimulus in man. Drug Dev Eval 1: 56–62

Hochrein H, Hapke HJ, Beck OA (1977) Fortschritte in der Pharmakotherapie von Herzrhythmusstörungen, I. Internationales Propafenon Symposion Fisher, Stuttgart

Ivancic R, Goldner V (1977) Propafenone in the treatment of extrasystoles – our experience. Drug Dev Eval 1: 131–144

Keller K, Meyer-Estorff G, Beck OA, Hochrein H (1978) Correlation between serum concentration and pharmacological effect on atrioventricular conduction time of the antiarrhythmic drug propafenone. Eur J Clin Pharmacol 13: 17–20

Rutsch W (1978) The influence of propafenone on ventricular premature beats. Herz/Kreisl 10: 183–186

Seipel L, Breithardt G, Both A (1975) Electrophysiological effect of the antiarrhythmics disopyramide and propafenone on the human cardiac impulse conduction system. Z Kardiol 64: 731–740

Wieser H, Philippi M, Schuler DF (1979) The antiarrhythmic effect of propafenone in reproducible ventricular beats. Herz/Kreisl 11: 71–76

Treatment of Severe Ventricular Arrhythmias with Propafenone

L. Ledain, N. Sourdille, J. P. Colle, J. Ohayon and P. Besse

Propafenone belongs to class 1 in Vaughan-William's classification of antiarrhythmic drugs. Several prior studies indicate that propafenone (P) is effective in suppressing chronic supraventricular and ventricular arrhythmias. The drug can be administered both intravenously and orally. The object of the following study was to determine the efficacy of P in treating severe ventricular arrhythmias and to compare the effects of intravenous and oral administration.

Methods

Patient Characteristics

We studied 23 patients, 50–75 years old. Of these, eight patients had chronic coronary artery disease, five had prior myocardial infarction, four had ventricular aneurysm, four had valvular disease, and two had no apparent cardiac disease. No patient had clinical congestive heart failure or altered hepatic and renal function and the serum potassium level was within the normal range in all cases. In the 14 patients of group A the arrhythmias were stable and permanent, with repetitive or paired premature ventricular contractions (PVCs) in four cases, bigeminy in three cases, frequent multiform PVCs in two cases, more than ten percent of the QRS complexes, and monomorph PVCs in five cases. In the nine patients of group B the arrhythmias consisted of paroxysmal atrial fibrillation or ventricular tachycardias.

Of the 23 cases, nine were resistant to another antiarrhythmic drug, which was discontinued 1 or 2 days prior to the study.

Study Design

The complete study included two control periods and three periods of P administration. The first 6 h were an initial control period to evaluate the number and complexity of PVCs. Patients then received 1.5 mg/kg P intravenously in 3 min. The efficacy was observed for 3. After that, a second control period of 3–24 h was observed to evaluate the spontaneous variation of PVCs. During the second part of the study, patients received intravenous P by continuous infusion over a 24-h period at a dose of 7 mg/kg. At the end of infusion, we changed to oral therapy, which consisted of either 150 or 300 mg P, three times daily at 8-h intervals. All patients stayed in the intensive care unit during the study, with continuous monitoring and tape recording. Each arrhythmia was analyzed by an ATREC system, which determined the number of PVCs and QRS complexes per h.

Clinical and Laboratory Examination

A cardiovascular physical examination was performed three times daily and blood pressure was measured every 2 h. A twelve-lead electrocardiogram was recorded every 8 h. All patients were questioned carefully with regard to symptoms and possible side effects. Laboratory determinations, including blood cell count, blood urea nitrogen, serum creatinine, bilirubin, serum transaminases, and electrolytes, were obtained on entrance into the study and after the treatment.

Results

Group A

Only the 14 patients in group A received the total P treatment. They were selected because of the stability of their arrhythmias. The spontaneous variation of PVCs from the first control period to the second and the variation with P are presented in Fig. 1. The spontaneous median change in PVCs was only. −13ofo, and the extreme variation among individual patients ranged from −40ofo to +30ofo. Thus, a partial therapeutic response was considered to be a reduction in PVCs exceeding 40%, and a full response was considered to be a decrease of more than 70%. Two patients in group A were con-

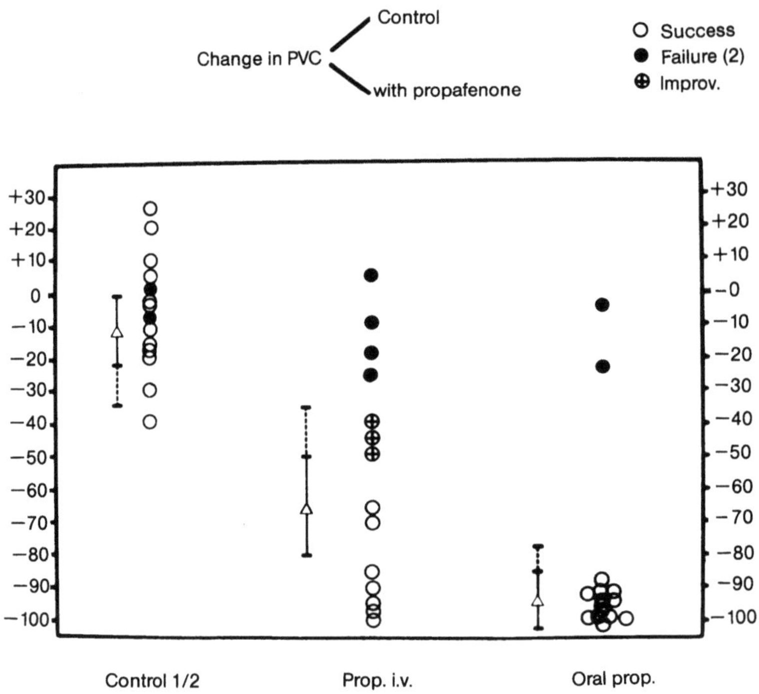

Fig. 1

sidered nonresponders to P. As shown in Fig. 2, the bolus injection and the continuous infusion failed to decrease the PVCs significantly. Oral therapy also failed for one patient, and the other showed a nonsignificant decrease. There were no unusual features in the clinical course of arrhythmias in these two patients; however, we could not determine their P serum concentrations and P resistance could not be confirmed. For five patients the effects were different with intravenous and oral P (Fig. 3). PVCs were suppressed 10–15 min after administrations of the bolus injection. The antiarrhythmic effect persisted for 30–50 min, then the frequency of PVCs returned to control levels in 1–2 h. The continuous infusion resulted in a 65% decrease in average hourly PVCs, which was statistically significant. But infusion never completely suppressed PVCs, and for two patients the PVC decreases were only 20% and 30%. However, oral therapy resulted in a decrease of at least 90% in average hourly PVC counts. The PVCs reappeared at the 8th and 16th h during oral therapy. For the last seven cases, P achieved total suppression and control of arrhythmias by either intravenous and oral administration (Fig. 4). An intravenous bolus totally suppressed PVCs in 10 min. Patients were free of PVCs for 30–60 min, after which time PVCs quickly reappeared and returned to the control level. It therefore appears that 1.5 mg P intravenously is effective after a delay of 10 min and for a duration of about 1 h. With infusion PVCs decreased progressively by 90% on average, and by 100% in five cases. Orally administered P maintained the full therapeutic response the following day.

It is of interest to consider the evolution of hourly PVC counts during the oral phase for the 12 responders (Fig. 5). The PVCs decreased during the first hour, but a full response was observed after the second. The lowest arrhythmia rate, representing the maximum antiarrhythmic effect, was found between the second and the sixth hour. The

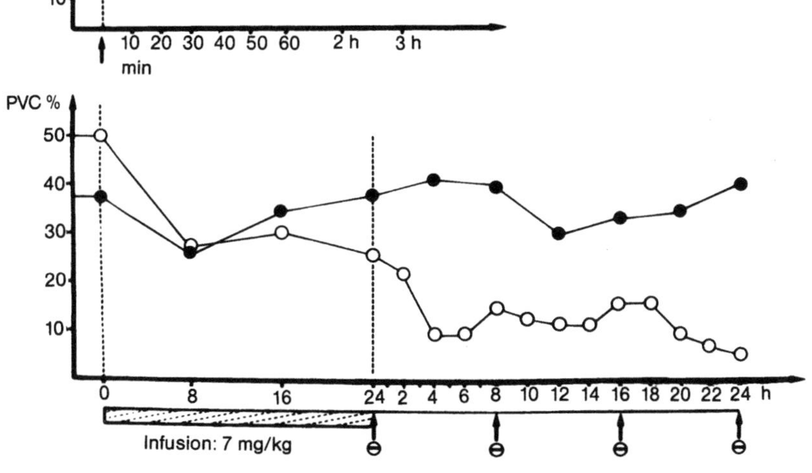

Fig. 2

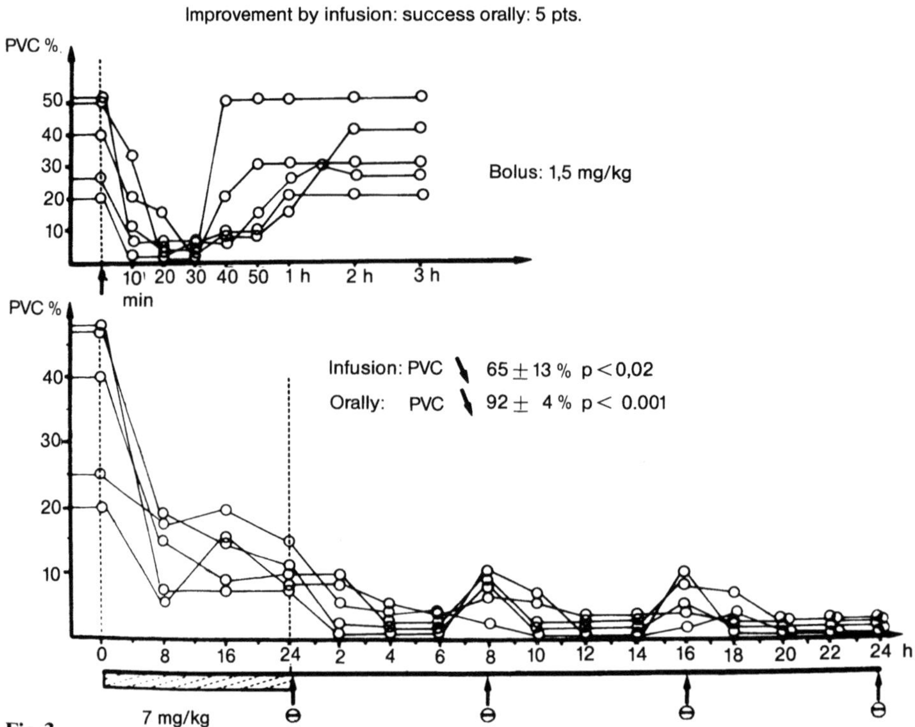

Fig. 3

PVCs reappeared and increased by 16% on average at the seventh and eight hours. Thus, the duration of the antiarrhythmic effect of one oral dose appears to be 6–8 h, three or four doses required daily. At the 15 th and 16 th hours the PVCs also reappeared, but at a lower rate. This suggests a progressive accumulation with prolonged therapy.

Group B

These nine patients presented paroxysmal tachycardia requiring urgent treatment; here the therapy was shorter. We tried to restore the sinus rhythm with 1.5 mg/kg intravenous P twice, with a 10-min interval. Of five cases of atrial fibrillation, P restored sinus rhythm in one and failed in four. Of four cases of ventricular tachycardia, P obtained complete reduction in two and only reduced the rate in the other two. The effectiveness of intravenous P in restoring sinus rhythm is therefore not convincing.

Electrocardiographic Changes and Side Effects

In our short-term experience with 23 patients P was generally well tolerated. There were neurological disturbances of mild dizziness in two cases, blurred vision in two, and mild tremor in one. Gastrointestinal complaints were frequent during the bolus injection

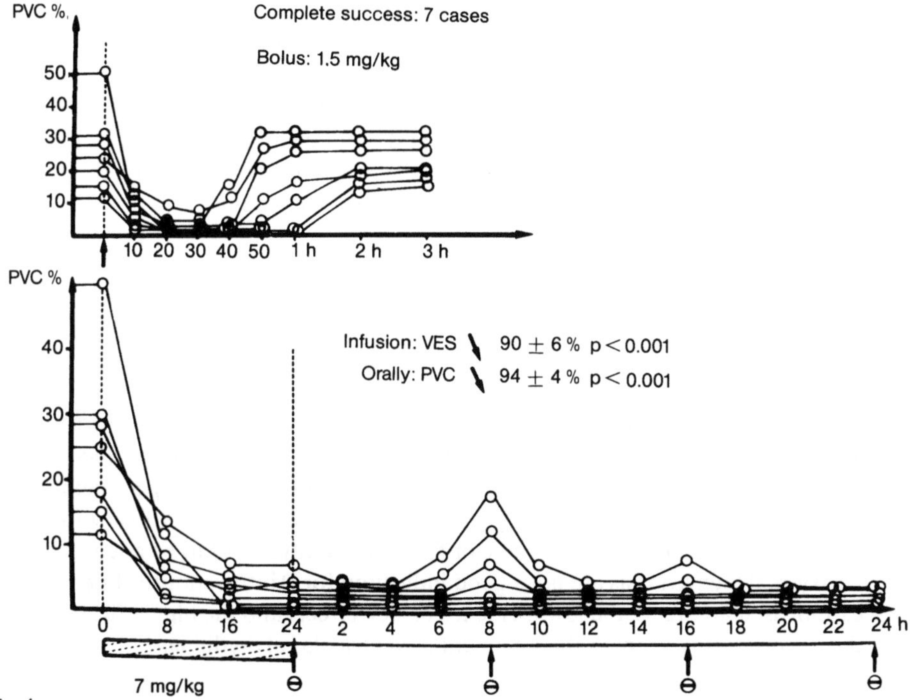
PVC %
Complete success: 7 cases
Bolus: 1.5 mg/kg
50
40
30
20
10
10 20 30 40 50 1 h 2 h 3 h
PVC %
Infusion: VES ↘ 90 ± 6 % p < 0.001
Orally: PVC ↘ 94 ± 4 % p < 0.001
40
30
20
10
0 8 16 24 2 4 6 8 10 12 14 16 18 20 22 24 h
7 mg/kg

Fig. 4

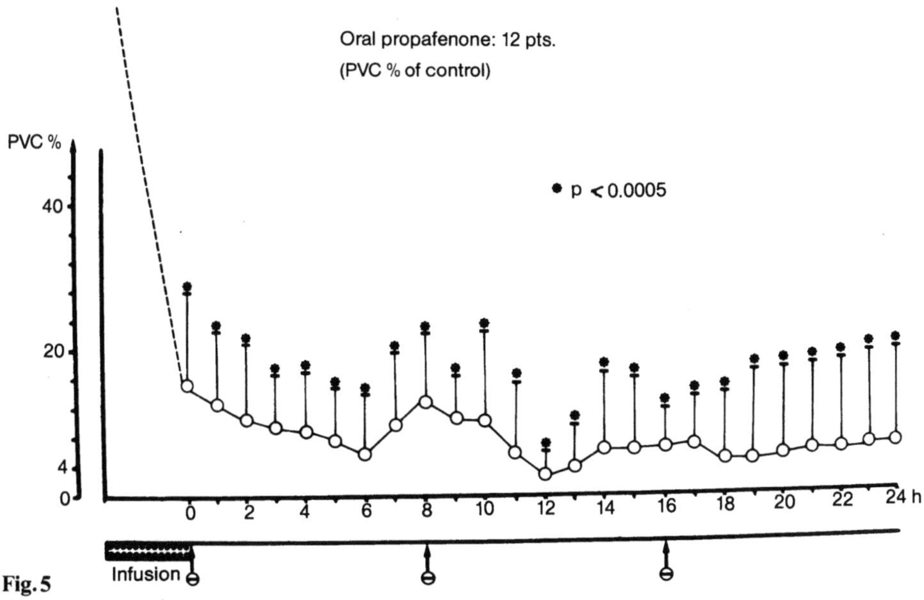
Oral propafenone: 12 pts.
(PVC % of control)
PVC %
• p < 0.0005
40
20
4
0
0 2 4 6 8 10 12 14 16 18 20 22 24 h
Infusion

Fig. 5

phase, including nausea and vomiting in six cases. We observed no blood pressure decrease and no cardiac failure. There was no disturbance of any biological parameter under control.

The electrocardiographic changes were moderate. The PQ interval increased by 17% on an average (160–180 ms). The QRS interval did not change in 12 cases, but two patients developed a left-bundle-branch block while receiving 900 mg P daily; the conduction disturbance disappeared with dose reduction to 600 mg daily.

Conclusions

Several conclusions can be drawn from our experience with P in severe ventricular arrhythmias. Intravenous P is fully effective in 50% of cases. Oral P is more effective, with a complete regression of PVCs in 85% of cases, but oral doses were larger than intravenous doses. The long half-life of P is a great advantage, maintaining efficacy for 6–8 h after one oral dose. A 150-mg dose three or four times daily seems to be adequate.

Paroxysmal tachycardias are not a good indication for P intravenously, but the minimal cardiovascular effects, the low incidence of side effects and the high efficacy of oral P make it a promising agent in the treatment of ventricular arrhythmias.

Use of Propafenone for the Prevention of Ventricular Hyperkinetic Arrhythmias in the Mitral Valve Prolapse Syndrome

F. Furlanello, G. B. Durante, P. Dal Forno, L. Frisanco, G. Mosna, R. Bettini, M. Disertori, G. Vergara, A. Del Favero and E. Stirpe

Sudden death has been reported to occurr in 1,4% of patients suffering from mitral valve prolapse (MVP). Ventricular hyperkinetic arrhythmias (VHA), also potentially malignant, are found in a substantial number of patients suffering from this syndrome. Thus effective antiarrhythmic treatment is necessary.

Propafenone is an important new antiarrhythmic agent which we have been using in clinical trials and electrophysiologic studies since 1978. Electrophysiological endocavitary studies have demonstrated that Propafenone markedly depresses infrahisian and intraventricular conduction as well as conduction in the accessory pathways of the Kent type.

Propafenone has already been reported as being effective in the treatment of VHA as well as recurring common ventricular tachycardia (RCVT).

We have studied the efficacy and tolerance of this drug in a selected population of patients with documented MVP and associated pronounced VHA.

The study population consisted of 17 patients whose age ranged between 18 and 61 years (mean 42), all were affected by MVP but one patient also had congestive cardiomyopathy. MVP was diagnosed according to phonocardiographic and echocardiographic criteria.

All patients had symptoms and entered the trial after at least two 24 hour ECG Holter recordings, which showed pronounced VHA with individual variability. In 6 patients these included chronic, polymorphous ventricular ectopic beats which had a tendency to occur in groups and to be repetitive with periods of non-sustained ventricular tachycardia.

All patients underwent maximal stress tests on the cycle ergometer which in 5 cases resulted in increased malignancy of the VHA.

The data of each patient were fed into a computer to facilitate easier intra- and interindividual comparisons.

In 10 patients previous treatment with antiarrhythmic agents proved ineffective when applied singly as well as when applied as a combination (max. 3).

The employed doses (after an adequate wash out period when patients had been on other antiarrhythmic drugs) were: 450 mg in 6 patients, 600 mg in 2 patients, 750 mg in 6 patients and 900 mg in 3 patients. The drug was given every 8 hours in all patients but 2 patients needed the drug four times a day. Follow-up ranged from 10 days (the drug was withheld for inefficacy and the patient left the trial) to 42 months (mean 16 months).

Cycle ergometer stress tests were performed on all patients within 15 days of the first administration of Propafenone and in contrast to what was observed before the onset of therapy none showed increased *malignancy* of the VHA.

24 hours ECG Holter recordings were performed within 15 days from the beginning of therapy and was subsequently repeated every four months.

Propafenone therapy achieved the complete disappearance of VHA in 3 patients and a greater than 75% reduction of the VHA in 10 patients as well as the disappearance of the indices of electrophysiological *malignancy* and of the episodes of non-sustained ventricular tachycardia. 3 patients had a less than 75% reduction of VHA.

Propafenone therapy was discontinued in two patients after 29 and 18 months respectively because of a bifascicular block (RAH + RBBB) in one patient and severe gastrointestinal side effects in the other.

From these results we suggest that Propafenone may be a useful drug for the treatment of VHA in the MVP Syndrome.

These results can be explained by the documented effectiveness of Propafenone on VHA without important extracardiac or cardiac side effects.

In particular Propafenone does not prolong the QTc interval which is often present in MVP Syndrome.

These first results need further confirmation. It is necessary to perform studies with larger populations and the extreme inter and intraindividual variability of VHA in the MVP Syndrome must be taken into account.

References

Disertori M, Vergara G, Dal Forno P, Inama G, Furlanello F (1981) Le Nuove Frontiere delle Aritmie Piccin p. 213
Swartz MH et al. (1977) Am J Med 62: 377

Beta-Blockers in the Elderly

Editors: E. Lang, F. Sörgel, L. Blaha
With contributions by numerous experts
1982. 29 figures. 17 tables. X, 107 pages.
ISBN 3-540-11682-6

Beta-blockers have attained a firm position in the treatment of both cardiovascular diseases as well as neuropsychiatric disorders. Their effectiveness in patients suffering from coronary heart disease, hypertension and hyperkinetic cardiac syndromes has long been proven. The development of new, selectively active beta-blockers has substantially reduced the number of possible side effects, thus enhancing their therapeutic safety. Because of the inevitability of side effects, however, beta-blockers habe been introduced only hesitantly in the treatment of the elderly.
The book is the first wide-ranging survey of the use of beta-blockers in older patients. The articles contained herein - written by pharmacologists, cardiologists, sports physicians, neurologists, psychiatrists and ophthalmologists - show that advanced age alone is not a contraindication for the use of beta-blockers and sympatholytic substances. The book also provides guidelines for the examination and determination of indications in the elderly.

Catecholamines and the Heart

Recent Advances in Experimental and Clinical Research

Editors: W. Delius, E. Gerlach, H. Grobecker, W. Kübler
1982. 149 figures, 49 tables. XIX, 383 pages.
ISBN 3-540-11119-0

Catecholamines and the Heart was the title of an international symposium convened in Munich in May, 1981, to evaluate recent studies into the sympathetic control of heart function in health and disease.
The papers delivered at the symposium, as well as the discussions which followed them, are contained in this book.
The papers cover three major topics:

- sympathetic innervation and adrenergic receptors in the heart
- biochemical and physiologic processes following stimulation or suppression of adrenergic receptors, and
- the pathophysiologic, clinical and therapeutic significance of adrenergic receptors in various types of heart disease.

Springer-Verlag
Berlin
Heidelberg
New York

Cardiomyopathy and Myocardial Biopsy
Editors: M. Kaltenbach, F. Loogen, E.G.J. Olsen
In cooperation with W.-D. Bussmann
With contributions by numerous experts
Corrected printing 1978. 203 figures, 56 tables.
XIV, 337 pages. ISBN 3-540-08474-6

Hyperthrophic Cardiomyopathy
The Therapeutic Role of Calcium Antagonists
Editors: M. Kaltenbach, S.E. Epstein
1982. 172 figures. XIV, 334 pages. ISBN 3-540-11065-8

Microcirculation of the Heart
Theoretical and Clinical Problems
Editors: H. Tillmanns, W. Kübler, H. Zebe
1982. 177 figures. XIV, 353 pages. ISBN 3-540-11346-0

Myocardial Infarction and Psychosocial Risks
Editors: J. Siegrist, M.J. Halhuber
With contributions by numerous experts
1981. 23 figures, 33 tables. X, 152 pages. ISBN 3-540-10386-4

Myocardial Infarction at Young Age
International Symposium Held in Bad Krozingen, January 30 and 31, 1981
Editor: H. Roskamm
1981. 83 figures. XII, 228 pages. ISBN 3-540-11090-9

Nitrates III
Cardiovascular Effects
Editors: P. Lichtlen, H.-J. Engel
1981. 326 figures. XX, 597 pages. ISBN 3-540-10761-4

Transluminal Coronary Angioplasty and Intracoronary Thrombolysis
Coronary Heart Disease IV
Editors: M. Kaltenbach, A. Grüntzig, K. Rentrop, W.-D. Bussmann
With contributions by numerous experts
1982. 210 figures. XVIII, 442 pages. ISBN 3-540-11219-7

Springer-Verlag
Berlin
Heidelberg
New York

MIX
Papier aus verantwortungsvollen Quellen
Paper from responsible sources
FSC® C105338

If you have any concerns about our products,
you can contact us on
ProductSafety@springernature.com

In case Publisher is established outside the EU,
the EU authorized representative is:
Springer Nature Customer Service Center GmbH
Europaplatz 3, 69115 Heidelberg, Germany

Printed by Libri Plureos GmbH
in Hamburg, Germany